## Praise for
## Ancient Herbs, Modern Medicine

"A valuable alternative perspective on health and illness."
*—Ted J. Kaptchuk, O.M.D.,*
*author of* The Web That Has No Weaver:
Understanding Chinese Medicine

"A wonderful description of Chinese medicine and its re-emergence in modern times."
*—Wayne B. Jonas, M.D.,*
*Director of Samueli Institute and*
*Former Director, Office of Alternative Medicine, NIH*

"With the increase of environmentally related illnesses, the integration of Chinese herbal medicine and Western medicine has become a necessity. Ancient Herbs, Modern Medicine introduces us to the future of medicine and the gentle arts of detoxification from our polluted environment."
*—David Steinman,*
*author of* Diet for a Poisoned Planet
*and co-author of* The Safe Shopper's Bible

"Ancient Herbs, Modern Medicine provides inspiring accounts of Chinese and Western medicine working together for the common goal of treating illnesses and enhancing human health. We are allowed a glimpse of the new medical system that is evolving—one that balances art and science, ancient wisdom and modern high technology, respect and compassion for the quality and value of life and high degree of effectiveness in eradicating diseases."
*—Ke-ji Chen, M.D.,*
*Editor-in-Chief of* The Chinese Journal of
Integrated Traditional and Western Medicine

# Ancient Herbs, Modern Medicine

## Improving Your Health by Combining Chinese Herbal Medicine and Western Medicine

Henry Han, O.M.D.,
Glenn E. Miller, M.D., and Nancy Deville

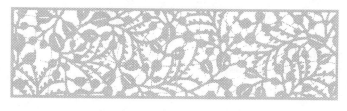

Bantam Books

**ANCIENT HERBS, MODERN MEDICINE**
A Bantam Book/January 2003

Published by Bantam Dell
A Division of Random House, Inc.
New York, New York

All rights reserved.
Copyright © 2003 by Nancy Deville, Henry Han, O.M.D.,
and Glenn E. Miller, M.D.
Illustrations copyright © 2003 by Jackie Aher
Cover design by Belina Huey

*Book design by Virginia Norey*

LIBRARY OF CONGRESS CATALOGING-IN-PUBLICATION DATA
Han, Henry.
  Ancient herbs, modern medicine : improving your health by
combining Chinese herbal medicine and Western medicine /
Henry Han, Glenn E. Miller, and Nancy Deville.
    p. cm.
Includes bibliographical references and index.
ISBN 978-0-553-38118-4
    1. Herbs—Therapeutic use. 2. Medicine, Chinese.
I. Miller, Glenn E., M.D. II. Deville, Nancy. III. Title.
RM666.H33 H36 2003
615'.321—dc21      2002026042

Bantam Books and the rooster colophon are registered trademarks of
Random House, Inc.

Published simultaneously in Canada

Ancient Herbs, Modern Medicine is meant to increase your knowledge of the Chinese approach to using plants for medicinal purposes. Because individuals and their medical histories inevitably vary, a physician or licensed herbalist must diagnose conditions and supervise the use of healing herbs to treat individual health problems. Herbs and other natural remedies are not substitutes for professional medical care. The authors and publisher of this book urge you to seek out the best medical resources available to help you make informed decisions. The authors and publisher strongly recommend that if you are taking Western drugs, you always tell your herbalist what medications you are taking. Likewise, always tell your Western M.D. if you are taking Chinese herbs.

The case histories in this book are true. In some cases, the names and some identifying characteristics of those mentioned in the case histories have been changed to protect the privacy of those individuals. Any resemblance in those cases to actual people is entirely coincidental.

To my parents, Dr. Huiwen Luo and Dr. Dewo Han, for their love and support and for being dedicated and open-minded doctors.
—*Henry Han, O.M.D.*

To my wife, Marjorie Gies, M.D., Ph.D., and to my children, Maggie and Dillon, for bringing greater meaning to my life.
—*Glenn E. Miller, M.D.*

To Cathy Quinn, Ph.D., my mentor and friend, for your love, wisdom and loyalty.
—*Nancy Deville*

# Acknowledgments

For the four years she devoted to this project, for her agenting skills, insights and friendship, thank you, Ling Lucas. To Danielle Perez, Senior Editor at Bantam Dell, for her journey across country and up the potholed, winding road to work out the organization of this book, thank you. Her attention to detail, editorial talent and encouragement were the driving force. She was a pleasure to work with and this book would not have been the same without her.

The execution of a book like this took a staff of hardworking individuals. First in line for thanks is Courtney Sampson, my assistant, who handled details of every facet of this project. De'in Sofley spent months interviewing, doing Medline research and transcribing interviews, often alone and self-motivated out in the field. Thanks to Reneé Perez for managing bookkeeping and miscellaneous and sundry details and to David Stanley, computer expert. Thanks to Derek Thiele, Esq., for his legal expertise. Many thanks to Pat Frederick for her editorial assistance from the very beginning of this project and to Sue Warga for her copyedit on the manuscript.

Many doctors of Chinese medicine, Western M.D.'s, scientists, and nurses contributed their expertise to this book. Glenn E. Miller, M.D., and Henry Han, O.M.D., took time away from their busy practices and businesses to write this book with me. Stephen Hosea, M.D., who is in private practice in the field of infectious diseases, was the first Western doctor who would talk to me about his opinion of and experiences with Chinese medicine. The contributions of Daoshing Ni, Lic. Ac., D.O.M., Ph.D., and Maoshing Ni, Lic. Ac., D.O.M., Ph.D., on the topics of spirituality, women and antiaging were invaluable and greatly enhanced the content of this book. Lorne D. Feldman, M.D. shared his story of healing and spiritual awakening.

For their contributions and cooperation, thanks to: Ke-ji Chen, M.D., internationally recognized authority on the integration of Chinese and Western medicines, for his knowledge of the history of Chinese medicine; Amy Birchum, a student of Chinese medicine, for creating the glossary of Chinese herbs; Soonae Choi, Lic. A., M.S., for creating the charts of Energetic properties of foods; Scott Blossom, Lic. Ac., for poring over the completed manuscript—his contribution and ideas are reflected in many pages of this book; Alex Soffici, M.D., and Mia Lundin, R.N., C.N.P., for their medical and hormone replacement expertise on women's health; Robin Marzi, R.D., expert in the fields of metabolism, women's health and fitness and sports nutrition, for her contribution to the subjects of antiaging and women's health; Sheldon Miller, R. Ph., for his insights on pharmacognosy; Kenneth Cohen, internationally renowned author, lecturer, health educator, China scholar and master of Qigong healing, and Francesco Garri Garripoli, author and lecturer on Qigong, for their contributions on Qigong; Gary Tunksy, Ph.D., for his unique take on cellular healing; David Steinman, nationally recognized authority on environmental toxins, for his help on this subject; oncology nurse and researcher Diane Fletcher, M.A., R.N., O.C.N., for her insights on research; Jo Ann Tall, Lic. Ac., for sharing her experiences with integrative medicine; Mary Enig, Ph.D., internationally recognized biochemist in the field of fats and oils and an authority on transfatty acids, for her contribution to the chapter on HIV; Michele Nichols, ashtanga yoga scholar, and Shelly Gault, who designed the meditation guidelines. Many thanks to Robin Monroe for her research on Chinese herbs in Chinatown in San Francisco and for creating the medicinal recipes in this book.

For those who spent many hours sharing your personal stories with me over a period of three and a half years, heartfelt gratitude for your generosity and time. Your stories are the glue that patched this book together and made it possible for others to understand how miraculous Chinese medicine can be.

Most of all, thank you to John for always being there.

*Nancy Deville*

# Contents

PART TWO

# Treating Common Illnesses

PART THREE

# Modern Plagues

PART FOUR

Health Maintenance and Excellence

# Foreword

Because I have devoted my life to bringing the integration of Chinese and Western medicine to the people of the Western world, I was honored to be asked to write the foreword to *Ancient Herbs, Modern Medicine*. Historically, Chinese medicine has been the only medical care system in China. Western medicine was not introduced into China until the seventeenth century and it did not play a significant role in health care until the past one hundred years. During this period of time, China developed a fully integrated medical system that employs both Chinese and Western medicines. Through this "experiment," we have learned that the tremendous conceptual gulf and differences between Chinese and Western medicines are not necessarily bad. In *Ancient Herbs, Modern Medicine* you will see that, in fact, where Western medicine is weak, Chinese medicine is strong, and vice versa. The integration of Chinese and Western medicines is the marriage of the art and science of healing, a balance of Yin and Yang.

In this age of ever accelerating information exchange, the integration of Chinese medicine and modern science is not only necessary but inevitable. For integration to occur, people must first learn about Chinese medicine. As more and more Americans are interested in learning about and using Chinese medicine, a book on the subject that is easy to read and understand is urgently needed—both for the layperson and to help educate Western medical doctors. *Ancient Herbs, Modern Medicine* fills this need.

When people are educated and are empowered to take care of themselves, and when doctors no longer fight over supremacy but instead come together in the spirit of cooperation to work for the benefit of all humankind, we will have a medical system that truly meets people's needs. This book is both an inspiration and a resource for those in the quest for this new health care system for our time, a medicine that brings together the best of both East and West, encourages personal transformation and facilitates the attainment of overall balance in people's lives. *Ancient Herbs, Modern Medicine* exemplifies the future of medicine in the Western world and serves as an encouraging sign that the tide of integration is beginning on American shores.

*Maoshing Ni, Lic. Ac., D.O.M., Ph.D.*
*Los Angeles, California*

# Preface

## Discovering Chinese Herbs

There was a time when I thought of Chinese herbal medicine as a primitive medical approach that no one with knowledge of modern medicine would consider using. Like many Americans, I had seen storefronts of Chinese apothecaries marked with indecipherable Chinese characters, where strange and even frightening-looking objects floated in jars. I imagined the doorways leading to darkened rooms where withered old men brewed up snake oil. I would venture to say that my attitude about Chinese medicine was shared by most Americans.

I did not equate Chinese herbal medicine with acupuncture, which I had used and advocated for most of my adult life. Acupuncture did not carry the same fraudulent stigma as Chinese herbal medicine. This was largely due to an event that occurred in China in 1971. While traveling with President Nixon on his first visit to China, James Reston, a *New York Times* journalist, had to have an emergency appendectomy. Instead of using narcotic painkillers, the Chinese doctors treated his postoperative pain with acupuncture. Reston returned to the United States and wrote a series of newspaper articles on his painless recovery. Americans took note and began searching out acupuncturists for treatment. Acupuncture proved effective; the word spread and demand increased. Since that time acupuncture has become synonymous with the legitimate part of Chinese medicine in the United States. Acupuncture has become relatively Americanized, with acupuncture clinics springing up across the country, most of them staffed by American-born and -trained acupuncturists.

In 1989, my husband and I settled in Santa Barbara, which is a mecca for alternative medicine. Over the next few years I became more educated about nontraditional medical approaches. I met a number of people who used Chinese herbs instead of over-the-counter drugs and often went to doctors of

Chinese medicine when they got sick. I decided to try Chinese herbs too. I remember getting my first sacks of herbs, roots and twigs and brewing them into a tea called a decoction. The bitter-tasting medicine was remarkably effective, and after my first positive experience both my husband and I became converts to Chinese herbal medicine.

As I began researching Chinese medicine to write this book, I learned that although we in the West think of acupuncture as being primary in Chinese medicine, Chinese herbs are in fact the most essential, most important aspect of Chinese medicine. Of course, no other medical approach comes close to Western medicine when it comes to diagnostic techniques, genetic research and other highly technological areas of science. You would not go to an herbalist in an acute health crisis; you would go to the emergency room and be cared for by Western-trained physicians. But Chinese herbal medicine has been proven to be effective for many chronic conditions that have eluded Western medicine.

Virtually every layperson I talked to about writing a book on Chinese medicine was eager to learn more about Chinese herbs. I did not find that same attitude among all Western doctors I spoke with. Herbal medicine has been traditionally viewed with suspicion and even contempt by a good portion of the Western medical establishment. Many in the medical community view practitioners who use Western drugs as scientifically minded and those who use herbs as witch doctors. Thinking back to my former reaction to the sight of Chinese apothecary storefronts, I understood this resistance.

As I continued to research, I learned that the active ingredients in more than half of the currently prescribed Western medications were originally extracted from natural substances.[1] This fact alone appeared to be the bridge that could eventually unite Western and Eastern medicines. True integrative medicine, wherein our Western medical community embraced Chinese herbs and worked collaboratively with doctors of Chinese medicine, seemed long overdue.

I found the ideal Western/Chinese collaborative relationship between Glenn E. Miller, M.D., a Midwest-born and -raised physician, psychiatrist and pharmacist, and Henry Han, O.M.D., a Chinese-born and -trained Doctor of Oriental Medicine. These two doctors, who were born, raised and trained at opposite ends of the earth, had begun referring patients to each other because they found that a combination of Western and Chinese medicines was more effective than Western medicine alone or Chinese medicine alone. Dr. Miller's

---

1. Many of these active ingredients are now synthesized, though the original source was from plants.

family history in pharmacognosy (the branch of pharmacology that deals with drugs in their crude or natural state) and Dr. Han's family history in Western medicine gave each doctor a well-rounded perspective on what integrative medicine could be like.

As I began writing this book with Dr. Miller and Dr. Han, I met other Western medical doctors who are using Chinese medicine within their practices. Western-trained oncologist Lorne Feldman, who survived kidney cancer, non-Hodgkin's lymphoma and kidney metastasis, now practices integrative medicine—a transformation due in part to his successful personal use of Chinese herbs.

Dr. Feldman led me to two other doctors of Chinese medicine who practice integrative medicine—Maoshing Ni, Lic. Ac., D.O.M., Ph.D., known as Dr. Mao, and Daoshing Ni, Lic. Ac., D.O.M., Ph.D., known as Dr. Dao. A close-knit family, the Nis trace their lineage in the Chinese medical healing arts back to the thirteenth century. Their father, Hua-Ching Ni, is the author of fifty books on Taoism and Chinese medicine. As sons of a renowned master physician, Drs. Mao and Dao were expected to step into their father's larger-than-life shoes. Their training began early in childhood, from memorizing old medical classics such as *The Yellow Emperor's Classic on Medicine,* or *Nei Jing,* to apprenticing in their father's busy clinic. Supplemental training included martial arts, Tai Chi, meditation and the study of the Chinese spiritual classic *I-Ching,* also called *The Book of Changes.* While others went to summer camp or vacations, they attended their father's "healing camp." It was only years later that they appreciated the wisdom of their family's tradition.

As a master of healing and spirituality, Master Ni was invited to teach Taoist philosophy and arts as well as Chinese medicine in the United States in 1975, and the family immigrated to the United States in 1976. Drs. Mao and Dao were trained in Chinese medicine in a traditional apprenticeship from father to son. Since their apprenticeship was not recognized in the early eighties in California, to obtain a license to practice they attended and obtained degrees from SAMRA University in Los Angeles. After graduating, Dr. Dao at nineteen years of age, and the following year Dr. Mao, at nineteen years of age, were the youngest people to ever practice Chinese medicine in America.

Dr. Mao returned to China to complete his postgraduate residency in Shanghai, at Zhong-Shang Hospital, a six-thousand-bed facility—the largest in the city—that served as the teaching hospital for the Shanghai Medical School (a Western-style medical school).

Dr. Dao completed his postgraduate residency in Dong Zhi Meng Hospital, in Beijing, and Xuan Wu Hospital, which is affiliated with the Beijing University of Traditional Chinese Medicine in Nanjing. In these prestigious hospitals, where doctors of Chinese medicine and Western medical doctors work side by side, Drs. Mao and Dao learned firsthand how these two medical traditions can be integrated to best serve patients' needs.

The brothers cofounded the Tao of Wellness clinic in Los Angeles, California, where Dr. Mao specializes in immunology, internal medicine and longevity and Dr. Dao specializes in general medicine, reproductive medicine and gynecology. They are highly regarded in the Western medical community and have worked hard to re-create the model of integrative healing they learned in China. They examine patients to arrive at a diagnosis according to Chinese medicine but, when appropriate, also refer patients to Western medical specialists to consult and obtain a detailed diagnosis through Western technologies to make sure they have all the information to create the best treatment protocol. Drs. Mao and Dao also cofounded the Yo San University, which offers educational training in Chinese medicine and actively promotes the integration of Chinese and Western medicines.

You may have heard about the integration of Chinese and Western medicines, or have read about doctors like Dr. Miller, Dr. Han, Dr. Mao and Dr. Dao, who practice integrated medicine. You may be curious about Chinese medicine, but your Western doctor may not be receptive. You may also have some feelings of doubt, thinking about the mysterious-looking apothecaries and the strange floating objects. This book is filled with real-life stories of people who struggled with chronic, degenerative and even terminal illnesses but found help with Chinese herbs. Many of these people were as skeptical about Chinese herbs as I had once been—as perhaps you are today.

Learning about and using Chinese herbs will change your life and your health for the better. Once you enter the door that formerly appeared strange and foreign, you will find yourself in the highly fascinating world of Chinese medicine, where you can heal and find a better quality of life by integrating your mind, body and spirit.

*Nancy Deville*
*Santa Barbara, California*

# Introduction

*A Western doctor, Glenn E. Miller, M.D.,*
*and a Chinese doctor, Henry Han, O.M.D.,*
*collaborate for a better medicine*

My career in Western medicine began with an interest in my family's background in pharmacognosy, which is the branch of pharmacology that deals with drugs in their crude or natural state. My father, two uncles and two cousins are all pharmacists. Growing up in the Midwest, I spent summers, weekends and holidays with my dad at his pharmacy. Before I could even see over the counter, my father would have me grind raw ingredients—many of which came from plant sources—in a mortar and pestle. My father would then put the ground powder into capsules, blend it into an ointment or mold it into suppositories. My father was a Scout leader who took me and my Scout troop on trails, pointed out plants and told us about their medicinal applications. I was fascinated that plants you might see on a trail could end up as raw ingredients in medications dispensed in pharmacies.

Throughout my childhood, as I continued to work with my father behind the counter in his pharmacy, fewer and fewer naturally occurring medicines were prescribed. Pharmaceutical manufacturers began growing into the behemoth companies they are today, and prescription drugs became the way of life in medicine and in the practice of pharmacy. Mortars and pestles, folded powder papers, ointment tubes and suppository molds were put on the shelf, destined never to be used again. Pharmacies that specialize in formulating compounded prescriptions dwindled in the United States to so few that physicians now have difficulty in finding one when the need for an individualized preparation arises.

I initially followed in the footsteps of my father and enrolled in pharmacy school. By the time I graduated from Drake University College of Pharmacy, they were no longer offering classes in pharmacognosy. We were not taught the preparation of natural herbs in the mortar and pestle. We were taught how to prepare and fill ointment tubes, but were informed that the chance of us ever having to do so "out in the real world" was rather low. The lack of attention to the properties of plants in pharmacy school did not dampen my interest. At the same time, my studies in pharmacy school were not enough for me. I knew I wanted to pursue a career in medicine.

In medical school, there was no place for my interest in the preparation and use of natural herbs. I attended one of the finest clinical medical training centers in the world at the University of Illinois College of Medicine, Chicago campus—and there it was all about mainstream Western medicine. It was not until I was in private practice in Santa Barbara that an opportunity arose for me to pursue my interest in natural herbs as medicine.

Throughout my career in medicine I have always had great respect for my patients' opinions and have advocated using whatever it took to give patients the best results. There were occasions when patients achieved positive results on medications I prescribed but suffered severe, and at times debilitating, side effects. When some of my patients began asking me about the interactions of various prescription medications they were taking with herbs they wished to take, my long-hibernating interest in natural herbs was awakened. I began researching so that I could accurately answer my patients' questions and address their needs. During the course of my research, I happened across Henry Han, O.M.D. (Oriental Medical Doctor), in my own backyard. When some of my patients told me about their positive experiences with Chinese herbal medicine in resolving their side effects, I realized I could treat many illnesses with Western medicine and the side effects could be alleviated with Chinese herbal medicine. Given my background, it seemed perfectly natural to me to use herbs in conjunction with Western medicines and treatment protocols. I began researching and studying Chinese medicine, referring patients to Dr. Han and collaborating with him on patients' treatment plans.

Dr. Han, who is the founder and chief physician of the Santa Barbara Herb Clinic and a specialist in internal medicine, was born in China and trained in Chinese and Western medicine in Beijing. When Dr. Han says, "To heal others is to heal myself," he speaks of an arduous journey in which his own life experience molded his philosophy about healing.

Dr. Han was born in 1958 in the People's Republic of China to parents who were Western-trained physicians; his father was a dermatologist and his mother a gynecological oncologist and surgeon (his sister later became an internist). After Chairman Mao claimed absolute control over the country in 1949, anyone who was not working-class was considered a potential antirevolutionary. The political turbulence, stirred by the development of a communist society, culminated in the Cultural Revolution in 1966. The campaign of Red Terror was set in motion to purge those suspected of being disloyal to the Party. Dr. Han's parents were among the educated professionals who were singled out and arrested.

Four years into the Cultural Revolution, his parents were exiled to the remote countryside in western China, and Dr. Han, then twelve years old, was allowed to go with them. Exile was meant to "reeducate" his parents through forced labor, yet their medical knowledge and skill were needed and called upon from time to time as they traveled through towns and villages where doctors rarely, if ever, visited. On occasion they asked their son to give them a hand when there was no nurse available to assist them.

Watching how Western medicine was practiced in dire situations left a deep impression on Dr. Han. He watched his parents incorporate Chinese medicine into their Western medical practice. The combined use of these two diverse medical systems came naturally for Dr. Han's parents partly because—in spite of their training in Western medicine—they were culturally accepting of Chinese medicine. By the majority of Chinese people the effectiveness of Chinese medicine is taken for granted and never questioned. Even in the second half of the twentieth century in the vast Chinese countryside Chinese medicine still shouldered most of the responsibility for health care. In addition, both of Dr. Han's parents had received some training in Chinese medicine as part of the institutionalized sponsorship by the government to promote the integration between Western and Chinese medicine.

As a boy, Dr. Han learned that, in many situations, the combined use of the two medicines seemed to work better than either one of the systems. Whenever he could, he spent hours hanging around herbal pharmacies to help process herbal formulas and satisfy his curiosity about the different colors, textures, shapes, smells and medicinal properties. There was magic in knowing that a plant was capable of healing an illness.

The Cultural Revolution officially ended in the fall of 1976 with the death of Chairman Mao. Dr. Han's family was reunited. In late 1977, Dr. Han enrolled in the Beijing University of Chinese Medicine. The training of the school was divided between traditional Chinese medicine (TCM) and Western medicine. Among his teachers were some of the world's most well respected Chinese herbalists and scholars of Chinese medicine.

Dr. Han then had the opportunity to go to the United States to study, and he chose the University of California in Santa Barbara. After Tiananmen Square Dr. Han became involved in student demonstrations in the United States, and it was therefore impossible for him to return to China. President George H. W. Bush issued a presidential order that provided protection for Chinese students. Dr. Han decided to stay in Santa Barbara and set up a practice there in 1989.

After meeting Dr. Han, my days of medical library and Internet research were over. Here was a master herbalist who was able to answer my questions. From the very beginning of our relationship, Dr. Han provided me with more and more enlightening information, not only providing assistance to my patients but fanning the flames of interest in integrative medicine. Through this interactive relationship I came to the understanding that there is more than one way to effectively treat patients. If Western medicine did not have the right or best answer, I was free to search for a better answer. When we integrated Chinese and Western medicines, the battle against disease had a much greater chance of being won.

Because Western and Chinese medicines can so effectively complement each other's weaknesses, the marriage of these two medicines makes sense. Chinese medicine, which operated independently from Western medicine for three thousand years, has been integrated with Western medicine in parts of China during the last two hundred years. In China, when a patient is evaluated, often both Chinese and Western medical approaches are considered. Sometimes Chinese medicine is more appropriate, sometimes Western. This integrated approach is widely accepted in China as a way of providing optimal medical care for the patient.

Dr. Han persisted in his goal of further integration. In his practice, whenever possible, he uses Western diagnostic laboratory tests in evaluating and monitoring patients' progress throughout the course of treatment. He continued to attempt to contact his patients' Western medical doctors, and slowly the barriers began to fall away. Today, many of the Western doctors of patients who shared their case histories for this book are now actively pursuing collaborative relationships with doctors of Chinese medicine, such as Dr. Han, as a result of the success their patients experienced with Chinese medicine. Dr. Han, Dr. Mao and Dr. Dao are a few of the doctors who now have Western doctors collaborating with them on patients' treatment plans, referring patients to them and even seeking Chinese medical treatment as patients themselves. These practices have become stellar models of how true integration can work for the betterment of medical care.

Our desire to share this model grew into the book you are now reading. Just as everything known about Western science could not be explained in one book, it would be impossible to fully explain every detail about Chinese medicine in one book. For that reason, *Ancient Herbs, Modern Medicine* will give you a basic understanding of the most important concepts of Chinese medicine, including theory and principles, acupuncture and herbs. Understanding these principles and medical modalities will enable you to understand your Chinese medical doctor when he or she explains your condition from a Chinese medicine perspective. You will also be able to talk to your Western medical doctor about Chinese medicine.

Chinese herbs come in two basic forms: raw, dried herbs that are individually prescribed and brewed into a tea called a decoction, and refined patent herbs that are standardized for certain conditions and come in pills, granules and tinctures. Patent herbal formulas are comparable to Western over-the-counter medications. Self-treating relatively mild or benign conditions or symptoms with patent herbal formulas can be safe and effective. Once you learn about herbs and are ready to try them, the appendices provide resources for you to find a Chinese herbal clinic in your area. If there are no clinics in your area, you can order herbs online at ancientherbsmodernmedicine.com.

In potentially life-threatening situations or when one is seriously ill, however, herbal formulas must be prescribed by a trained and experienced herbalist. To maximize the benefits of your treatment, your herbalist and Western physician should collaborate and communicate throughout the course of your treatment. If you are taking Western drugs, always tell your herbalist what medications you are taking. Likewise, always tell your Western M.D. if you are taking Chinese herbs.

Chinese medicine fills a need sorely felt in today's world. The efficacy of Chinese medicine can rival that of Western medicine—and for many chronic illnesses, Chinese medicine is actually more effective and a better choice. This is why in the modern era of advanced science and technology, this ancient medicine has not only held its ground but remains vital and is gaining increasing acceptance worldwide.

The strength of Chinese medicine comes from three thousand years of treating illnesses and promoting health. The core of its wisdom is sophisticated theory and philosophy, which has provided Chinese medicine with its characteristic of gentleness, its holistic approach to illness and health and its strong emphases on quality of life and prevention.

We believe that by promoting the marriage of the best of the West and East, the emerging health care model for the new millennium can have a better balance between art and science, ancient wisdom and modern high technology, respect and sensitivity for the wholeness and quality of life and a high degree of effectiveness in eradicating diseases.

*Glenn E. Miller, M.D.*
*Santa Barbara, California*

# Ancient Herbs,
# Modern Medicine

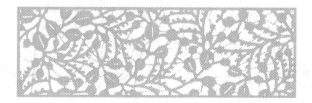

# PART
# ONE

### Understanding the Basics
### of Chinese Medicine

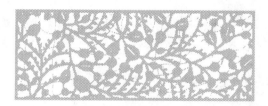

# 1

# Chinese and Western Medicines, Past and Present

*How these medicines evolved in different directions and how they can come together*

When Wang Qingren, a doctor of Chinese medicine, attended public executions in 1797, tagging along to the gravesites, then returning in the shadow of night to perform autopsies, his clandestine activities served an honorable purpose. In the early seventeenth century an Italian explorer and missionary had brought into China the book *Method of the West,* which had provided the first glimpse into Western medicine. After that, Western medical literature was further introduced into China via Christian missionaries. Performing autopsies helped Dr. Wang verify some of the knowledge of anatomy that he had learned from his reading.[2] Unlike his Western counterparts of that era who freely attended gross-anatomy classes, Dr. Wang was forced to work under a cloak of secrecy because of the Chinese cultural veneration for the body as a whole.

The restrictions Dr. Wang worked under began centuries earlier. The history of Chinese medicine reaches back to the dim and ancient past where the distinction between myth and historical facts is blurred, food and medicine were interchangeable and shamans, high priests, witches and doctors all provided medical care. Thousands of years before written language, the knowledge of Chinese medicine was passed through oral retelling of tales and legends.

The concept of wholeness in Chinese medicine took form through legendary discussions and dialogue between Emperor Huang Ti (the Yellow Emperor) and his physician Qi Bo (circa 2697 to 2205 B.C.). Nearly two thousand

2. In Chinese, the surname is actually the first name. Jane Doe would be Doe Jane in Chinese.

years later (circa 200 B.C.) *Nei Jing*, or *The Yellow Emperor's Classic of Internal Medicine*, was written down in eighteen volumes.[3] It is said to contain the bulk of those discussions, including information on medicinal herbs, anatomy, medical theory, acupuncture, spirituality, life force, Yin and Yang. (Many of the major Chinese terms are capitalized throughout this book to define them as specific Chinese medical terms and in some cases to differentiate them from similar Western terms.) *Nei Jing* thoroughly explored the synergistic relationship between man and nature and health and illness to further define the concept of wholeness.

Taoism is a philosophical system derived chiefly from the *Tao-te-ching*, a book traditionally ascribed to Chinese philosopher Lao-tze but believed to have been written in the sixth century B.C. Taoism, a central influence of Chinese medicine, stated that "the heaven and the human are one" and described an ideal human condition of freedom from desire and of effortless simplicity, achieved by following the Tao (path)—the spontaneous, creative, effortless path taken by natural events in the universe. The notions of Qi (the life force) and Yin and Yang—which are the foundation of Chinese medicine—are inherited from Taoism.

In addition to these influences, within a hundred years of Confucius's death in 479 B.C., a system of ethics for the management of a well-ordered society began to develop from his teachings. So powerful was Confucius's influence that by the Han Dynasty (140 to 85 B.C.), Emperor Han Wu Di issued two decrees, "Banishment of all other schools" and "Favor only that of Confucianism," making Confucianism the sole official national philosophy and effectively forbidding all other social codes of behavior. One of Confucianism's main tenets was that the *whole* body was sacred and should remain complete throughout life and death.

Because of the veneration for the body as a whole, Confucianism opposed the practices of anatomical study and surgery, which would maim the body or corpse. These restrictions—which continued over many centuries—forced researchers such as Wang Qingren underground. While Western medicine continued delving into and learning from the human body's organs, tissues and bones in order to diagnose and treat illness, Chinese medicine evolved in the opposite direction, developing methods of diagnosis via external means such as observing, touching and listening to the patient.

---

3. *Nei Jing* is attributed to the Yellow Emperor but it is believed to be a collection by numerous doctors and scholars.

In primitive times, throughout the world, disease was considered to be the result of a malevolent spell cast by an angered enemy, of displeasing a god or of inviting an evil spirit into one's body. Medicine consisted of magic and religious rites with witch doctors and sorcerers. For Western medicine, the transition from superstition to science was a gradual process, extending over centuries. When Greek physician Hippocrates, the so-called father of modern medicine, was born (circa 460 B.C.), medical thought had only partially discarded magic and religion as a basis for healing. As did the Chinese medical bible *Nei Jing,* Hippocrates rejected supernatural belief systems. He spoke disparagingly of the "charlatans and quacks" who perpetuated such beliefs and urged the exploration of disease as a natural phenomenon that could be observed and investigated. Like doctors of Chinese medicine, Hippocrates focused on the effects of food, occupation and environment in the development of disease. Understanding that mind and body were connected, he said, "Our natures are the physicians of our diseases." But by the seventeenth century, French mathematician and philosopher René Descartes introduced the premise that the body and the mind were *entirely separate,* which was quickly and heartily embraced by Western science as absolute truth. To explain why this premise was so readily accepted could take volumes of conjecture and discussion. Perhaps explaining the working of the human body, although incredibly daunting, at least seemed possible. To accept the mind as part of the system would have made the task virtually impossible. Another reason may have been that the mind seemed connected to the soul and, to the highly religious society of the day, separating the two was both logical and reverential.

Ancient Chinese, desiring to present themselves to their ancestors as whole, feared decapitation as capital punishment. This core reverence for the wholeness of the human being encouraged the development of a mind/body-oriented medicine. At the same time, due to the belief in the separation of mind and body, Western medicine proceeded to develop a "headless" medicine.

Western medicine generally revolved around folk medicine until scientific breakthroughs in human anatomy and physiology, knowledge of infectious agents, drugs and therapeutic procedures began to occur in the nineteenth and twentieth centuries. The discovery of microorganisms such as bacteria and fungi led first to the germ theory of disease in the mid to late 1900s, which precipitated major scientific advancements. Continued advances have removed Western medicine far from its humble origins.

Unlike Western medicine's dramatic and exponentially exploding development, Chinese medicine has not needed to change very much from its original philosophy of wholeness and balance. One change that has begun to occur over the past two hundred years is Chinese medical doctors' interest in capitalizing on Western scientific knowledge and technologies. This change occurred very slowly and initially with great resistance.

When in 1830 Chinese doctor Wang Qingren used his newfound knowledge of human anatomy to write a book attempting to correct some erroneous assumptions of anatomy made by ancient Chinese scholars, critics accused him of magnifying confusion. Because the Western concept of physical organs does not have much significance in Chinese medicine, they said that it did not matter where the organs were located. At the same time, as Western medicine progressed, physicians and scientists viewed Chinese medicine as charlatanism and the notion of any kind of credibility was considered preposterous. This disdain from both sides kept the line drawn in the sand.

Integration, however, took on a life of its own and proceeded tenaciously, however haltingly. The first Western medical clinic was established in China in 1827, the first Western medical hospital in 1834. By the beginning of the twentieth century Western medical hospitals were starting to spring up in the larger cities. From the mid-nineteenth century to the early 1950s a rudimentary form of integrative medicine began to develop in China. Both Chinese and Western medicine were used, but in a side-by-side fashion instead of a truly combined, integrated use.

Unfortunately, one of the consequences of this approach is that those who were trained in Western medicine began to advocate the abandonment of Chinese medical theories entirely. They wanted to use Chinese herbs as Western doctors used drugs. In other words, they looked for effective herbs, isolated the active ingredients and extracted those from the natural substance to use only the isolated ingredient as Western medicine does. For example, in the 1920s the active ingredient, ephedrine, in the Chinese herb Ma Huang—which has been used in China for nearly four thousand years—was isolated and used to treat asthma and similar conditions. But this was not integration.

In his early seventies, Ke-ji Chen, M.D., is an internationally recognized authority on the integration of traditional Chinese medicine and Western medicine.[4] "Until the early seventeenth century China had been decidedly more advanced technologically compared to the Western world," Dr. Chen said. In

4. Ke-ji Chen, M.D., is president of the Chinese Association of Integrated Traditional and Western Medicine, professor and chief researcher of the China Academy of Chinese Medicine, editor-in-chief of the *Chinese Journal of Integrated Traditional and Western Medicine* and academician of the Chinese Academy of Sciences.

fact, by 1523 B.C. a writing system with two thousand characters was in use in China (in the West an alphabet emerged in Greece circa 800 B.C.). The Chinese discovered the orienting effect of lodestones, from which they pioneered the navigational compass around 101 B.C. In 105 B.C. a Chinese eunuch refined the process of papermaking. Gunpowder was believed to have originated in China in the ninth century. These are only some of the accomplishments by ancient Chinese. "But the momentum was lost around the early seventeenth century for cultural and historical reasons," Dr. Chen said. "When Europe emerged from the long dormancy of the Dark Ages, it was thrust forward through the Renaissance, which stimulated scientific knowledge and discoveries. In the meantime the deterioration—socially, culturally and scientifically—in China continued and culminated in a series of defeats by foreign powers that resulted in the collapse of the Ching Dynasty [1644 to 1908]. China's entrance to the modern era came with tremendous pain. China had had a brilliant past and civilization but had been left far behind."

By the turn of the twentieth century, the young and elite intellectuals of China took it upon themselves to redeem the country. "They were so pained and blinded by the humiliation and hurt pride that the country had suffered in the past several hundred years that they could not see anything valuable in Chinese tradition," Dr. Chen said. "In search of an answer they pondered what it was about the West that gave it power and vitality. A prevalent sentiment among the Chinese intellectuals was that it would best serve China to do away with tradition and adopt the ways of the West. It was against this background that the abandonment of Chinese medicine was proposed. The trend was so extreme that in the 1920s the nationalist government had banned Chinese medicine entirely. Within three months, the decision caused a tremendous outrage from the Chinese people of all classes, and the ban was lifted."

In 1949, Mao Tse-tung established the People's Republic of China. Seventeen years later, the turbulent political atmosphere erupted in the Cultural Revolution and the Red Terror swept over China. Those in power turned a blind eye as marauding bands of crazed teenagers pillaged the country, arresting and imprisoning high-ranking government officials and persecuting so-called intellectuals and antirevolutionaries. While most of China's culture was dismantled, by 1954 Chairman Mao Tse-tung officially recognized Chinese medicine as "the legacy of the motherland." From that point on, Chinese medicine was fully reinstated and endorsed by the government.

However, as a result of this influence, Chinese medicine evolved into two different schools. Traditional Chinese medicine continues to integrate mind,

body and spirit in a true spiritual sense, relying on an ancient form of meditation called Qigong to build self-awareness, unity of mind and body and ultimately enlightenment. The school influenced by the Communist regime in
China uses Chinese medical modalities such as herbal medicine and acupuncture in more of a nuts-and-bolts fashion. Eschewing a belief in spiritual unity,
this more clinical practice of Chinese medicine views the mind/body connection in a more scientific and psychological manner.

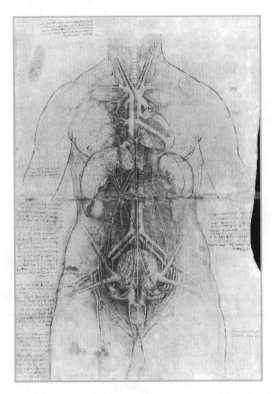

*Figure 1*
*Leonardo da Vinci (1452–1519)*
*Anatomical study of the principal organs*
*and arterial system of a female torso*
(Used by permission of The Royal Collection
© 2002, Her Majesty Queen Elizabeth II)

Western medicine sees the human body as a collection of physical components such as bones, fluids, organs, tissues, cells, DNA and molecules. Chinese
medicine does not delve into tangible components but rather views the body's
patterns of Energy as part of a greater whole that is constantly in motion and

constantly seeking balance. While the material dimension of a living being is made of the same elements that make up all tangible substances, what gives a living being life is the Energy within. Energy is formless, though we all know it exists. In Chinese medicine, the pattern of Energy within the body (and its environment) is referred to as Qi (pronounced *chee*). Broadly speaking, Qi is the integration of Yin and Yang. In other words, instead of being made up of materials, the human body is made up of Yin and Yang Energy—two opposing yet mutually dependent forces. Yin Energy is water, cool, calm, passive, and Yang Energy is fire, warm, active, aggressive.

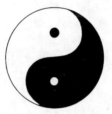

*Figure 2*
*Within the traditional Yin/Yang symbol, black and white holes*
*signify that Yin is part of Yang and Yang is part of Yin.*

Chinese medicine evolved from the belief that true health results from balancing the entire system. In Western thought the word *system* is thought of in compartmentalized terms, such as the system of the human body, the endocrine system, the nervous system and so on. Other examples are the solar system, Freud's system of psychological functioning (superego, ego and id), the U.S. system of government and a computer system. Chinese medicine considers human beings (who are composed of an interconnected mind *and* body) and their environment to be part of the same system, or part of a whole. Yin and Yang, and their constant fluctuations, dictate the balance of this whole. These constant fluctuations of Energy occur within a never-ending circle of nature, so that all occurrences have a consequence, sometimes positive and sometimes negative.

Meridians are invisible channels in your body in which Qi (the integration of Yin and Yang Energies) flows. Meridians do not correspond to any known physiological structure in Western medicine. They are not like the Western concept of the circulation system, the nervous system or lymphatic system.

Meridians are a complex web of channels that branch out to smaller and smaller Meridian channels that become as minuscule as capillaries. Qi continually flows through these channels to create the wholeness of your body.

Because Qi permeates the universe, Meridians connect your internal body with the outside universe as well.

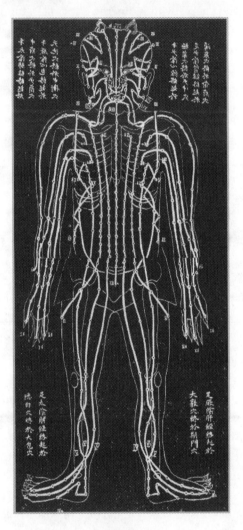

*Figure 3*
*Ancient illustration of the*
*Meridian system*

In diagnosing and treating illness, Western medicine uses sophisticated scientific technologies to attempt to pinpoint the exact cause—whether it be bacterial, viral, cancerous cells or another tangible cause. Chinese medicine does not need to isolate tangible causes of disease in order to treat illness.

From a Chinese medicine point of view, your Qi flows through the Meridian system of your body. Yin and Yang Energy form an infinite number of patterns within your body. For example, the Heart, Liver, Spleen, Kidneys and Lungs have individual Yin and Yang Energy. (The following chapters describe the Five Energetic Systems based on these organs.) Moreover, each human has his or her unique Energy balance. This pattern of Energy is constantly in motion and strives to be in balance. The balance is achieved as the Energy movement delivers nutrients and oxygen to nourish the body, and also removes toxins and metabolic waste. Toxins result from various sources: environmental (such as pesticides and carbon dioxide), biological (such as bacteria and viruses), biochemical (such as mercury, lead or other heavy metals and alcohol) and physical (such as radiation and cigarette smoke). Metabolic waste is the end product of metabolism—in other words, imagine each cell to be like a living being that must eliminate waste.

If the equilibrium of Qi is upset for any reason, there will be a slowing down of the Energy flow and the toxins and metabolic waste will not be sufficiently removed. When Qi becomes weakened, blocked or stagnated, this Energetic imbalance will result in illness and disease. To arrive at a diagnosis, the Chinese doctor compiles a complete picture of you as a whole being (more will be said about the methods of diagnosis in chapter 3). Chinese medicine then uses herbal medicine, acupuncture and other ancient healing methods to get Qi moving and correct the imbalance that caused the problem. Chinese medicine places all of its emphasis on the fact that you and all of your systems—body and mind—are a whole, interconnected and interdependent.

By the twentieth century in the West, biomedical theory had been designated the one true path to health. But several decades ago, consumer confidence in Western medicine began to wane. The cultural revolution in this country in the sixties and seventies helped shift the attitudes of the public from utter reliance on and belief in the medical system to one of questioning, personal exploration and self-confidence. In the eighties and nineties, as health care payment systems and time constraints dictated by insurance companies increasingly limited the effectiveness of physicians and weakened traditional patient-doctor bonds, the movement was pushed along.

In 1993, Harvard Medical School physician and researcher David Eisenberg, M.D., and his colleagues published the results of a survey that showed that in 1992 one in three respondents had used at least one alternative or nontraditional therapy. A second survey published in 1998 indicated that between 1990 and 1997 total visits to alternative providers increased 47 percent, from an estimated 427 million in 1990 to 629 million in 1997. More people paid visits to alternative-care providers than to all allopathic (Western-style) primary-care providers. Annual expenditures for alternative-medicine services increased 45 percent, to $12 billion.

Responding to this trend, in 1995 Beth Israel Deaconess Medical Center created the Center for Alternative Medicine Research and Education, which is associated with Harvard Medical School. Dr. Eisenberg was appointed director, and Ted J. Kaptchuk, O.M.D., author of the classic comprehensive guide to Chinese medicine, *The Web That Has No Weaver,* was named associate director. The center studies the scientific and medical dimensions of complementary and alternative treatments as well as the legal, ethical and economic implications of these therapies. The research of Drs. Eisenberg and Kaptchuk and others at the center encourages interaction between Western doctors and their patients. This research also recognizes the tremendous influence of public demand for alternative medicines, and that as a result there are increasingly more courses in alternative medicine offered in Western medical schools.

In addition, research on complementary/alternative treatments within universities and medical schools is becoming more commonplace. Since natural substances, such as herbs, currently cannot be patented, many pharmaceutical companies have little interest in promoting the research of traditional Chinese medicine. Oncology nurse and researcher Diane Fletcher, M.A., R.N., O.C.N., from the University of Pittsburgh Cancer Institute, said, "Research on Chinese herbs has been going on for thousands of years in China. Even though there has been a significant amount of research published there, it usually is not up to Western scientific standards for design, implementation and reporting of results. So in one sense, research on Chinese herbs in the U.S. is light-years behind, but in another sense we need to do our own research according to our own standards. But it can take years to get results, and then studies must be replicated to further prove or disprove those results."

The government responded to this need in 1998 and formed a division of the National Institutes of Health called the National Center for Complementary and Alternative Medicine (NCCAM). The government has subsequently given the NCCAM millions of dollars of funding for research studies. Across the United States, many academic institutions are starting to organize and conduct research on Chinese herbs. At the same time, many Western physicians and other health care practitioners are incorporating Chinese medicine into their practices. No doubt the eighteenth-century Chinese doctor Wang Qingren would have found great satisfaction in seeing the line in the sand becoming blurred and integration naturally occurring.

The following four chapters describe the basics of Chinese medicine. If you find this material too dense to read all at once, you may want to skip to Part Two, which contains case histories and health programs for a variety of conditions, and revisit these chapters later.

# 2

# Qi, Yin and Yang

*Healing is restoring the balance between Yin and Yang*

In 1962 Binrong Ma was a whiz kid mathematician who had graduated at the top of his class from the prestigious Fu Dan University in China. In 1965, as the Red Terror overtook China, Professor Ma was sent to the countryside and assigned the job of raising pigs. In 1975 Ma was allowed to return to the Capital University of Medical Science, where he was assigned to study Chinese medicine. Three years later, an epidemic of hepatitis B swept across China. Hepatitis B is a chronic systemic illness, caused by a viral infection, that results in extensive inflammation and necrosis (death) of liver cells. It is profoundly debilitating and in some cases evolves to cirrhosis (scarring of the liver) and liver failure. Hepatitis B, which is transmitted by exposure to blood or by intimate contact, was spreading across China like a firestorm. Hospitals in the larger cities, such as Beijing and Shanghai, were full of sick people.

Because Western medicine had not yet developed a vaccination against hepatitis B, the epidemic could not be effectively halted by Western medicine. Chinese medicine was known to be effective in the treatment of hepatitis B, but treating so many ill people with Chinese herbs was impossible because Chinese medicine is not designed to be standardized like Western medicine. Western medicine begins by diagnosing an illness; once the diagnosis is clear the basic treatment is almost always the same for everyone. Chinese medicine, on the other hand, recognizes different patterns of imbalances or subtypes within the same diagnosis. The treatment is individualized according to the person's subtypes and other aspects of the individual's uniqueness. The efficacy of treatment depends upon how specifically the treatment plan can be tailored to address each patient's individuality. To prescribe herbal medicine during a hepatitis epidemic would require thousands of practitioners to observe and probe people for information, organize signs and symptoms into patterns of imbalances and formulate individualized herbal prescriptions. There were not enough experienced herbalists to go around. Even if doctors worked day and night, the epidemic would move faster than they could diagnose and prescribe.

Professor Ma was called upon to join an elite task force that included Dr. Yubo Guan, a doctor of Chinese medicine who was a specialist in treating liver disease. The team was sequestered and instructed to develop a traditional Chinese medicine (TCM) artificial intelligence system in hepatitis B, which would use a computer program to simulate Dr. Guan's diagnostic and liver/hepatitis treatment expertise. Using the old TQ16 computer that did computation and calculation by punching holes in an infinitely long paper belt, after weeks of working, often at night, the team successfully developed a single program. This program diagnosed thousands of sick people on an individual basis and was able to generate over a hundred thousand different herbal formulations, quickly arresting the epidemic.

Herding Chinese medical diagnostic principles into a computer program was like chasing mercury. To understand the complexity of the variables within the hepatitis B diagnosis and the treatment methods offered by Chinese medicine, a deeper understanding of the basic concepts of Chinese medicine is useful, beginning with the Vital Substance Qi.

## Qi

In a cosmic sense, Qi is viewed as the basic substance (mass or matter), as well as the Energy necessary to create the physical world, which includes all living things. As explained by Western science, throughout the universe mass can be converted to energy, and energy can be converted into mass—for example, the food we eat is converted to energy, and burning wood creates the energy of heat. From a Chinese medicine perspective, Qi is the singular common bond that exists and connects all living things, thereby being able to pass back and forth and interact. In fact, Qi is not only the common bond between all living things but also the commonality shared by all existence. Qi cannot be created or destroyed, it can only be transformed from one form to another.

Qi supports and sustains your body's life functions such as breathing, metabolism, thoughts and feelings, but it is also the life function itself.

The basic properties of Qi

- Qi is dynamic in nature, in that it is constantly moving (circulating) and changing (transforming).
- Qi is always striving to attain balance and harmony.
- Qi involves the constant movement of Yin and Yang, two mutually dependent opposites.

The creation of Qi

Qi is derived from three sources:

- Qi is genetically inherited. Your genetically inherited Qi is made up primarily of Kidney Energy and determines your constitutional uniqueness and strength. (The Five Energetic Systems, comprising of Heart, Lung, Spleen, Liver and Kidney Energies, are explained on pages 25–27.) *Note: When names of organs are capitalized, they denote the Chinese medicine Energetic system. Organs in lowercase denote organs in the Western sense.*
- Qi is acquired internally through your body's functional activities, such as converting nutrients from food sources via digestion. This source of Qi is made up primarily of Spleen Energy.
- Qi is acquired from the air (oxygen) via Lung Energy.

Once integrated within your body through the actions of these three sources, Qi is then distributed throughout your body and to all other Energetic systems in order to sustain their functions and activities.

The basic movement of Qi

- *Ascending.* Qi distributes and spreads nutrients and oxygen throughout your body as it ascends.
- *Descending.* Qi passes down metabolic waste and toxins for elimination, and can also deliver nutrients as it descends.
- *Inward/Outward.* Qi supports and strengthens your body through inward movement. Qi disperses nutrients and expels toxins through outward movement.
- *Circulating.* Qi circulates. In other words, Energy or the Life Force circulates within your body.

The basic functions of Qi

- *Powers the circulation of Energy.* Qi is the source of the dynamics within your body.
- *Regulates the Energy movement.* Qi acts as the traffic controller, directing the various Energy systems throughout your body.
- *Nourishes your body.* Qi delivers nutrients throughout your body.
- *Detoxifies your body.* Qi removes toxins and metabolic wastes from your body.
- *Protects your body.* Qi guards against the invasion of External Causes and protects against Internal Causes. (External Causes and Internal Causes are explained on pages 33 and 36.)
- *Maintains all organs, blood and bodily fluids within the physical systems to which they belong.* Qi maintains blood within the circulatory system to prevent hemorrhaging and keeps your internal organs suspended appropriately to prevent them from sagging—for example, a prolapsed uterus.
- *Energizes your body.* Qi keeps your body Energized by maintaining the back-and-forth transformations of Qi and the metabolism of your body.


Classification of Qi

- *Primordial (Yuan Qi).* The most fundamental and important Qi. It is primarily genetically inherited. It can be strengthened or depleted throughout the course of life. It provides the most important part of vitality. It nourishes and supports all the other specific Energetic systems. It dictates growth, development and aging.
- *Ancestral (Zong Qi).* Originates from within the region of your chest (lungs and heart), and is closely connected to the air you breathe. Its main function is to support breathing and blood circulation.
- *Protective (Wei Qi).* The Qi created from nutrients by Spleen Energy, supported and enhanced by Kidney Energy, and distributed by Lung Energy. It is active and circulates primarily along the exterior of your body to protect against the invasion of External Causes.
- *Nutritive (Ying Qi).* This is the Qi most intimately associated with the Vital Substance of Blood. It circulates along blood vessels. Its primary function is to deliver nutrients to and throughout the body.
- *Meridian (Jin Qi).* This is the Qi that circulates within the Meridians. It connects all of the Energetic systems and parts of your body into an inte-

grated whole. It nourishes, regulates and detoxifies. This is the Qi that acupuncture primarily works through.

◦ *Organ (Zang Fu Qi).* This Qi belongs to and carries the functions of each individual major and minor Energetic system. In a Western sense, this Qi empowers the physiologic functions of each organ.

## Vital Substances: Blood (Xue), Fluid (Jin Ye), Essence (Jing) and Shen

*Blood (Xue):* The primary function of Blood is to nourish. The concept of Blood within Chinese medicine is similar to that of blood as defined by Western medicine. The only significant difference is that Blood has an intimate connection with Qi. In Western medicine blood circulation is considered mechanical in nature. In Chinese medicine Blood circulation is powered and carried by the movement of Qi. In Chinese medicine, like Western medicine, Blood is the substance that circulates throughout the blood vessels.

Blood is created primarily from nutrients extracted from the food you eat and is converted by Spleen Energy, transported to Lung Energy and combined with your Primordial Qi, which is then powered into the circulatory system. During this circulation all five major Energetic systems—Heart, Lung, Spleen, Liver and Kidney—are involved in maintaining Blood's movement and distribution.

*Fluid (Jin Ye):* Fluid within Chinese medicine encompasses all of your bodily fluids (except blood), including secretions such as gastric juices, tears, saliva and perspiration. As in Western medicine, Chinese medicine recognizes that Fluid contains many other substances that are important to your body. Thereby, it also has nourishing properties. The Fluid of your body is continuously interconnected with Blood.

The creation of Fluid is initially accomplished through the function of Spleen Energy. Spleen Energy extracts and absorbs Fluid from the ingestion of water and foods. These absorbed Fluids are transported to Lung Energy, which distributes them throughout your body. During this process Kidney Energy is involved in Fluid regulation and distribution. The Small Intestine Energetic system and the Large Intestine Energetic system (explained on page 27) are also involved. The Small Intestine separates the pure Fluid from Impurities, and the Large Intestine reabsorbs some Fluid.

A disharmony of Fluids produces visible or invisible Phlegm and Dampness.

*Essence (Jing):* Essence is an entirely inherited, specific part of Kidney Energy that governs reproduction and development. Although it is inherited, your Jing can be strengthened or depleted during the course of life. It is confined within the Kidney Energy system.

*Shen:* In a broad sense, Shen is spirit without a religious affiliation. For example, an individual who has the presence of good health, balance and harmony as well as the radiance of health is said to "have the Shen." A Chinese medical doctor is trained to observe the patient's Shen. If someone is gravely ill but still has Shen, it means he or she will survive.

In a specific sense, Shen is all of the mental and psychological functions and activities of an individual. In the Chinese culture, if your Shen is blurred, it means that you are not alert. Generally, the more Shen one has, the more balanced one's body will be. Shen is closely associated with Heart and Kidney Energies. In order for Shen to be created and sustained there needs to be a balance of the Vital Substances Qi, Blood, Fluid and Essence as well as a balance of Kidney and Heart Energies.

## Yin and Yang

In Chinese medicine, optimal health is achieved through a state of balance and harmony that involves body, mind and environment.

Harmony is determined by the balance between Yin and Yang. Yin and Yang are the most basic concepts used by Chinese philosophy to characterize the world and life. To ancient Chinese sages, Yin and Yang were the essence of existence and changes. Everything embodies Yin and Yang, and the interactions and movement between Yin and Yang provide a dynamic source for the occurrence, development and shifting of all things. Yin and Yang are a pair of mutually dependent opposites.

Originally, Yang, meaning "the sunny side of the mountain," represented the positive or active aspects. Yin, meaning "the shady side of the mountain," represented the negative or passive aspects. Yang is heat, light, day, summer, vigor, masculinity, upwardness, exterior and function. Yin is cold, dark, night, winter, stillness, femininity, downwardness, interior and substance. A common conceptualization of Yin and Yang in Chinese medicine is water (Yin) and fire (Yang).

## The nature of Yin and Yang

- *Yin/Yang polarity (direct opposites) is omnipresent.* This polarity exists in all things or phenomena.
- *Yin and Yang are opposite yet interdependent.* Yin and Yang define each other and are relative to one another. Up would have no meaning without down; cold is definable only in relation to heat. The Equator is hot in relation to the North Pole, yet it is cold in relation to the surface of the sun. This relativity also determines that there are no absolutes—everything is relative. There is no distinct or separate black and white, yes and no, normal and abnormal, or sick and healthy.
- *Within Yin there is Yang, and within Yang there is Yin.* For instance, male is Yang and female is Yin. A woman's body's functional activity is Yang and her substance, the physical structure, is Yin. Within her body, the exterior is Yang and interior is Yin. Internally, her Energetic systems can be again divided into Yin and Yang Energetic systems depending on their structure and functions.
- *The Five Energetic Systems are Yin.* Liver, Heart, Spleen, Lung and Kidney are mostly solid organs that store Vital Substances, which are Qi, Blood, Fluid, Essence and Shen. The minor Energetic systems are Yang: Gall Bladder, Small and Large Intestines, Stomach and Urinary Bladder are mostly hollow and responsible for transporting and eliminating impurities from the Vital Substances. Each Yin organ, in turn, has its own aspect of Yin and Yang. (The Energetic systems are further explained on pages 25–30.)
- *Yin and Yang are always striving for balance.* Western medicine observes homeostasis as the body's adaptive responses that attempt to return the body from an abnormal state back to the status quo. From a Chinese medicine point of view homeostasis in the human body is maintained by the perpetual dance of Yin and Yang. There is a constant and normal rhythmic or cyclic fluctuation of Yin and Yang. At the same time, Yin and Yang are always trying to engage each other, ensuring that the other does not get too far away. This is why day always follows night, and after winter there will be a summer. It is natural for humans to sleep during the night (for Yang to merge into Yin) and become awake during the day (for Yang to emerge from Yin). We also need rest and relaxation (Yin) after a period of exertion and stress (Yang).
- *Yin and Yang transform into each other.* This is true under normal conditions of health and in abnormal conditions of disharmony (illness and

death). For example, to sustain any functional activity (Yang) in your body, your body needs to consume certain nutrients (Yin)—thus the process of Yin transforming into Yang. On the other hand, energy (Yang) is spent to assemble the building blocks of your ever-renewing body structure (Yin)—thus the process of Yang transforming into Yin. When the transformation does not proceed properly or proportionally, it will lead to imbalances, which are illnesses or death; for example, dehydration (weakened Yin) due to a high fever (excess Yang), or hypothermia (weakened Yang) resulting from overexposure to cold (excess Yin). With severe exposure to cold, the person may go into shock—Yin and Yang disconnection due to a radical transformation of Yang to Yin. The person may even die—Yang ceases to exist due to complete transformation of Yang to Yin.

The focus of healing is to support the inner propensity of Yin and Yang striving for balance. To assist in your understanding of the many variables of Yin and Yang it is useful to also understand disharmonies, excess imbalance and deficiency imbalance. Once Yin and Yang are defined many other concepts of secondary importance within Chinese medicine can then be determined.

## Yin and Yang excess and deficiencies

- *Physical.* Symptoms that are degenerative, recessive, weak and lowering body temperature or causing a cold feeling are considered Yin. Symptoms that are inflammatory, expressive, agitated and elevating body temperature or causing a hot feeling are considered Yang.
- *Emotional.* Depression, sadness, withdrawal and lack of motivation are Yin. Anxiety, anger, aggression and mania are Yang.
- *Personality traits.* Reserved, introverted, calm, steady and reticent are Yin. Ostentatious, extroverted, excitable, volatile and outspoken are Yang.
- *Constitution.* A person whose body tends to run on the Cool side, who likes to dress warmly and prefers warm weather, has more of a Yin constitution. The person whose body tends to run on the Hot side, who likes to dress coolly and prefers cool weather has more of a Yang constitution.

## Imbalances between Yin and Yang have eight scenarios

- *Yin deficiency, also known as deficient Heat imbalance.* When Yang is normal but the person can exhibit some Yang symptoms because there is not enough Yin Energy to balance the Yang.

* *Yang deficiency, also known as deficient Cold imbalance.* When Yin is normal yet the person exhibits some Yin symptoms because there is not enough Yang Energy to balance the Yin.
* *Yin excess, also known as excess Cold imbalance.* The person shows pronounced Yin symptoms but without any weakness.
* *Yang excess, also known as excess Heat imbalance.* The person shows pronounced Yang symptoms but without any weakness.
* *Yin deficiency/Yang excess.* The person shows pronounced Heat symptoms along with Yin weakness.
* *Yang deficiency/Yin excess.* The person shows pronounced Cold symptoms along with Yang weakness.
* *Yin and Yang deficiency.* The person can exhibit a general weakness and fluctuate between deficient Heat and Cold symptoms.
* *Yin and Yang excess.* The person can have Heat and Cold symptoms at the same time or alternately without any discernible weakness. This is demonstrated in certain types of common cold or flu as well in malaria, when the person can fluctuate between fever and chills.

Since each Yin organ of the Five Major Energetic Systems has its own Yin and Yang aspects, and can have all the above imbalances, as the illness can involve any number of them, the possible combination of imbalances among the Five Energetic Systems is 32,768 ($8^5 = 32,768$). This is derived from the fact that each of the Five Major Energetic Systems can experience eight different possible imbalances between Yin and Yang. If we take into consideration imbalances of Yang organs of the Six Minor Energetic Systems and the different Pathogens that can interact with the Five Energetic Systems, the possible conditions of imbalances will quickly reach an astronomical number.

## The Five Element Theory

In the development of Chinese medicine, once Yin and Yang were in place, the next important concept to be determined and defined was the Five Element Theory.

Western medical science is literal. In other words, doctors read lab reports or use other black-and-white diagnostic methods to determine a diagnosis and treatment plan. Chinese medical concepts cannot be explained in a literal fashion. It is extremely difficult for Westerners to fully understand the symbolism Chinese medicine uses to diagnose and treat illness. Unlike Western medicine,

Chinese medicine never evolved a scientific language. In part, the Chinese language does not readily invent new words as does the English language, which adds some two thousand new words each year. Also, Chinese medicine does not place great emphasis on technology. Rather, it developed a philosophical, symbolic and metaphoric emphasis. Today, Chinese medicine continues to use the same ancient language of its origins.

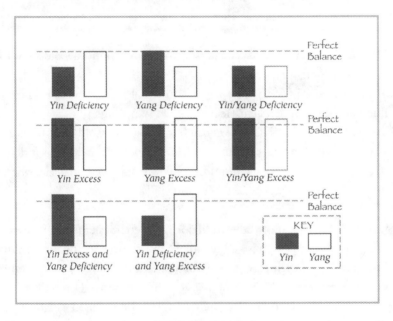

*Figure 4*
*The eight variables of Yin and Yang*

The Five Element Theory was first formed in China at about the time of the Zhou dynasty (867 to 255 b.c.). Historically, it arose from observations of the natural world made in early times by people in the course of their lives and productive labor. Wood, fire, earth, metal and water were considered to be five indispensable materials for the maintenance of life and production, as well as representing five important states that initiated normal changes in the natural world. In other words, all phenomena in the universe correspond in nature to either wood, fire, earth, metal or water, and these elements are in a state of constant motion and change.

The primitive concept of the Five Elements was later developed into a more complex theory, which, together with the theory of Yin/Yang, served as a conceptual tool for understanding and analyzing all phenomena. In traditional

Chinese medicine the Five Element Theory served to guide clinical diagnosis and treatment. Modern Chinese medical practitioners are finding the Five Element Theory to be archaic and limiting and are increasingly relying on the Five Energetic Systems instead.

The Five Energetic Systems evolved to some extent from the Five Element Theory. There is good reason to think that the Five Energetic Systems began to gain prominence and the Five Element Theory began to lose its grip on the mainstream of Chinese medicine around 1115 to 1368 B.C. (Jing-Yuan era).

The shift from the Five Element Theory to the Five Energetic Systems was a gradual process. In fact, the Five Element Theory is still in use today in Chinese medicine, but the use has become confined to specific areas of practice, such as certain styles of acupuncture.

## The Zangfu

The complexities that perplexed the Chinese experts during the hepatitis epidemic of the 1970s included the role of the Zangfu, which is a collective name for the solid Yin organ systems of the Five Major Energetic Systems (Lung, Heart, Spleen, Liver and Kidneys) and the hollow Yang Organ systems of the Six Minor Energetic Systems (Small Intestine, Large Intestine, Gall Bladder, Bladder, Stomach and San Jiao [Triple Warmer]), explained on pages 27–30.

## The Five Energetic Systems

### The Yin Organs

The Yin Organs, also known as the Zang or the Five Major Energetic Systems, encompass the Kidney, Heart, Lungs, Spleen and Liver Energies. The notion of balance and wholeness is the heart and soul of Chinese medicine; the Yin/Yang theory provides the bones and skeleton; the Energetic systems are the flesh and blood of Chinese medicine. The Five Major Energetic Systems provide the medium through which the Yin and Yang interactions can flow.

*Kidney Energy:* Provides the most important part of your vitality by storing and generating Jing (Essence). Kidney Energy is responsible for sexuality and reproduction, structural integrity and functions of the bones. It also serves a major part of cognitive functions such as memory, concentration and the capacity to process information. Kidney Energy regulates bodily fluids. Kidney Energy dictates growth and development. The fluctuations of the life cycle—conception, birth, adolescence, old age and death—are dictated by Kidney Energy. It is also responsible for part of the function of breathing, specifically deep inhalation. The strength of your Kidney Energy is reflected in the state of your hair (lustrous versus dry and brittle). Kidney Energy is particularly connected to the ears, in that many disorders affecting the ears are treated by harmonizing Kidney Energy. Emotional connections are fear/courage. Kidney Energy is associated with the minor Energetic system of the Urinary Bladder. This association determines that the disharmony of each system can affect the other system.

*Heart Energy:* Provides the main dynamic source for blood circulation. Heart Energy is closely associated with Shen. Your Heart Energy is reflected in the state of your complexion (glowing and vibrant versus dull and dry). The Heart is connected with the tongue, in that many disorders of the heart are reflected in the appearance of the tongue and, conversely, some disorders affecting the tongue are treated by harmonizing Heart Energy. Emotional connections are happiness/agony. Heart Energy is associated with the minor Energetic system of the Small Intestine.

*Lung Energy:* Responsible for breathing. Lung Energy is closely associated with Qi, particularly in that Qi connects our body with the environment. Lung Energy is involved in the distribution of nutrients and Fluid and is also part of the regulating process of blood circulation, which is similar to the ideas of Western medicine. Lung Energy is reflected in the state of your skin (moist and firm versus dry and wrinkled). Lung Energy is particularly connected to the nose, in that the nose is the gateway to the lungs. Many External Causes affect the lungs via the nose, and the majority of disorders and symptoms involving the nose are treated by harmonizing Lung Energy. Emotional connections are sorrow, grieving and chronic worry. Lung Energy is associated with the minor Energetic system of the Large Intestine.

*Spleen Energy:* Represents a major part of the digestive function; not just for food but also for Fluid assimilation and regulation. It is responsible for providing nourishment for the entire body. It also controls circulation by regulating blood coagulation. Spleen Energy determines the strength of the muscles and functions of the limbs. Spleen Energy is reflected in the state of your lips (moist and plump versus dry and cracked). The Spleen is connected to the mouth, in that many disorders affecting the mouth are treated by harmonizing Spleen Energy. Emotional connections are pensiveness and profound or obsessive thoughts. Spleen Energy is associated with the minor Energetic system of the Stomach.

*Liver Energy:* The great regulator of our body. It regulates Energy flow and circulation, digestion, emotions, fluid and menses. It stores and releases Blood. Liver Energy is reflected in your fingernails and toenails (smooth and strong versus cracked, ridged and brittle). The Liver is connected to the eyes, in that many disorders affecting the eyes are treated by harmonizing Liver Energy. Liver Energy determines the strength and flexibility of the body's tendons and ligaments. Emotional connections are anger/sadness. Liver Energy is associated with the minor Energetic system of Gall Bladder.

# The Six Minor Energetic Systems

## The Yang Organs (Fu)

In addition to the Yin Organs, there are the Yang Organs—called the Fu or the Six Minor Energetic Systems. The Six Minor Energetic Systems actually come closer to relating to the organ of similar name, in terms of their functional similarities, than do the Five Major Energetic Systems.

*Small Intestine Energy:* Associated with Heart Energy, Small Intestine Energy stores and transports foodstuffs and helps to separate the Purity (nutrients) from the Impurity (digestive waste) within the foodstuffs.

*Large Intestine Energy:* Associated with the Lung Energy, the main function of Large Intestine Energy is the transportation and elimination of digestive waste.

*Gall Bladder Energy:* Associated with Liver Energy, Gall Bladder Energy stores and releases bile, and assists in digestion, which is identical to the function as Western medicine conceives of it.

*Urinary Bladder Energy:* Associated with Kidney Energy, Urinary Bladder Energy stores and eliminates urine, which is identical to the function in Western medicine perspective.

Figure 5 — Zang Xiang System: The Functions and

| Major Energetic System (Zang) | Associated Minor Energetic System (Fu) |
| --- | --- |
| Kidney Energy system | Urinary Bladder<br>Main function: Stores and eliminates urine |
| Liver Energy system | Gall Bladder<br>Main functions: Stores and releases bile;<br>    assists digestion |
| Heart Energy system | Small Intestine<br>Main functions: Stores and transfers foodstuffs;<br>    separates the Purity from the Impurity in<br>    foodstuffs |
| Spleen Energy system | Stomach<br>Main functions: Stores and transports foods;<br>    assists in digestion |
| Lung Energy system | Large Intestine<br>Main function: Transports and eliminates<br>    digestive waste |

# Connections of the Major and Minor Energetic Systems

| Main Functions | Connections | Dominant Emotions |
| --- | --- | --- |
| Stores and generates Jing | Bones | Fear |
| Governs development, reproduction and sexuality | Ears | Fright |
| | Genitals/anus | |
| Provides vitality | Hair | |
| Regulates fluid | Teeth | |
| Assists inhalation | Saliva | |
| Nourishes and supports brain and some cognitive functions | | |
| Regulates Qi and Blood movements | Tendons/ligaments | Anger |
| | Eyes | Sadness |
| Stores Blood | Nails | |
| Regulates emotions | Tears | |
| Regulates digestion | | |
| Regulates menstruation | | |
| Governs Blood circulation | Blood vessels | Happiness |
| Stores Shen | Tongue | Joy |
| | Facial complexion | |
| | Sweat | |
| Governs digestion and assimilation | Muscles | Pensiveness |
| | Mouth | Worry |
| Provides nutrients for body | Limbs | |
| Assists fluid metabolism | Lips/gums | |
| Contains and prevents bleeding | | |
| Governs breathing | Skin | Sadness |
| Assists Qi generation | Nose | Grief |
| Supports immune system | Mucus | |
| Assists distribution of nutrients | | |
| Assists fluid regulation and Blood circulation | | |

*Stomach Energy:* Associated with Spleen Energy, Stomach Energy stores, transports and assists in the digestion of food. After food has left the stomach, Stomach Energy moves Purities downward through your gastrointestinal tract to the small intestines, and ultimately the large intestine. As Stomach Energy pushes downward the Purities are extracted by Spleen Energy, which moves these Purities upward and distributes them to nourish your body.

*San Jiao (Triple Warmer):* The Triple Warmer is not an actual organ-based Energetic system, but rather a functionally based activity through which most of the major and minor Energetic systems are integrated. Through its functional activity the metabolism of nutrients and Fluid is accomplished.

## Zang Xiang System/Theory

*Zang* means "Organ" (in an Energetic sense), and *Xiang* means "sign" or "manifestation." The Zang Xiang system is the functional connection of an Energetic system in its entirety. It is the Energetic web that weaves together a major Energetic system with its associated minor Energetic system. Zang Xiang theory is the study of how the harmony or disharmony of internal Energetic systems reflects or expresses itself outwardly.

# 3

## Diagnosis

*Everything that goes on within you
can be seen on the outside*

The region of Lin Xian in central China is about forty miles across and in the 1960s boasted a population of seventy thousand. The region had garnered the attention of the Chinese government and the World Health Organization as having the highest rate of esophageal cancer in the world with a consistent 15 percent of the adult population dying of this cancer. In 1964 the Chinese government and the U.N. sent a team to study this problem. The team was made up of pathologists, surgical oncologists and gastrointestinal and infectious diseases experts. To be politically correct, they invited a few doctors of Chinese medicine to join their field research.

The team set out to examine and diagnose everyone in the county over the age of twenty-six, approximately 50,000 people. The time and cost were exorbitant. Among the diagnostic procedures was an endoscopy in which a balloon was inserted into the patient's stomach, inflated and then gently pulled out to collect cell samples from the esophagus. As patients arrived to be examined, one of the doctors of Chinese medicine often made remarks such as, "Oh, he's okay. Don't bother with him." Or, "He really looks bad." The doctor's assessment was almost always consistent with the balloon endoscopy, which baffled the Western doctors. When they questioned him, they learned that the doctor of Chinese medicine had based his opinion on examining the patients' tongues.

The field team, still skeptical, organized an independent comparative study, which concluded that the Chinese doctor's diagnosis was nearly as accurate as the balloon endoscopy. At the researcher's request, the doctor taught the entire

team how to examine tongues, which sped up the diagnostic process tremendously.

The doctor of Chinese medicine understood what Chinese medicine has
known for thousands of years: *Everything that goes on within you can be seen on
the outside.* If you truly understand the significance of the concept of wholeness, then it logically follows that every aspect of your mind, body and spirit
will affect and be reflected in every other part of your mind, body and spirit.
From asking questions and observing, the doctor can organize all of the information into a meaningful pattern of harmony or disharmony to arrive at a diagnosis and treatment plan.

## Zheng

The objective of diagnosis in Chinese medicine is different from the objective or goal of diagnosis in Western medicine, which focuses primarily on gathering information in order to arrive at a specific diagnosis so that treatment can
be determined. In Chinese medicine, the outcome of collecting, analyzing and
integrating data from history gathering and examination of the patient is
aimed at determining the Zheng. Zheng is a comprehensive assessment of the
nature of the patient's condition that weaves together all the relevant information about the condition into a meaningful pattern, including (1) the Causes
(explained below), (2) the patient's state of Qi—strong or weak, or one of the
many states in between, (3) the circumstances such as location and season, (4)
personal data such as constitution and temperament and (5) lifestyle factors.

In Chinese medicine as in Western medicine, physicians are taught to follow
the Law of Parsimony. When there is more than one complaint or symptom
your doctor tries to find the most simple, singular answer that accounts for all,
or the majority, of the signs and symptoms. For example, if you have a
headache, sore throat and runny nose, chances are that you do not have a brain
tumor, throat cancer and allergies, but rather have the flu.

## Causes of Disease

The causes of disease from a Chinese medicine perspective are organized
into the following major categories: External Causes, Internal Causes, Non-
Internal Causes, Non-External Causes. (These terms are capitalized throughout
to define them as Chinese medical terms.)

External Causes

When identifying the causes of illnesses, Chinese medicine refers to External Causes: Wind, Cold, Summer Heat, Dampness, Dryness and Fire. External Causes do not refer to the actual physical entities of wind, cold, heat, dampness, dryness or fire but rather imply that a given Cause shares the properties of these phenomena. In other words, Wind does not mean that your body is invaded by a gust of wind. Rather, the Cause shows some similar properties of those of wind, such as being transient and changeable, appearing and disappearing quickly. Wind, Cold, Summer Heat, Dampness, Dryness and Fire are symbolic. A disease is typically caused by a combination of several Causes.

*Wind:* In nature, wind is swift, mobile, changeable and strikes suddenly. Consider the flu, which is often caused by the External Cause Wind. It invades your system with sudden onset of illness, and the symptoms can also change rapidly. The condition can begin with a sore throat. By the time you receive medication for your sore throat the symptoms may have moved into your chest.

*Cold:* Associated with degeneration and a decrease in metabolism. In nature cold is contracting, congealing, stiffening and tightening. A patient suffering from flu can also suffer from chills, tight muscles and stiff joints.

*Summer Heat:* Characterized by a pronounced inflammation, accelerated metabolism and hyperactivity. For instance, a patient with acute pneumonia with high fever, profuse sweating, thirst, dehydration and agitation and even delirium would be said to be suffering from the External Cause Heat.

*Dampness:* Connected with properties such as abnormal accumulation of fluid or moisture, swelling, heaviness, sluggishness and a stubborn and protracted course of illness. Dampness can be seen in the case of fungal or candida infection, or certain dermatological conditions that are characterized by pronounced swelling and oozing caused by an infectious agent as well as watery diarrhea, edema (water retention) and phlegm accumulation in the lungs or nose.

*Dryness:* Dryness mainly damages your body's Fluid—such as symptoms that can be seen in certain types of bronchitis where the patient has dry cough, accompanied by pronounced dry mouth, throat, lips and nostrils.

*Fire:* Fire has a property similar to Summer Heat, except that it is much more extreme. Many infections are considered to present an element of Fire. Fire is present when there is localized swelling, redness and the area is hot to the touch, such as with mumps, and the bodily discharge can become discolored or pustulant.

*Li Qi:* Any External Cause may also be considered Li Qi, if aside from exhibiting typical properties of other External Causes, it is highly contagious, evolves rapidly and causes the same or a very similar pattern of severe symptoms among different patients. Smallpox, typhus, tuberculosis and HIV would all be considered to be Li Qi. External Causes that have the condition Li Qi are usually also characterized by Heat or Fire.

*External Toxins:* External Toxins are chemical and biological toxins such as environmental pollutants, viruses and bacteria. Water polluted with human waste would be considered an External Toxin. External Toxins can appear in any season, although they tend to appear more with the warm weather.

*Relative Proportions:* It is important to determine the relative proportions of the various causatory factors involved before designing a treatment program. Successful treatment requires precise recognition of various proportions, combinations and interactions of External Causes and/or Toxins. The herbalist must refine his or her senses to recognize the interactions among different Causes, as well as among the interactions between the Causes and the patient's Qi. Herbal formulas are tailored exactly to the diagnosis of relative proportions to ensure maximum results and minimum side effects.

In Chinese medicine, for example, when diagnosing and treating arthritis, the various Causes involved, the relative proportions of the Causes and the state of Qi are determined.

Different symptoms of arthritis are caused by various External Causes.

- *External Wind:* Arthritic symptoms that are somewhat fleeting and changeable in nature. The pain moves from joint to joint.
- *External Cold:* Significant pain that remains localized in a particular joint(s); the pain is clearly aggravated by cold environment and/or weather.
- *External Dampness:* The patient suffers joint swelling and edema.
- *External Heat:* The patient's arthritis causes notable redness and inflammation.

A patient with symptoms of 60 percent Wind, 20 percent Cold, and 20 percent Dampness will be treated with a different approach than an arthritis patient with 60 percent Cold, 30 percent Dampness, and 10 percent Wind. In chronic arthritis the state of the patient's Qi would invariably be weakened or damaged, which needs to be considered when planning treatment strategies.

This is a simplified explanation of diagnosis using relative proportions. Regardless of the illness, an experienced and talented Chinese doctor uncovers a complicated web of interactions involving many factors, which may be immediately evident or extremely subtle.

*The Association Between External Causes and the Seasons:* External Causes are often associated with the seasons. When the Energy of the season becomes abnormal or excessive, it can lead to imbalances. For example, Wind is predominantly seen in the spring, Cold in winter, Summer Heat and Fire in summer, Dampness in the late summer and early fall (called Long Summer in Chinese medicine) and Dryness in fall.

When weather becomes erratic, such as when the temperature becomes unseasonably warm in winter or cold in summer, people's bodies can be thrown out of balance. This abnormal change can create an incubator effect, providing the invading External Cause a highly favorable environment in which to flourish. It is often the case that when there's a sudden cold spell during the summer, there is an outbreak of infectious disease. This is known in Chinese medicine as "untimely Energy." For example, when a flu hit hard in late summer and early fall in Beijing in the 1960s, many industries had to close down because two-thirds of their employees were sick. The government intervened and established many temporary sidewalk stands to make enormous amounts of herbal formulas to pass out to people on the street. The teas, called decoctions, were made from a classic formula designed to treat the flu. But the formula did not work very well and people continued coming down with the flu.

The government consulted a well-respected herbalist, Dr. Pu Fuzhou. Dr. Pu understood that the original classic formula, created about 1,800 years ago, was proven effective and often used to treat upper respiratory infection with a high fever. But the particular virus that was going around China at the time had a strong element of Dampness because of the time of the year in which it occurred. Dampness in nature is heavy, stubborn and clinging. It tends to attach to or become entangled with other Causes and make them difficult to clear. Dampness was not considered in the design of the original formula. Dr. Pu added just one herb—Cang Zhu (Red Atractylodes), which is traditionally used to resolve Dampness—to the original classic formula, which dramatically improved the efficacy of the formula. This story demonstrates how a Cause that is associated with a certain season can interact with the human body, thereby altering the disease pattern.

Internal Causes

In addition to External Causes, there are also Internal Causes. These are psychological in nature. The Internal Causes were described by the Chinese medical classics as the Seven Emotions: Anger, Joy, Sadness, Grief, Pensiveness, Fear and Fright. These emotions represent a wide range of inner states. They are, by themselves, neither good nor bad. But when excessive or out of control, they can lead to imbalances and illness.

Non-Internal, Non-External Causes

Between Internal Causes and External Causes is the third category, called Non-Internal, Non-External Causes. This category includes Constitutional Factors, Lifestyle Factors, Intermediate Causes and Unforeseen Events.

*Constitutional Factors:* Each individual has a unique configuration of Yin and Yang balance, with a slight tilt one way or the other. This defines your Energetic individuality. A minor imbalance does not necessarily mean illness. In fact, it is very rare to see a person with a picture-perfect balance. However, a constitutional tendency toward imbalance can interact with an illness, influencing how it manifests and even determining the direction the illness will evolve. For example, when someone with a Warm constitution is invaded by a Cold Cause, although initially he or she will experience symptoms reflecting the nature of the Cold Cause, after a short time his or her Warm constitution will interact with the nature of the Cause, and the person will show signs and symptoms of Heat. This is known as the theory of "conformity and transformation," which stipulates how disease and different constitutional types interact.

Your unique constitution impacts the way you get sick. Everyone has his or her unique constitution. Some of us run Hot, others Cold. Some are robust and others are delicate. Your constitution will affect the way your illnesses develop, progress and resolve. Let's say that you have a constitutional imbalance and do not have enough cooling Energy to balance the warming Energy. This is the most commonly seen constitutional type in the West. When you come down with a flu caused by the External Causes Wind and Cold, after a day or two your constitution (Yin deficiency) and the natural Causes characteristic of influenza (Wind and Cold) will interact and change the entire picture of your illness. Your Yin deficiency (warm body temperature) will begin to turn the characteristic Wind and Cold disharmony into a Wind and Heat disharmony.

In this case, the initial Wind and Cold symptoms, such as congestion with clear nasal discharge, pronounced chills and body ache, would disappear quickly, and the person would soon develop Heat symptoms, such as sore throat, more pronounced fever, and yellow or discolored nasal discharge and Phlegm.

Conversely, if a person with a Cold constitution is invaded by a Wind and Heat Cause, the symptoms that are characteristic of Heat, such as sore throat, discolored discharge and more pronounced fever, would soon conform to the patient's basic constitution. The sore throat would disappear within a day or two, the discharges would turn white and thin and the degree of fever might lessen, replaced by pronounced sensitivity to cold or draft, possibly with achiness all over or a stiff neck or tightness in shoulders and upper back.

If the External Cause and your basic constitution are opposite, the External Cause can be altered by your constitution. That is why we all may feel lousy when we have the flu, but we feel lousy in different ways.

Some people have a significant constitutional weakness in a certain area that makes them vulnerable to specific illnesses. A person's constitution is also important in health maintenance and disease prevention. If your lifestyle agrees with your system by helping to correct your original imbalance rather than aggravating it, you will then have a relatively healthy life. But if your lifestyle goes against your constitution, it will eventually lead to illness. A Chinese doctor can predict which direction your health is heading in the future based on your constitutional tendency, and can take steps to prevent illness from occurring.

External Causes and Internal Causes interact with your unique body constitution. In addition, Chinese medicine recognizes that the evolution of illness depends on the relative strength of the External Cause and its ability to cause illness and the power of your immune system to heal your body. Everyone is different—a fact that is extremely important in Chinese medicine.

From a Western medical point of view, many conditions are single diseases that are caused by a definitive cause, for example, the flu virus. In other words, everyone receives the same diagnosis and everyone is treated similarly. But in Chinese medicine the flu can be classified in several categories and herbal formulas are widely varied.

Historically, Chinese medicine recognized that the flu is caused by an External Cause that it is contagious and evolves rapidly. Wind is often a major factor in flu, because the nature of flu is to strike suddenly and to change rapidly. From the Chinese medical point of view, there are many different types of flu. Symptoms common to all types of flu are fatigue, congestion, runny nose, fever and chills. But there are many types or variables. Each type depends on the nature of the External Causes and the interactions of your unique composition.

*Lifestyle Factors:* This includes dietary patterns, stress levels and stress management and excess or indulgence due to lack of moderation and discipline. For example, eating sweets and oily foods tends to generate Damp stagnation. Eating overly hot and spicy foods can increase internal Heat. Overeating Cooling or cold foods will slow down your Energy movement.

*Intermediate Causes:* At various stages, some diseases can create or generate disease-causing substances—such as stagnation of Blood and Phlegm—that cause other illnesses. Others are Internal Toxins, which are mostly due to abnormally accumulated metabolic waste. Much metabolic waste is toxic to the human body and needs to be regularly eliminated from the body. For example, according to Western medicine, urea is an end product of protein metabolism, and highly toxic to the body. It is eliminated through urination. If for any reason it becomes abnormally accumulated in the body, it will cause serious problems. Similarly, a patient with severe constipation can have headaches and mood fluctuations due to the reabsorption of toxins simply because the fecal matter stayed inside the body for too long.

*Unforeseen Events:* Illnesses caused by unforeseen events such as accidents and injuries are different from illnesses caused by External or Internal Causes for obvious reasons, but they can nonetheless cause severe damage to the structure and Energy of a healthy person. Therefore they are considered one of the causes of illnesses and can be treated based on exactly what is damaged.

## Diagnosis

Diagnosis in Chinese medicine includes an assessment of the Vital Substances that make up the human body: Yin, Yang, Qi, Jing (Essence), Blood, Fluid and Shen. Recognizing and identifying the patterns of imbalance or disharmony is referred to as Bian Zheng, or Differentiation of Patterns of

Disharmony. Bian Zheng is the most important process and method of diagnosis in Chinese medicine, during which doctors collect information and weave it into a meaningful pattern, and upon which the treatment is targeted. The Eight Principles of Differentiations are:

Yin, *Interior, Cold, Deficiency*
Yang, *Exterior, Heat, Excess*

The Cold and Heat here refer to Energetic temperature. They are the result of imbalances between Yin and Yang and are different from physical temperature.

The theories of Chinese medical diagnosis and treatments are founded on thousands of years of knowledge and experience. The Chinese method of diagnosis relies heavily on the senses, which is what makes the practice of Chinese medicine such an art. The more experience a doctor of Chinese medicine has, the more refined his or her senses become. The traditional Chinese medical diagnostic procedure follows what is called the Four Examinations: Inquiring, Looking, Listening/Smelling and Touching. The Four Examinations determine the pattern of harmony and disharmony. An examination will take between thirty minutes and one hour.

## The Four Examinations

*Inquiring:* When you see a doctor of Chinese medicine, your evaluation will begin with in-depth questions about yourself, not just your current complaints or symptoms. The doctor will listen to you—which for many is perhaps one of the most appealing aspects of Chinese medicine. Chinese medicine believes that you are the best judge of how you feel, and values your symptoms as much as the physical signs.

The doctor of Chinese medicine will question you thoroughly about your main complaint.

◆ *How did your problem start?* Is your problem consistent or intermittent? Has it been getting worse over time? Does it have a pattern? What makes your problem worse or better? Has your initial problem led to other symptoms or problems? How are you handling the problem emotionally?

◆ *How is your family's health?* How is your parents' health? How is your grandparents' health? Are you aware of any family history of disease? These questions help to evaluate your constitutional strength or imbalance and dictate prognosis to some degree.

- *Do you have any children?* This question can evaluate Jing (Essence) in certain situations, such as when an individual is having infertility problems.
- *How is your energy/vitality?* This is to evaluate if your Qi is sufficient or deficient. People's Energy has differing patterns. Some people's Energy is better in the morning and goes down as the day progresses. Others have a hard time getting up in the morning, but their Energy picks up later in the day. These different patterns have significance in Chinese medicine. There are physical and psychological Energies. Even though they often go hand in hand, they can become independent of each other.
- *Does your body generally run on the Cold or Warm side?* This question is directed at evaluating your Yin and Yang balance or imbalance. So that this question is not mistaken to mean fever or chills, your Chinese doctor will also ask: How many covers do you use at night? Do you dress warmly or coolly? Do you prefer warm weather or cool weather? Do you prefer warm drinks to cool drinks?
- *Do you feel thirsty or have a dry mouth?* This question evaluates the level of Fluid. You can be thirsty and have a dry mouth, thirsty and not have a dry mouth or have a dry mouth and not be thirsty. Everyone is different, and these variables in dry mouth and thirst provide information about your particular Imbalance. Thirst and dry mouth are two different symptoms even though they often appear together. Different combinations of their presence can have different clinical meanings. For example, in certain types of Yin deficiency the patient can have dry mouth but does not want to drink.
- *Do you sweat easily? Do you have spontaneous sweating or night sweats? Do you hardly sweat at all?* This question also evaluates the level of Fluid and balance between Yin and Yang, assesses the state of Wei Qi and can indicate imbalances with Energetic systems.
- *How is your breathing?* Do you have any shortness of breath? Any cough? Any bronchial irritation? Any feeling of phlegm in your throat? Do you have to clear your throat? Do you have any wheezing? This question evaluates Lung Energy.
- *How is your appetite?* Does food appeal to you? Do you have any cravings? Do you have any nausea, stomachache, heartburn? If you have stomach pain, does your pain have any pattern? Does food make it better or worse? Does physical pressure, such as massage, make it better or worse? Does applying heat help or make it worse? This question evaluates Spleen and Stomach (digestive) Energy.

- *How is your digestion?* Do you have any indigestion, gas and bloating, burping, abdominal cramping or distension? This question evaluates Spleen (digestive) Energy.
- *How is your diet? What do you typically eat?* These questions evaluate your Energetic pattern of your food in relation to your constitution or your imbalances.
- *Are your bowel movements regular?* Any diarrhea or constipation? Is your elimination complete? This question evaluates Stomach, Spleen and Intestine Energies.
- *Is your urination frequent?* Do you have any irritation or pain? What is the color of your urine? This question evaluates the function of Bladder and Kidney Energies.
- *How is your sleep?* Do you have any difficulty falling asleep or staying asleep? Is your sleep restful? Do you have nightmares? This question evaluates your Heart, Liver and Kidney Energies and your Shen.
- *How are your emotions and moods?* How is your stress level? Do you experience any mood fluctuations? Do your mood fluctuations have any patterns? Do you feel irritable, anxious or depressed? This question evaluates your Heart, Liver and Kidney Energies and your Shen.
- *How is your sex drive?* Has there been any change? Does sexual intercourse affect your energy level? Are you sexually active, and how often do you have sex? This question evaluates your Jing (Essence) and the level of your Kidney Energy.
- *How is your cognitive functioning?* How is your mental clarity, concentration and memory? How is the speed of your information processing? How is your sense of centeredness? This question evaluates your Jing (Essence) and your Shen.
- *Do you exercise?* What kind of exercise do you do? How much and how often? This question evaluates Qi, Blood, Kidney and Liver Energies and your Shen.
- *(If you are female) Are your menstrual cycles regular?* How many days is your cycle? How long does your period last? How is the flow—light, moderate or heavy? Any clotting? Any abdominal cramping? Any PMS? This question evaluates Liver, Kidney, Blood Energies and your Shen.

**Looking:** The Chinese doctor also learns about you by observing your body build and body language, movement, appearance and complexion, behavior, tongue, eyes, ears, palms, hair, fingernails, tears, sweat, phlegm, nasal discharge, vaginal discharge, vomit, urine and feces. Traditionally, because Chinese homes did not have bathrooms with sinks and running water next to the bedrooms, people used chamber pots. In old times, doctors came to patients' homes, and it was natural for the doctor to examine the contents of the chamber pot. Today, when necessary, a Chinese doctor can ask a patient to collect a specimen. The doctor is also able to observe certain body fluids such as perspiration while examining a patient. In addition, your doctor will look at your Shen.

Since it is beyond the scope of this book to cover all of these areas, we will focus on observing the tongue, which is central to Chinese diagnosis.

### Observing the tongue

Observing the tongue is one of the most important diagnostic methods of Chinese medicine. The doctor looks at the form, including the size and shape, color, texture, movement, coating and moisture. Tongue diagnosis takes a lot of experience and a trained eye. A healthy tongue is pink, neither too red nor too pale. It is not puffy or too thin. It looks flexible yet firm, straight and steady. It has a uniform, transparent thin white coating. It is moist but neither too wet nor too dry. It fits comfortably and moves freely within the mouth.

Some tongues are relaxed or steady and some tongues are edgy or quivery. Some tongues look fresh and pinkish, and some tongues look "old" or purple. There are, obviously, a lot of variables. Some abnormalities do not necessarily mean that there is a problem. Some imbalances are constitutional and define your unique constitution.

The first part (tip) of your tongue reflects the balance and imbalances of your Heart and Lung Energy. The middle part of your tongue reflects your Spleen and Stomach Energy. The back part of your tongue reflects your Kidney and Urinary Bladder Energies. Both sides of the middle section reflect the Liver and Gall Bladder Energy.

You may wish to learn the basics of tongue examination to observe on your own or to better understand what your Chinese doctor sees on your tongue. Begin by looking at your tongue in natural light. Keep your tongue relaxed.

### Size and shape

◆ *Swollen, enlarged, puffy:* Indicates Qi deficiency. Sometimes the tongue will be so swollen that it will have teeth marks or indentations along the edges. When Qi is deficient, Fluids accumulate abnormally, and the tongue is one of the first places where this abnormal accumulation of Fluids (Dampness) can be seen.

* *Flabby:* Indicates Qi deficiency. Your tongue has a group of muscles that maintain a proper posture. When there is an underlying Qi deficiency these muscles lose their ability to maintain the muscle tone and your tongue becomes flabby, lies against your lower palate and becomes imprinted with teeth marks.

* *Hard or ridged:* This is a sign of extreme Heat or Cold in an illness that is caused by an External Cause.

* *Small, thin:* If your tongue is small, thin and pale then you are severely Blood and Qi deficient. If your tongue is small and thin but scarlet and dry then you are either severely Yin deficient or extremely Fluid deficient (dehydrated).

* *Small or shriveled:* This is a sign of Yin deficiency.

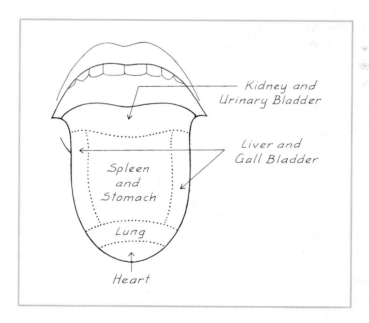

*Figure 6*

*Color*

* *Red:* Indicates Heat.
* *Pale:* Indicates Cold or Blood deficiency.

- *Scarlet:* Indicates both Heat and severe Yin deficiency.
- *Purple or dark:* Indicates stagnation or excess Cold.

### Texture

- *Old or aged:* Indicates Heat or stagnation.
- *Tender or frail:* Indicates Qi and Blood deficiencies.
- *Cracks or fissures:* Indicates Yin deficiency.
- *Strawberry-like appearance:* Indicates Heart or Stomach Heat.

### Movement

- *Trembling:* If your tongue is trembling and pale, you have Heart and Spleen Energy deficiency or Qi and Blood deficiency. If your tongue is scarlet and trembling, you have Heat that resulted in Internal Wind.
- *Off center to one side:* Indicates Liver imbalance and/or Blood deficiency or both, which can lead to Internal Wind and stroke.
- *Darting:* Can indicate either impending stroke or children who are cognitively underdeveloped (Jing and Shen deficiency).
- *Lolling:* Indicates Qi exhaustion.

### Coating

- *White coat:* Indicates Cold or superficial illness.
- *Yellow coat:* Indicates Heat or internal illness.
- *Gray coat:* Gray and moist indicates Cold and Damp. Gray and dry indicates that Heat has damaged Fluids.
- *Black coat:* Indicates extreme Heat or extreme Cold or extreme stagnation.
- *Thick coat:* Indicates that the External Cause is more pronounced or the illness is more severe. When the coating changes from thick to thin, it means that the illness is resolving.
- *Thin coat:* Indicates that the External Cause is less pronounced and the illness is mild. When coating changes from thin to thick, it means that the illness is progressing and becoming more severe.
- *Density:* The degree of stickiness or denseness indicates the amount of internally accumulated Dampness.
- *Peeled coat:* Indicates Yin deficiency. A peeled coat is the area of the surface

of the tongue that has a geographic look and where the texture of tongue underneath looks raw and without any coating.

- *Partially peeled coat:* Indicates Qi and Yin deficiencies.
- *Wet coat:* Indicates abnormal Fluid accumulation.
- *Dry coat:* Damaged Fluid or Yin deficiency or excess Heat.

*Evaluation of body language, posture and self-presentation*

A person's body language reflects what is going on internally. Your Chinese doctor (like your Western doctor) will get a general impression of you by how you present yourself. Whether you are thin or heavy, slouched over or erect, pointed in your speech or mumbling, strong or weak, physically fit or out of shape, hyper or sedate are all factors that will give your Chinese doctor an impression of you as a whole.

**Listening:** Like your Western doctor, your Chinese doctor listens to the quality of your voice. Some people have big voices, some quiet, some clear, some hoarse. Some people articulate and are precise, others are scattered and fumble for words. The strength of your breathing, rhythm and rate are all important. Listening also includes the sounds of your digestive tract, heartbeat, coughing, wheezing, hiccups, burping, sniffling and sneezing.

**Smelling:** Smelling includes the detection of unusual odor not only from bodily discharge but also from the patient's breath and overall body scent.

**Touching/Palpating:** Touching as a means of diagnosing involves two methods. One method is to palpate the body. Certain information about the nature of the imbalance can be acquired through feeling the patient's temperature (hot or cold), muscle tone (hard or flaccid), moisture (clammy or dry), tenderness (whether physical pressure helps or aggravates pain or discomfort), any abnormal masses and around certain acupuncture points or along the fourteen Meridians.

Pulse

Another important method of diagnosis is taking the pulse. Traditionally in China, pulse taking is such a prominent diagnostic method that seeing a doctor is often referred to as "having my pulse taken."

In Western medicine, the main purpose of pulse taking is to find out the patient's pulse rate. In Chinese medicine, doctors look for much more than that. Pulse taking requires a great deal of training, experience and sensitivity.

The pulse is taken on both wrists, as each side reflects different aspects of the body. The pulse is taken at three different positions on each side along the radial artery near the wrist about one and a half to two inches apart—the width of the middle three fingers held snugly together. At each position, three different depths of pressure are exerted. This results in a total of eighteen pulses taken.

Aside from the pulse rate, the Chinese doctor also feels for the depth, strength, width, shape, rhythm and length of the pulse. Classically, there are twenty-eight pulse "characters." Pulse character is the distinctive feel discernible by a trained practitioner, and gives a particular diagnostic significance, such as a strong or weak pulse.

The sixteen most common pulse characteristics are:

- *Floating or superficial pulse.* Distinct or apparent at the surface, less so with moderate or deep pressure. Indicates early stage of invasion by External Causes.
- *Deep or sinking pulse.* Only palpable at a deep level. Indicates the imbalance or disharmony is internal.
- *Slow pulse.* Slower than normal rate. Indicates internal Cold.
- *Rapid pulse.* Faster than normal rate. Indicates internal Heat or certain weaknesses.
- *Thin or thready pulse.* Small in width yet distinct. This can also be described as narrow in width. Indicates Blood deficiency. Can also indicate Yin deficiency.
- *Large or big pulse.* Broad in width yet distinct. This can also be described as wide in width. Indicates excess of any condition such as Heat, Cold, Qi or Blood or Phlegm stagnation, to name a few.
- *Empty pulse.* Large but lacking strength. Indicates Qi and Blood deficiency.
- *Full pulse.* Large yet forceful. Large refers to the width of the pulse. Forceful means the property opposite of weakness. So the full pulse is the combination of these two characters. Indicates pronounced excess of any condition, such as Heat, Cold, Qi or Blood or Phlegm stagnation, to name a few.

- *Wiry pulse.* Feels taut and distinct. Indicates Liver Energy imbalance or pain or stagnation.
- *Slippery pulse.* Feels slithery and fluid. Indicates excess of Dampness or Phlegm and Dampness.
- *Choppy pulse.* Opposite of a slippery pulse. It feels catchy, scraping, rough and uneven. Indicates Blood stagnation or deficiency.
- *Tight pulse.* Taut and full like a stretched rope. Indicates excess Cold, stagnation.
- *Soggy pulse.* Soft and nebulous, lack of distinction. Indicates Qi and Blood deficiency/Damp accumulation.
- *Irregular/knotted pulse.* Slow and skips beats irregularly. Indicates Heart Yang deficiency/Cold excess; Heart Qi and Blood stagnation.
- *Intermittent pulse.* Skips beats at a regular interval. Indicates serious Heart disharmony. Depleted condition of all the Energetic systems.
- *Hurried pulse.* Racing, skips beats irregularly. Indicates excess imbalance disrupting Heart, Qi and Blood.

## The Importance of Integrating Western and Chinese Medical Diagnoses

Western medicine tends to value science above symptoms. Because Western medicine is a more crisis-oriented medicine, most diagnostic tests are designed to pick up the signs of acute illness. In diagnosing chronic illness, Chinese medicine has the advantage because it recognizes signs before an illness becomes a crisis and can therefore take steps to prevent that crisis.

When an illness occurs, even though it may appear that it affects a certain part or aspect of your body, it is really affecting you as a whole, and your body and mind react as a whole. Western medicine tends to focus on and identify the part of the body that is most affected. Yet the information your whole body gives out in reaction to an illness is different from the information extracted from a singular area. This information inevitably involves the combined reactions of all the parts that are affected, such as your organs, immune system, nerves, endocrine system and circulatory system, as well as your emotional and psychological reactions. This combined information contains the essence of your body's imbalance and is the basic content of the Zheng—the objective of Chinese medical diagnosis. While this information is valuable, so is the information garnered by Western medical technologies. By using both Western and

Chinese diagnostic methods to gather different types of information, diagnosis and treatment would clearly be more effective and comprehensive. We can have a medical system that has the analytical power of modern technology combined with heightened sensitivity for human beings with all their complexities and subtleties.

# 4

## Acupuncture

*Connecting the interconnected systems
of the body with acupuncture*

Czechoslovakia was entombed in ice in January 1965 when Jitka Gunaratna, then twenty-one, left home for the tropical country of Ceylon (now Sri Lanka) to set up housekeeping with her husband, a native of that country.

Five years after arriving in Ceylon, Jitka became interested in studying acupuncture. "My husband, Piryasiri, had suffered with migraine headaches for many years," Jitka said. "He had tried all sorts of treatments—medications such as vasodilators, analgesics, traction, physiotherapy. We learned about a doctor with the formidable title of Lord Pandit Raja-Guru Professor Doctor Sir Anton Jayasuriya, who practiced acupuncture with very good results. So Piyasiri went to him. He usually had a migraine at least once a week, and the attack was so severe that sometimes he could not work at all. After the initial acupuncture treatment, he had a migraine only once, and it was very mild. That encouraged him to continue. He was treated twice a week for three weeks and then once a week for a month, then once a fortnight for another two months. After that he went in for a treatment once a month if he felt a migraine coming on. After a year his migraine problem disappeared, and he has never had the problem again."

Acupuncture is a Chinese medical technique that has been developed and refined for over three thousand years. Acupuncture consists of inserting a number of very fine steel needles into the skin at specific Meridian points. In ancient China needles were made of stone, animal bones and bamboo. Over the millennia, it was observed that stimulating certain points on the body's surface could have therapeutic effects. These observations and experiences accumulated through both trial and error and clinical experimentation, and eventually developed into the sophisticated and unique treatment system we know as acupuncture.

The majority of acupuncture points lie on the body surface along the thirteen Meridians. Eleven Meridians, each corresponding to a major or minor Energetic system (Liver, Heart, Spleen, Lung, Kidney, Gall Bladder, Small Intestine, Stomach, Large Intestine, Urinary Bladder and Triple Warmer), are distributed symmetrically on the body. There are two additional Meridians along the body's centerline, one along the front (called Ren) and the other along the back (called Du). Meridians form the network of channels or passageways by which Qi travels.

The thirteen major Meridians branch out to smaller channels. This branching out continues until the channels eventually become as minuscule as capillaries. This is how Meridians connect every part of the human body. In fact, Meridians, and the Qi that travels inside them, are the foundation for the wholeness of your body. For example, when you stimulate your Liver Meridian, it can affect all of the functions of the Energetic system to which the Liver is linked. The fourteen major Meridians and all the connecting channels have acupuncture points close to the body surface, for a total of 365 acupuncture points.

It is often of great interest to Westerners that an ailment on one part of the body requires needling in a distant site. For example, the treatment of many different types of headaches can be achieved by placing acupuncture needles in certain points in the feet and legs. Indigestion can be treated with acupuncture points on the bottom of your feet. Hemorrhoids are treated by needling a point on the head. The proven efficacy of acupuncture only further demonstrates that the body is indeed a whole interconnected system.

To understand how acupuncture works, think of a garden hose. Water can freely run through it unless there is an obstruction. If the obstruction is small then the water flow will be only slightly altered. If the obstruction is more severe, the water flow will be severely altered. If the hose is crimped, water pressure (Qi energy) builds up. When the crimp is straightened out, the water will burst forth, removing any obstruction (Qi stagnation). When the obstruction is removed, the water (Qi Energy) will once again be allowed to flow freely. This is the way acupuncture works. The obstruction in Meridians causes the Energy to flow slower, which results in a dysfunction in the Energy system that is associated with the Meridian. Acupuncture stimulates and regulates Qi flow, which removes the obstruction so that Energy can flow with regularity and the Energetic system can be made to resume its normal function.

Acupuncture points are Energetic junctures close to the surface of your skin that are access points to your internal Energy system. Think of these points as tiny valves where Qi is drawn in and out of your body's Energy flow. All acupuncture points are points on your body surface where there is lowered electrical resistance and a higher concentration of sensory and tiny nerve structures underneath the skin. These areas are more sensitive or more responsive to a physical stimulation. Acupuncture needles are inserted into these specific channels to influence your body's Energy flow, or Qi, thus allowing your body to balance and heal itself. Think of acupuncture needles as conduits through which we can strengthen deficient Qi or disperse stagnant Qi.

For the treatment of a chronic disease with a deficiency of Qi, needles are put into selected points to draw in or increase Qi. There are also cases where it is necessary to move excess Qi out of the body. For example, an infection from a toothache is an excess of Qi. Draining excess Qi from the imbalanced site can be accomplished through acupuncture. In the case of stagnation, Qi is dispersed or unblocked but not drained. Needles are inserted and then stimulated repeatedly for a longer time. The stimulation is provided by manually lifting and thrusting the needles, or by electrostimulation, which is explained below.

One cannot needle the body indiscriminately and hope to hit a specific acupuncture point along a Meridian channel. To know which Meridian point to needle, you must first identify which Meridian system is affected. This is where the in-depth diagnostic methods of Chinese medicine come into play. Each patient must be treated as an individual to determine the exact Energy system(s) affected.

Because acupuncture is used to reestablish harmony within your Energetic systems, it can be used for a vast range of illnesses and pain disorders and also to provide effective anesthesia during certain surgical procedures. In the case of chronic pain, acupuncture stimulates the release of endorphins, which are your body's internally produced substances similar to opiates (pain relievers). Research in the United States has focused on the use of acupuncture in pain relief and analgesia, to counteract the side effects of chemotherapy, and as an aid in reducing the cravings of former smokers and drug addicts.

The Acupuncture Clinic of Lord Pandit Raja-Guru Professor Doctor Sir Anton Jayasuriya in Kalubowila Colombo South General Hospital treated 150 to 200 patients every day. After Piyasiri Gunaratna's successful treatment for migraine headaches, Jitka became interested in acupuncture and enrolled to train under Jayasuriya at his institute, Medicina Alternative. Following graduation she stayed on at the clinic for the next twelve years, working as Jayasuriya's assistant.

"Professor Jayasuriya was constantly studying new ways of curing his patients without any harmful side effects by applying natural methods of holistic medicine," Jitka said. "He made acupuncture anesthesia available in Sri Lanka and saved the lives of countless patients who were not candidates for traditional anesthesia." In 1979 Columbo South General Hospital performed over seven hundred major surgical procedures using acupuncture anesthesia alone. Jitka assisted Jayasuriya on many such surgeries.

"After working at the clinic I was leaving the clinic quite exhausted," Jitka said. "I started giving myself tonification treatments with acupuncture in the afternoon before I started to treat my private patients. Tonification points act as a pick-me-up. They are typically used after a long illness and for many other conditions, such as hypotension, loss of appetite, anorexia and anemia. I was using them to get a boost of energy during a long day—but suddenly I got pregnant! I was thirty-five years old, and after seventeen years of marriage it was a bit of a surprise." (Acupuncture can improve ovarian function. See chapter 17 for a case history on infertility and acupuncture.)

Since it was Jitka's first baby and she was an older mother, her obstetrician decided it would be best delivered by Cesarian section. In 1977, Jayasuriya had performed the first acupuncture anesthesia during a Cesarian section in Sri Lanka; the infant girl was given the name Zusanli—the name of an acupuncture point. Jitka was found to be an appropriate candidate for acupuncture anesthesia. About 2 percent of the population is not suited to acupuncture analgesia. A patient is considered not suitable for acupuncture anesthesia if he or she does not feel the so-called acupuncture sensation—numbness, heaviness, slight pressure or tingles along the Meridian—when needled.

## The difference between acupuncture as analgesia and acupuncture as anesthesia

An analgesic alters the perception of pain, such as acetaminophen or aspirin minimizing the pain of a headache. An anesthetic creates a total loss of the sensation of pain, such as the drugs that are given during surgery to induce a deep sleep, or novocaine to numb and eliminate pain during dental procedures.

There are three key components to acupuncture as an analgesic and an anesthetic. First and foremost, acupuncture is extremely effective in killing pain. It is also somewhat effective in producing sedation. Although capable of effectively relaxing skeletal muscle, acupuncture is often unsatisfactory in its ability to relax smooth muscles, which line many organs. This is why the majority of acupuncture analgesia is utilized in neck, facial and skull operations, which do not require the stretching of large muscle organs. Acupuncture is often utilized in brain and neck surgery and dental procedures because the patient needs to be awake and conscious or because of the proximity of the surgery to the brain stem.

For surgery, acupuncture is also used in individuals that have a known history of allergy or intolerance to traditional anesthetics. However, because of the large smooth-muscle groups and organs found within the abdomen and pelvis, such surgeries rarely incorporate acupuncture as the sole anesthetic; rather, it is most often used as an adjunct to conventional anesthetics. The use of acupuncture as an adjunct allows for a lower dosage of chemical/conventional agents, thus providing a safer procedure for those patients with sensitivities to these agents. Acupuncture is also now used as anesthesia for childbirth. Unlike conventional anesthesia, acupuncture anesthesia does not lower blood pressure or depress breathing.

## Electroacupuncture

On her delivery day Jitka was taken to the operating room, where Jayasuria gave her ten needles—some were stimulated by high-frequency electric current.

A high-frequency stimulator is an electronic device designed for administering acupuncture anesthesia. It sends electronic pulsation with a very high frequency through electric wires connected to the acupuncture needles. The intensity and frequency required for acupuncture anesthesia are hard to sustain if they are to be provided manually.

Electrical stimulation is used during operations by way of a high-frequency stimulator, which makes the operated area numb when connected to selected needles. When using acupuncture anesthesia during surgery, it is essential to put some of the acupuncture needles alongside the incision. These needles are connected to the high-frequency stimulator. The other needles connected to the stimulator depend on the area operated upon—the head, chest, abdomen, pelvis—and of course the experience and knowledge of the acupuncturist.

Surgery is not the only condition in which electroacupuncture is utilized. Electroacupuncture can be used in nearly all situations in which traditional acupuncture is used. Most often it is used in the situation where the primary treatment focus is on dispersing Qi rather than tonifying. The flow of Qi is stimulated by connecting acupuncture needles to the small DC charge of an electroacupuncture stimulator. The needles are connected in pairs and several pairs can be connected at the same time. The frequency and strength of the electric pulse is monitored by the acupuncturist to achieve the desired effect without discomfort to the patient.

Using electroacupuncture for anesthesia, it takes about twenty minutes to achieve the induction state. Because the patient needs to get used to the stimulation and because he or she is fully conscious, it is necessary to work gently and to constantly adjust the stimulation. That is one reason why operations using acupuncture anesthesia are more demanding of the surgeon's skill. The surgeon must be gentle and quick, and the acupuncturist must constantly communicate with the patient and decide how to manage the stimulation as to not allow any discomfort. Such techniques, therefore, are not suitable for long operations, especially those where some force must be used, such as orthopedic operations where saws, hammers and chisels are used.

During Jitka's surgery, after a twenty-minute acupuncture induction period, at 8:30 A.M. the obstetrician started to work. "At 8:48 my son was born, and at 9:05 I was back in my bed," Jitka said. "Five days later I attended a dinner organized by my husband at a restaurant in Colombo. There is nothing else I can say about my recovery. The whole affair was less stressful than a common cold."

Jitka and her family fled Sri Lanka under death threats during the bloody civil war in 1989. They settled in the Czech Republic, where Jitka is a visiting lecturer at the Institute for Postgraduate Studies for medical doctors. There she has organized a successful postgraduate training course in acupuncture.

The Acupuncture Clinic of Lord Pandit Raja-Guru Professor Doctor Sir Anton Jayasuriya and the acupuncture institute he founded, Medicina Alternative, in Colombo, Sri Lanka, are among the most important acupuncture institutions in the world. Jayasuriya has never deviated from his philosophy that acupuncture treatments should be free. Rich and poor are always treated free of charge; students of acupuncture who attend Medicina Alternative are charged tuition. Most acupuncture clinics in the United States, unless funded by charitable organizations, charge between $25 and $125 per treatment.

## What You Can Expect When You Go
## for an Acupuncture Treatment

When you go to a Chinese doctor for acupuncture treatment, your treatment will be no different than if you were being treated in China. Your treatment will begin with the Four Examinations, Inquiring, Looking, Listening/Smelling and Touching, to determine your pattern of harmony and disharmony. This will give your doctor a comprehensive picture of your problem. Your doctor will then explain your imbalances and the treatment plan he or she advises.

You will be situated in such a way as to facilitate the effectiveness of the acupuncture treatment. Often this takes the form of lying or sitting on an acupuncture table. Other times you may be encouraged to walk around while the needles are in place. A caring acupuncturist will provide a tranquil atmosphere in a private room, with the temperature warm enough and with soothing music to enhance your relaxation. The acupuncturist will then dart needles into the acupuncture points that are appropriate for your treatment. This is mostly painless and can, in fact, be unnoticeable. Usually four to twenty needles will be inserted.

The insertion depth of the needle depends on two main factors: 1) Depth and needle insertion techniques are designed to engage Qi. This engagement is known as deqi. The patient experiences sensations of numbness, heaviness, distension or radiating tingles. The acupuncturist, on the other hand, experiences a subtle heaviness or pulling beneath the tip of the needle when deqi is achieved. 2) The thickness of the tissue at the acupuncture point. On thin muscles such as areas around the skull and close to the bones around the wrist the needles are inserted horizontally or obliquely to avoid the bone. On thick muscles and in areas where there is low risk of damage to underlying anatomical structures, needles are typically inserted at a depth of 1 to 1.5 cun (see Figure 7). Tiny needles (0.5 cun in depth) are utilized for areas such as fingers, toes, head, face and particularly the ears. On the other hand, an acupuncturist might use unusually long needles (up to 8 cun) for areas such as the hip.

Once a needle is inserted, the wire handle is twirled or the needle is lifted and thrusted until the feeling of deqi is achieved. It is necessary for the patient to feel the deqi when the needle is inserted. Since some patients are not as receptive, it is necessary to repeatedly stimulate the needles. For the sensitive person it is enough to leave the needles in place after insertion, without manipulation, for fifteen to thirty minutes. In the treatment of chronic disorders it is often advisable to use less manipulation of the needles, as strong stimulation tends to disperse Qi.

## Cun

A standardized unit of measure is not ideal for locating the correct acupuncture point(s) because of wide variations (individual differences) of physical height, weight and breadth. Also, the difference in gender and age will affect the correct point locations. The cun—a relative measurement—takes into account the individual's unique size. Therefore, each individual is measured only against him or herself. In Chinese medicine this distance is "the inch (unit) that follows your body." For each individual's body the relative distance is functionally constant, but this constant distance varies from person to person. A cun is therefore determined by measuring the distance between a person's distal and medial crease on their middle finger or the broadest part of the thumb at the level of the distal joint.

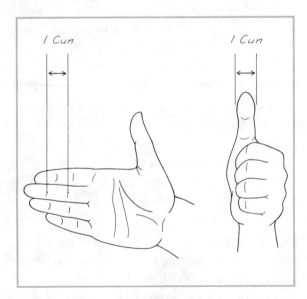

*Figure 7*

At the end of an acupuncture treatment you may feel euphoric, relaxed and drowsy, or you may feel energized, with the relief of pain and other symptoms.

Although many conditions are improved by one acupuncture treatment, it usually takes a series or course of treatments to heal. Often herbal formulas are included in the treatment plan.

## When Acupuncture Is Not Recommended

- Hemophilia
- Severe psychosis
- Drug or alcohol intoxication

Also, certain points are contraindicated in pregnancy, as they can cause miscarriage.

It is important to note that acupuncture can be useful in treating the symptoms of AIDS as well as the side effects of drugs used to treat HIV and AIDS, and to strengthen the immune system.

Strict hygienic protocols including the use of sterile, disposable needles are practiced by reputable acupuncturists.

## Choosing Your Acupuncturist

Just because you have tried acupuncture does not mean you had a quality experience with acupuncture. An acupuncturist may know the points, but that does not mean he or she can effectively treat you. Acupuncture is an art form that some people master and others do not—no matter how well intentioned. Moreover, the relationship between the acupuncturist and patient is extremely important. The right match between acupuncturist and patient is an important aspect of your healing process. A good rapport between you and your acupuncturist will ease any anxiety you may feel about your condition or about the actual acupuncture procedure. "A patient who has confidence and is relaxed is more likely to respond better to the treatment," Jitka said. "Acupuncture is a very personal type of healing in which an acupuncturist and a patient exchange their own vital energy—Qi." Because of the interaction of Qi during an acupuncture treatment, it is important that you experience a sense of rapport and safety with your practitioner. Feelings of tranquility, respect and confidence must be achieved. If you sense that your practitioner is rushed, distracted, upset or not fully present, postpone your treatment or look for another practitioner with whom you feel comfortable. Fortunately, there are now many excellent and compassionate acupuncturists to choose from.

By the same token, any practicing acupuncturist will tell you how very draining some patients can be. "I call them octopuses," Jitka said. "As an acupuncturist, one feels like one is being wrapped and sucked by their tentacles." Dr. Mao, who is the cofounder of the Tao of Wellness clinic in Santa Monica, California, said, "There is power in the exchange of Vital Energy or Qi. There is certainly Energy transference in clinical situations. When you are in practice you cannot avoid so-called toxic people. I practice and teach my students how to shield oneself from taking on a patient's anger and also how to cleanse oneself of negativity at the end of every working day. It is a mental, spiritual and Energetic practice of gathering protective Energy, so that one doesn't pick up negative Energy from patients."

See page 425 for resources to find an acupuncture clinic in your area.

## Moxabustion

Moxabustion involves burning dried mugwort leaves directly over acupuncture points to allow the heat to penetrate the areas around acupuncture points along the channels that influence Qi and Blood flow. Moxa is made of the aromatic herb mugwort (Chinese: Ai Ye), a member of the Artemesia family of herbs, many of which have medicinal qualities.

Moxa is dehydrated mugwort leaves, which are treated, pulverized into a cotton-ball-like consistency—similar to the newsprint filling in padded mailing bags—then molded into a cone or stick that looks somewhat like a cigar. A moxa cone can be wrapped around the metal shaft or handle of the acupuncture needle or placed on a slice of dehydrated herb such as ginger, which is then placed directly on an acupuncture point and burned. A moxa stick is lit and the red glowing end held about one inch over specific acupuncture points, or over acupuncture needles that are inserted into points. The doctor of Chinese medicine will hold the moxa until your skin is warm, then draw it away, repeating this process for several minutes to half an hour.

Mugwort goes into Liver, Spleen and Kidney Energy Meridians. Moxa's basic function is as a warming agent that promotes Energy flow. It is used to treat Cold or deficient imbalances and alleviate certain types of pain.

Moxa burns slowly, giving off a musty smoke. Some people find the smoke disagreeable because it lingers in hair and clothing. Smokeless moxa is available, and although hard to light, it is still often used. Moxa can be used on infants, children or adults who are afraid or cannot tolerate acupuncture needles.

Other forms of moxa include long thin sticks that resemble ordinary incense sticks, used as described above. Also, moxa can be burned in a box that is placed over an acupuncture area. Moxa can be wrapped around the metal handle of an acupuncture needle before the needle is inserted into a specific acupuncture point. The moxa is lit, warming the needle and penetrating the channel.

Moxa is suitable for use at home by the layperson. You can purchase moxa in various forms in many herbal stores, from your Chinese herbal clinic and online at ancientherbsmodernmedicine.com.

## Acupressure as Another Alternative to Needling

Acupressure is based on the same principles as acupuncture, though the pressure of touch is used instead of needles. The fingertip, *not the pad,* of the finger(s) is used when exerting pressure. Whenever possible, the tip of the thumb is used because the thumbs are able to exert more and sustained pressure. The amount of pressure applied should be moderate, yet enough to create a significant sensation of Qi. If too little pressure is applied, you will only feel the sense of touch. If too much pressure is applied, you will feel notable pain. A little bit of soreness or tenderness actually is just about the right amount of pressure. Once the correct amount of pressure is being applied, while maintaining constant pressure one can make very small circular motions—so small they are hardly perceptible—with the applying finger(s), without lifting the finger(s). The duration of applied pressure should be maintained for at least one minute at a time, but no more than three minutes. This procedure can be repeated on the opposite side immediately. This process can be repeated back and forth between sides several times.

## Simple Acupressure Treatments You Can Apply to Yourself

### Headache

To treat a headache with acupressure, follow the two steps in the order presented: Cuan Zhu point and Tai Yang point. Alternate the two pairs of points several times by pressing each pair for about one minute at a time.

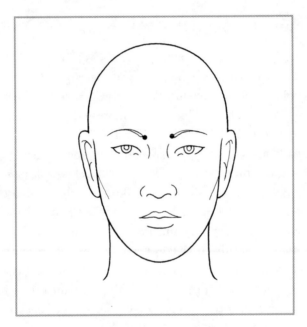

*Figure 8*
*Cuan Zhu Point*

*Step One*

◈ *Cuan Zhu point:* Simultaneously using the tips of both thumbs, with the palms facing inward toward each other, press the points located at the very inner area (closest to the bridge of the nose) of the eyebrows.

*Step Two*

❖ *Tai Yang point:* Simultaneously using the tips of both thumbs with the palms over your forehead and the pads of the remaining fingers lightly touching the center of the forehead, apply pressure to the slightly concave and some-what softer area of the temple located approximately one and a half to two inches on a line extending from the outer corner of your eyes toward your ears.

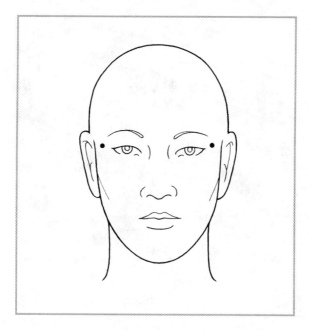

*Figure 9*
*Tai Yang Point*

## Nausea

To treat nausea (motion or morning sickness) with acu-pressure, follow the two steps in the order presented: Hegu point and Nei Guan point. Alternate the two pairs of points several times by pressing each pair for about one minute at a time.

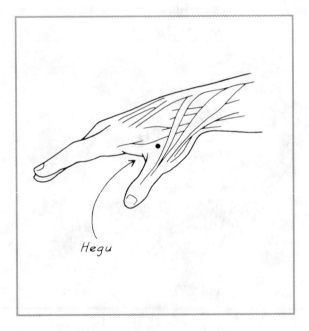

*Figure 10*
*Hegu Point*

*Step One*

* *Hegu point:* With one hand resting palm toward your stomach, use the tip of the thumb of the other hand to apply pressure at a point located between the base of the thumb and base of the index finger.

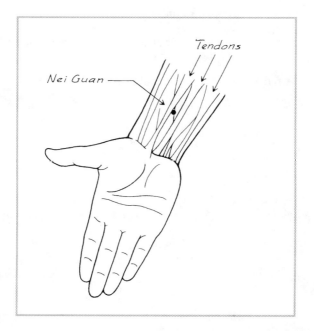

*Figure 11*
*Nei Guan Point*

### Step Two

◈ *Nei Guan point:* With one arm bent and palm facing upward make a fist. You will notice two major tendons running alongside each other, from the base of your hand
through the middle of your wrist. Using the tip of the
thumb of the opposite hand, apply pressure to a point between these tendons approximately two finger widths
down from the most distal (closest to the palm) crease line
of the wrist.

### Stomachache

To treat a stomachache or abdominal cramping with acupressure, use Zu San Li point. Press this point for about one minute, release, and repeat several times.

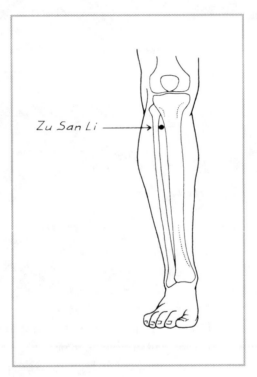

*Figure 12*
*Zu San Li Point*

⬩ *Zu San Li point:* Follow the ridge of the tibia (shinbone) all the way up to the top of the tibia, located just below the patella (kneecap). You will notice that the head of the tibia forms a T shape with the ridge of the shinbone. One index finger width toward the outside of the leg from the shinbone ridge and one index finger width down from the outer aspect of the top of the T is the acupressure point. Using the tip of either thumb, exert pressure on this point.

Eyestrain

To treat eyestrain due to overuse (this is also good for pre-serving and promoting good eyesight) use the following four pairs as a group in the order presented: Jing Ming point, Cuan Zhu point, Chen Qi point and Tai Yang point. Maintain pressure on each pair of points for about one minute before moving on to the next pair. Repeat the steps once if necessary.

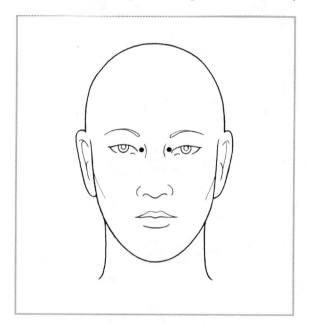

*Figure 13*
*Jing Ming Point*

*Step One*

◈ *Jing Ming point:* Using the tips of the thumb and index finger, apply pressure to a pair of points located between the bridge of the nose and the inner corner of each eye, just above the eye itself. You will notice that you are applying pressure in such a way as to feel the bony upper part of the eye socket.

*Step Two*

❖ *Cuan Zhu point:* Simultaneously using the tips of both
thumbs, with the palms facing inward toward each other,
press the acupressure points located at the very inner area
(closest to the bridge of the nose) of the eyebrows.

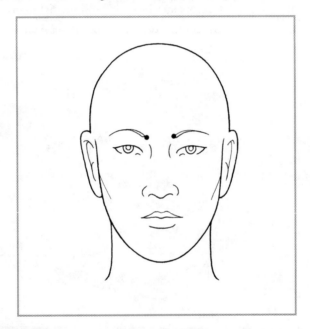

*Figure 14*
*Cuan Zhu Point*

*Step Three*

◈ *Cheng Qi point:* Apply pressure to a point located straight down from the pupils of your eyes and straight across from the top of each nostril where it flares out from the ridge of the nose. Use the tips of the index or middle fingers to apply pressure to both sides simultaneously.

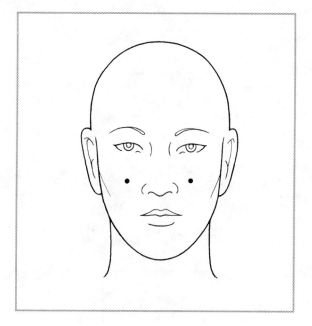

*Figure 15*
*Cheng Qi Point*

*Step Four*

◈ *Tai Yang point:* Simultaneously using the tips of both
  thumbs with the palms over your forehead and the pads of
  the remaining fingers lightly touching the center of the
  forehead, apply pressure to the slightly concave and somewhat softer area of the temple located approximately one
  and a half to two inches on a line extending from the outer
  corner of your eyes toward your ears.

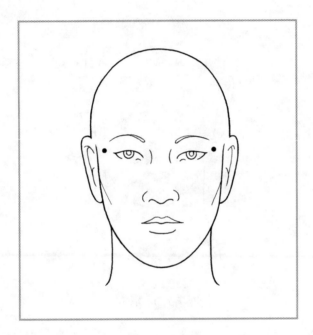

*Figure 16*
*Tai Yang Point*

### Anxiety and tension

To treat anxiety and tension with acupressure, follow the three steps in the order presented: Shen Men point, Nei Guan point and San Yin Jiao point. Maintain pressure on each pair of points for about one minute before moving on to the next pair.

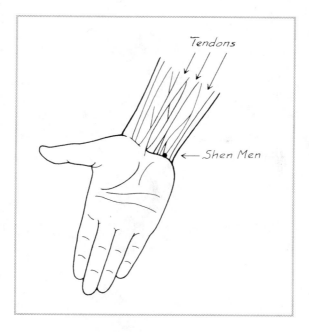

*Figure 17*
*Shen Men Point*

*Step One*

◈ *Shen Men point:* Using the tip of the thumb, apply pressure to a point on the opposite wrist located along the first wrist crease closest to your hand, approximately one and a half index finger widths from the outer edge (pinky side) of the hand.

*Step Two*

◈ *Nei Guan point:* With one arm bent and palm facing upward, make a fist. You will notice two major tendons running alongside each other from the base of your hand
through the middle of your wrist. Using the tip of the
thumb of the opposite hand, apply pressure to a point between these tendons approximately two finger widths
down from the most distal (closest to the palm) crease line
of the wrist.

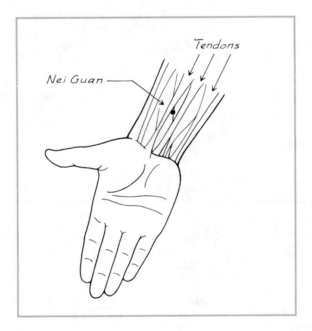

*Figure 18*
*Nei Guan Point*

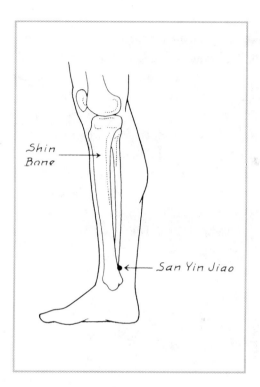

*Figure 19*
San Yin Jiao Point

*Step Three*

◈ *San Yin Jiao point:* This is where the Spleen, Liver and Kidney Meridians cross. This point is located on the inner aspect of the lower leg approximately three index finger widths above the inner bulge of the ankle bone, just beneath the tibia, in the soft area between the tibia and the lower part of the calf muscle.

## Seeds

The entire body is represented in acupuncture points on the ear. Auricular (ear) acupuncture is a branch of acupuncture that treats disharmonies or illnesses by needling exclusively acupuncture points on the ear. Some acupuncturists use seeds instead of needles. The seeds of the Wang Bu Liu Xing plant (Vaccaria) are often used, while others prefer to use stainless steel beads. Seeds are attached to surgical tape and adhered to certain specific acupuncture points on the ear. For example, certain points can be used when you feel anxious, stressed or experience cravings from withdrawal from cigarettes, sugar, caffeine or other stimulants; stimulating the seeds with the tips of your fingers can provide relief. The seeds are commercially available, but the application points have to be very precisely located. The seeds are best attached by a trained acupuncturist.

# 5

## All About Herbs

*The various forms and formulations of herbs*

Westerners have grown up with medicine that comes in sanitary, often hermetically sealed packages with enclosures only the scientifically trained can read and understand. Western medicines are sugarcoated, perfectly formed pills and capsules in childproof and tamperproof containers. Sterile drugs are administered via tubes directly into a vein or given as an injection. In comparison, especially if one is unprepared, Chinese herbal medicine appears earthy and primitive. Chinese herbs have been likened to a bird's nest or a sack of sticks and twigs and bark and often come as a surprise when a person goes for their first visit to a Chinese doctor.

## The Roots of Western Pharmacology

Although we in the West have grown used to a more removed presentation when it comes to medicine, the fact is that Western pharmaceuticals developed directly from herbology. The roots of Western pharmacology extend as far back as the Ebers Paprus, Egyptian compilations of medical texts circa 1550 A.D., which contain seven hundred magical formulas and folk remedies. In the first century A.D., the Greek physician Dioscorides wrote the first Western pharmacological treatise, a listing of herbal plants used in classical medicine. Before the early ninth century the doctor and pharmacist were one and the same. The herbalist both prescribed and prepared medical compounds. "When I went to school we had a yearlong course called pharmacognosy, the study of plant life and how it relates to human beings and their health," said Sheldon Miller, R. Ph. (father of Dr. Glenn E. Miller), who earned his pharmacy degree in 1952. "In those days, many of our medications were from herbs, plants, trees, shrubs and so on. Before I graduated from pharmacy school I apprenticed in a drug-store. We had what they called masquerading jars—five-gallon glass jars in which you weighed out a certain amount of tree bark or roots or whatever you were working on. You would add a dilutant such as alcohol or water. The jars would be turned every twenty-four hours. That was my job, picking them up and turning them over. As far as herbs are concerned, we were one step removed from the actual harvesting process. In those days, you were grinding and mix-ing and folding and filling."

Mr. Miller remembers when medicines were one step removed from their plant sources—indeed, it has been only since the late eighteenth century that pharmacology has developed with advances in chemistry and biology that en-abled drugs to be standardized. Western pharmacology recognized that a natu-ral substance can contain many ingredients, not all of which are responsible for its medicinal effect. Researchers first isolated the ingredient from a plant source that was thought to have the primary healing property for a given condition. Active ingredients are the constituents within the natural substance responsible for a particular biological effect. Isolating the specific active ingredient(s) re-sponsible for a therapeutic effect has been the focus of Western medicine.

The next step was to determine or standardize how much of the ingredient to prescribe. In the early nineteenth century, chemists began to make exciting progress in isolating active ingredients—aspirin (from the bark of willow trees), morphine (from the seeds of poppy flowers), strychnine (from the poi-sonous Nux Vomica tree), quinine (from the bark of the cinchona tree), peni-cillin (from molds on grains) and many others—from their crude plant sources. In the twentieth century, and particularly since World War II, pharma-cological researchers developed a vast array of new drugs. Since that time, more drugs have been made by chemical synthesis—many of which are chemical im-itations of plant medicines. However, a quarter of modern prescription drugs still come from plant sources.

## Isolated Active Ingredients and Side Effects

Two thousand years ago, Chinese medical scholars became aware of active ingredients and actually isolated a number of them from mineral sources. However, they quickly noted the problem of side effects and by the late third century, decided to stay with the use of whole natural substances, which con-tain ingredients that are meant to interact synergistically and to counteract potential side effects. (See chapter 15 for more on isolated active ingredients, side effects and whole natural herbs.)

## The Roots of Chinese Herbology

The first important figure in Chinese herbology was the divine husbandman Shen Nong, who is believed to have lived around five thousand years ago. Shen Nong is mentioned in dozens of books dating as far back as 607 B.C. He is said to have discovered the medicinal properties of herbs by systematically trying herbs himself, sometimes with toxic or adverse reactions, compelling him to quickly find an antidote.

Around the time of Christ, Chinese scholars of herbology began sorting out the knowledge in herbology that had accumulated up to that point. These works eventually led to the writing and compilation of the book *Shen Nong's Herbal Materia Medica*. The book has three volumes, containing 365 medicinal substances. More than 60 percent of these 365 medicinal substances are still in use today. *Shen Nong's Herbal Materia Medica* established the basic theory of herbology. It defined the relationships of herbs in a formula and their roles, such as primary, secondary, assisting or facilitating herbs. It explained that the nature of interactions among different herbs in a formula can be synergetic, counterbalancing or contradicting. There are also magnified toxicities, in which case the combination or interaction is to be avoided. The book described the flavors, Energetic temperatures and toxicity of herbs. In addition, under each herb, the book indicated the natural habitat, growing conditions, harvest time, method of processing and method of how to identify the quality of herbs and recognize the genuine species.

## Chinese Herbs

In Chinese medicine there are well over eight thousand herbs known to have medicinal qualities. Only about five hundred are commonly used. While not all the substances used in Chinese herbal medicine are technically herbs, the use of the word is standard in Chinese medicine. Herbal formulas contain combinations of roots, seeds, grains, flowers, berries, fruit peel, bark, leaves, stems, kernels, wood, shells, nuts, minerals, pollen, resin, seaweed, clay, fossilized bones and occasionally animal parts or proteins.

## The Regulating Property of Herbs

Western medicine, such as blood pressure medication, is generally intended to target one specific biological function. For example, a drug can lower blood pressure. But if you take too high a dose for you, or if you are exquisitely sensitive, the drug will reduce your blood pressure to below normal. While Western doctors often pinpoint one specific problem and prescribe one drug for that problem, Chinese herbalists rarely prescribe a single herb but rather combine herbs to achieve a regulating function. Many herbs can *normalize* a biological function—that is, the same herb that is prescribed to lower the blood pressure in hypertensive people can also raise it in hypotensive individuals. That is the wonder of many herbs. In addition, most herbs provide a wide margin of safety, so you do not usually have to worry about overdosing.

Blood sugar regulation is another example of how Western medicine and Chinese medicine approach an imbalance differently. Patients with hypoglycemia (low blood sugar) or hyperglycemia (high blood sugar) are given different medications by Western medicine. However, in Chinese medicine the same group of herbs can effectively normalize blood sugar, raising or lowering it as the need may be.

## The Basic Medicinal Properties of Herbs

The basic medicinal properties of herbs are characterized through the theories of Five Flavors, Four Temperatures, Basic Energetic Tendencies and Meridian Affinities.

### Five Flavors

The basic Energetic properties used to characterize herbs are Sour, Bitter, Sweet, Acrid and Salty. Bland and Stringent were added to the original list, but the term Five Flavors remains to this day.

> Sour: *Any property that is contracting, holding or pulling back is considered Sour.*
> Bitter: *Any property that is clearing or drying is considered Bitter.*
> Sweet: *Any property that is tonifying or harmonizing or that soothes urgency is considered Sweet.*
> Acrid/Pungent: *Any property that disperses or promotes movement of Vital Substance is considered Acrid.*

Salty: *Any property that is softening (of hardness or any mass) or purging is considered Salty.*

Bland: *Any property that is draining (Dampness) or promotes urination is considered Bland.*

Stringent: *Any property that is contracting, holding or pulling back yet is stronger than Sour is considered Stringent.*

## Four Temperatures

The Four Temperatures (different from physical temperature) used to characterize properties of herbs are Cool, Cold, Warm and Hot. Neutral was added to the list later on.

Cool: *Any herb that can counteract or decrease Heat disharmony.*

Cold: *Similar to Cool but stronger or more extreme.*

Warm: *Any herb that can counteract or decrease Cold disharmony.*

Hot: *Similar to Warm but stronger or more extreme.*

Neutral: *Neither Warm nor Cool. Appropriate to be used for disharmonies other than Heat or Cold in nature.*

## Basic Energetic Tendencies

The Four Basic Tendencies of Energetic movement of herbs are Ascending, Descending, Floating and Sinking.

Ascending: *Any herb that is Energetically uplifting, dispersing or expelling, opening up orifices, or inducing vomit.*

Descending: *Any herb that is Energetically purging, draining, clearing, calming, dissolving or constricting.*

Floating: *Similar to Ascending but primarily affects upper part of the body.*

Sinking: *Similar to Descending but primarily affects lower part of the body.*

## Meridian Affinities

In Western pharmacology, when you take a drug it will most often evenly distribute throughout your body with the exception of areas such as the brain and placenta, where the body has protective barriers that prevent certain substances from reaching brain and fetal tissue. In Chinese medicine each herb is intended to target particular aspects of your body's Energetic system. It does this by entering specific Meridians. This is known as the herb's Meridian Affinity. For example, if a doctor considers your problem to be related to Liver Energy, he or she will prescribe herbs that target your Liver Energetic system. Although the herbs were used to target this Energetic system, they will also go into other Meridians as well. It is very rare for an herb to only go to one single Meridian. The majority of herbs and herbal formulas target multiple Meridians. On the other hand, of ten thousand known medicinal herbs, only two or three go into all fourteen Meridians.

## The Art of Herb Combining

Each one of the herbs in a Chinese formula has multiple active ingredients that result in various effects on the body. When combined, these herbs can potentially produce a nearly infinite number of interactions.

In every formula there are four essential types of herbs. The *primary* herb acts as the chief therapeutic agent for the main illness or symptoms, and it is usually in the largest dose. The *secondary* herb or herbs reinforce the therapeutic effect of the primary herb for the main disease or symptom. It can also act as the chief therapeutic agent for the secondary disease or symptoms. The secondary herb or herbs can be one, a group or several groups depending on the complexity of the patient's condition.

The third type, the *assistant* herb, reinforces the primary or secondary herbs and counteracts or reduces the toxicity and side effects of these herbs. The assistant herb can be used to buffer any harsh qualities of the primary or secondary herbs if these herbs are too strong for a particular patient.

The fourth herb, the *facilitator,* may not have any direct therapeutic effect but facilitates the actions of other herbs. The facilitator herb increases the digestibility of all the herbs and increases the synergistic effect of the formula. The facilitator herb also helps deliver the therapeutic properties of the other herbs to the site of the disease. A good example is a patient suffering from attention deficit disorder; the facilitator herb can act upon the blood brain barrier to allow the delivery of the therapeutic properties of herbs to the brain. The cardinal principle of designing an herbal formula is to maximize the positive synergistic medicinal effects while minimizing the undesirable actions and interactions.

When herbs are combined there are many factors to take into consideration. The practitioner must consider that when one factor changes, many other changes may also occur in the body. Sometimes there are very complex interactions. For example, when you drive to work, you have to consider a lot of factors. Your goal is to get to work within a certain time. Sometimes by taking a longer route you can actually get there faster. The distance is not the only factor that you take into consideration. There are traffic conditions, weather and so on.

Herbs are selected based upon your specific Chinese diagnosis. For example, if you have Yin deficiency, an herb that nourishes Yin Energy will be part of your formula. If you have Yang deficiency, an herb that strengthens Yang Energy will be part of your formula. If you have Yang excess, an herb that is Cooling in its Energetic nature will be part of your formula. If you have excess Yin, an herb that is Warming in its Energetic nature will be part of your formula. These are only a few examples.

The art of herb combining is referred to as herbal formulation. All of the elements must work toward a common goal. If you look at one or two herbs individually, you may not recognize how they would help a certain condition, but when looked at in combination their purpose becomes clear. It is possible to create an herbal formula that generates new properties that cannot be derived from individual herbs. In herbal formulation, one plus one plus one does not necessarily equal three. For example, there is a classic formula used to treat anxiety disorder that contains only three herbs: wheat barley, date and licorice. Individually, none of these three herbs can reduce anxiety, but when combined they are very effective. That is the synergy of herbs.

## Eight Strategies

The principal treatment strategies or methods in herbal therapy, referred to as the Eight Strategies/Methods, are: Clearing, Dissolving, Harmonizing, Inducing Vomiting, Purging, Sweating/Releasing Exterior, Tonifying and Warming. Draining and Moving were added to the list later.

> Clearing: *The herbal treatment strategy to eliminate Heat or Toxin. Any herb that has this type of effect is considered a Clearing Heat or Clearing Toxin herb.*
> Dissolving: *The herbal treatment strategy to disperse certain stagnations, soften hardness or masses, or assist digestion of old,*

undigested foods. It is usually used for abnormally accumulated Qi, Blood, Phlegm, Fluid and foods that cannot be eliminated through Clearing or Purging. Any herb that has this type of effect is considered a Dissolver.

Harmonizing: *The herbal treatment strategy to regulate or balance certain relationships or disharmony. It is usually used in the situations where neither simply eliminating nor strengthening is appropriate. Any herb that has this type of effect is considered a Harmonizer.*

Inducing Vomiting: *The herbal treatment strategy to induce vomiting. It is usually used for helping the body to expel Toxin or abnormally accumulated Foods, Phlegm or Mucus. Any herb that has this type of effect is considered an Emetic (a substance taken to induce vomiting).*

Purging: *The herbal treatment strategy to clean Stomach and Intestines or induce diarrhea. It is usually used to eliminate stagnations that settled in the digestive tracts such as abnormally accumulated foods, fecal matter, Blood, Phlegm and Fluid. Any herb that has this type of effect is considered a Purgative.*

Sweating/Releasing Exterior: *The herbal treatment strategy to create or induce perspiration. It is usually used for early stages of imbalances caused by External Causes. Any herb that has this type of effect is considered an Exterior Releaser.*

Tonifying: *The herbal treatment strategy to strengthen or support Vital Substance. It is usually used for conditions of deficiency. Any herb that has this type of effect is considered a Tonifier or Tonic.*

Warming: *The herbal treatment strategy to counteract Cold disharmonies or certain stagnations. Any herb that has this type of effect is considered a Yang Warmer or Yang tonic.*

Draining: *The herbal treatment strategy to promote urination. It is usually used for edema (abnormal Fluid accumulation) or certain types of Dampness. Any herb that has this type of effect is considered a Diuretic.*

Moving: *The herbal treatment strategy to promote or invigorate the movement of Qi, Blood, Fluid and foods. It is usually used for stagnation. Any herb that has this type of effect is considered a Mover.*

## The Style of the Herbalist

Chinese herbalists have two basic styles. Classical herbalists begin by identifying a classic formulation that best approximates the patient's needs. The herbalist modifies the formula to fit the patient's unique condition. Creative herbalists, such as master herbalist Henry Han, O.M.D., use only the core ingredients from classic formulas and modify them accordingly. In situations when classic formulas do not come close enough to meeting the patient's needs, the creative herbalist will design a formulation from scratch. In time, the creative herbalist compiles an inventory of innovative, unique formulas. The creative herbalist's style allows him or her to be sensitive to newly emergent illnesses that often do not fit with classic formulas and to create highly effective formulas. Dr. Han's creativity in designing formulas has resulted in his reputation for treating difficult illnesses.

## Classic Herbal Formulas

There are some fifty thousand herbal formulas that have survived the test of time, although only about five hundred are commonly used, classic formulas. Throughout history, an enormous number of herbal formulas have come and gone. How a particular herbal formula withstands the test of time is in many ways similar to a process of natural selection. If an herbal formula does not adequately address a health problem, it will fall out of use after a while. It is a testament to their effectiveness that many reliable classical herbal formulas were created hundreds of years ago.

## How to Prepare a Decoction from an Herbal Formula

Herbal formulas are brewed into a tea called a decoction to extract the medicinal qualities. The best cooking pots are ceramic or glass. Stainless steel is acceptable. Do not use cast iron, aluminum or copper pots as they will transfer these metals into your herbs as well as alter the therapeutic qualities of the herbs you are brewing.

&#9830; Use bottled or filtered water rather than tap water, which is treated with chemicals and fluoride. The preferred filtering method is reverse osmosis, a method in which water is forced through a semipermeable membrane that separates contaminants from the water.

- Begin by soaking your herbs in enough water to cover them by about one-fourth to one-half inch for a minimum of fifteen minutes, a maximum of overnight (eight hours). Soaking herbs too long will cause them to ferment and rot.
- Bring the herbs in the same water they have been soaking in to a rolling boil. Turn down the heat to a low simmer and cook, covered, for twenty to thirty minutes. Your herbalist will advise you of the variations in cooking time depending on your formula.
- Strain the herbs and reserve the liquid.
- Pour fresh water over the herbs to cover them by about one-fourth to one-half inch. Repeat the cooking process.
- Strain the herbs again and combine the two batches of liquid. This will be your tea for one day, divided into two or three equal portions depending on your herbalist's instructions. Warm tea over low heat or drink at room temperature.
- For certain conditions, your herbalist will prescribe herbs that require longer or shorter cooking times. These herbs will be packaged separately and will come with special cooking instructions.

It is best to drink your herbal tea one hour before eating on a relatively empty stomach so that your body can best absorb the herbs. Most people find Chinese tea a bitter medicine to swallow but feel the healing benefits are worth putting up with the unpleasant taste. If the tea is a little hard to digest, you may drink it one hour after eating, or add a few slices of fresh ginger to the herbs while cooking. If the tea upsets your stomach, tell your herbalist. He or she can adjust your formula to eliminate these or other side effects.

## Growing, Harvesting and Processing Herbs

Dried herbs are primarily imported to the United States from mainland China. About 30 percent of the herbs we receive in the United States are cultivated; the rest are grown wild. There are people in China known as herb collectors who make a living collecting herbs in the wild. Each region of China is known for producing certain indigenous herbs. Indigenous, wild-grown herbs are often of superior quality to herbs that are cultivated—even if they are cultivated in their indigenous area. These wild herbs, in general, have a higher concentration of active ingredients and are less likely to be exposed to environmental contamination. Organically cultivated herbs have become available in recent years.

A preliminary visual inspection is done by experts, who inspect raw herbs to make sure they are the correct species and also for freshness and quality. Moldy or otherwise undesirable herbs are discarded. A quality herbal supplier puts herbs through a finely tuned scientific test process to ensure the presence and desired amount of active ingredients. A variety of factors influence the quality of herbs. For example, if herbs are not properly harvested or the climate or soil conditions have been significantly altered, quality can suffer. Improper drying or cleaning methods can also influence quality. Herbs should also be tested for herbicides, pesticides, heavy-metal contaminants or any other harmful substance. Poor-quality and tainted herbs are discarded. Herbs are then put through a preliminary process where they are thoroughly cleaned under running water for a period of time and then sun-dried. The next step is to cut or crush the herbs into smaller pieces in order to maximize surface area. This allows for the optimal extraction of active ingredients when the herbs are eventually combined into a formula and brewed into a decoction.

For certain raw herbs, traditional treatment methods are required to maximize the therapeutic effect while minimizing toxicity. One example is Ban Xia (Pinella), which cannot be used in its raw form due to its strong toxicity. It is first soaked and then cooked in ginger juice to neutralize its toxicity. Each herb is treated individually with established practices developed over thousands of years.

Each dehydrated herb is priced based upon its traditional cost of production, grade of quality, availability and weight. As in Western pharmacies, many herbal apothecaries may add a filling fee for the dispensing of the herbs. The overall cost of a package of dehydrated herbs (one day's dose) ranges from $3 to $15 depending on the type and quantity of herbs your formula contains.

## Patent Formulas

In ancient times, herbs were ground into powder and mixed with honey, as a preservative, and formed into pills. A person had to eat quite a few of these "pills" since the herb powders were not concentrated. Today, dried herbs are processed into patent formulas. The process occurs in a clean room to guard against environmental contamination. Dried herbs are brewed into a decoction in softened and purified water free of heavy metals. The decoction is put through various drying and concentrating processes to create an extract, which can then be compressed into tablets or put into capsules or other dosage forms.

The patent formulas that have already been combined and put into tablet or capsule form obviously cannot be altered or customized. However, loose freeze-dried granules and tinctures (liquid herbs) made up of one single herb can be customized by combining these patent herbs to arrive at a formula that is more suitable for a particular patient. In order to fully customize a formula, each of the herbal ingredients must be available in individual form so that the herbalist can pick exactly the right herbs and combine them in precisely the correct ratios.

The use of patent formulas has several benefits. First is convenience. Patent formulations available as tablets, capsules and tinctures can be obtained without a written formulation. There are a good number of classic patent formulas that can easily be found at most Chinese apothecaries, herbal stores or online herbal stores. Second, if the user makes a mistake in determining the selection of patent formula, it usually will not lead to any significant harmful consequences. Third, although patent formulas are meant for minor illnesses—similar to the intended use of Western over-the-counter drugs—if someone is suffering from a more serious illness and cannot obtain a customized dried herbal formula, patent formulas can be used in the interim.

It is labor-intensive to customize herbal formulations. An herbalist is required to select all the necessary herbs and relative ratios. He or she must communicate this list to the herbal pharmacist. The herbal pharmacist requires time to accurately fill each formula. The cost of maintaining custom herbs in inventory and filling customized formulas can be two to three times as great as the cost of the herbs themselves. For these reasons, patent formulas are quite a bit less expensive than customized herbal formulas. A patent formula can run between 50¢ and $3 per day.

Patent herbs come from China, Taiwan, Hong Kong and Korea and are even made in the United States. Making patent formulas is considered an art in China, where herbs are selected, harvested and processed into extracts through strictly guarded traditional Chinese medical standards to ensure the quality. Two years ago, the Chinese government mandated that all herbal manufacturers meet Good Manufacturing Practices (GMP) standards.

## Where to Buy Herbs and Other Supplements

The Western constitution differs from the Asian constitution. Westerners eat a high-calorie, high-carbohydrate, red-meat-heavy diet, which is Warming, compared to the low-sugar, rice-and-vegetable-based diet of the East, which is Cooling. Lifestyle is another major factor that influences constitution. The pace of life and stress level in the West are notably higher than in the East. Influenced by Chinese medicine, Chinese culture places a great deal of emphasis on moderation and discipline. Westerners have a strong tendency to do things all the way in work and play.

These differences account for the Chinese constitution being Cooler (Yang deficiency or Yin excess), with the Western constitution being Warmer (Yin deficiency or Yang excess). In addition, the Energetic systems of these two constitutions are somewhat different. In China, the most common deficiency seen is the Spleen Yang deficiency. In the United States Kidney Yin deficiency along with Liver Energy stagnation are more prevalent.

Formulas created for the Asian population may not be optimal for the opposite Western constitution, or a higher dosage may be required. For these reasons, Dr. Han is continually researching and creating formulas that are optimal for the Western constitution. You can purchase these formulas—traditional patent formulas as well as formulas containing both Chinese herbs and Western nutraceuticals—online at ancientherbsmodernmedicine.com. (Nutraceuticals are natural substances that, when taken in specific doses, have positive therapeutic effects.)

Self-treating relatively mild or benign conditions and symptoms with patent herbal formulas can be safe and effective. In potentially life-threatening situations or when one is seriously ill, however, herbal formulas *must* be prescribed by a trained and experienced herbalist. To maximize the benefits of your treatment, your herbalist and Western physician should collaborate and communicate throughout the course of your treatment. If you are taking Western drugs, always tell your herbalist what medications you are taking. Likewise, always tell your Western M.D. if you are taking Chinese herbs. References on pages 423–430 will help you find a Chinese herbalist to treat you on an individual basis.

# PART
# TWO

## Treating
## Common Illnesses

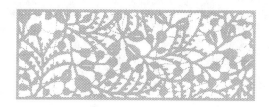

# 6

## Chronic or Recurrent Illnesses

*Chinese medicine is more effective than Western medicine
when it comes to treating most chronic conditions and
illnesses such as gastroesophageal reflux disease (GERD)*

Most women do not approach the milestone of their fiftieth birthday with resounding joy. Stephanie Wilbur, however, was ecstatic. She was getting married for the first time in her life to a man she had met as a dance partner. She had wanted to find someone who could dance Cuban salsa, and word came back through friends that Morris had grown up in New York amid Puerto Rican rhythms and liked to dance the mambo, which is the basic step for South American dance. A year later, after an introduction followed by monthly rendezvous—where the couple would demurely meet, then spend the rest of the evening dancing hot Latin dances—they fell in love.

A frantic summer of wedding plans, a dream wedding and two weeks of glorious honeymoon behind her, Stephanie was sweating it out in Morea, French Polynesia. It was winter in the South Pacific, and flu was sweeping the island. It was a long flight home with a 102-degree fever. Inexplicably, her illness dragged on for one year, and then two. Other health problems that she had had in the past—heartburn, laryngitis, sinus infections and bronchitis—recurred with a vengeance. Ultimately, she could not work and was forced to shut down her family therapy practice. She was deeply depressed and having panic attacks that lasted for hours on end. "I was sure that I was going to die. I couldn't leave the house. I couldn't do anything."

At fifty-six years of age, Stephanie has salt-and-pepper hair hanging halfway to her waist, penetrating brown eyes and a pleasant face. "I understand now that my wedding was a huge precipitating factor in my getting that sick," Stephanie said. "Being married to Morris was probably the first time in my life that I ever felt safe enough to collapse."

In the years before Morris, Stephanie had been no stranger to ill health. She had had a lifelong struggle with gastrointestinal problems, especially chronic esophageal reflux. She was conceived in the forties, "when everyone smoked and drank a lot during pregnancy and nobody cared." An only child, Stephanie sat at the dinner table night after night under a thick blue fog of cigarette smoke as her parents fought. "There was a lot of anxiety, tension, fighting, screaming, yelling—either my mother or my father getting up and leaving the table and not coming back. I was so anxious I would eat as fast as I could. As early as six years old, I thought that it was normal to leave the table with a feeling of nausea or stomach pain. I remember having the sensation that food wasn't moving down my throat quickly enough." On top of the gastrointestinal problems that Stephanie developed as a child in the smoke-filled home, she endured hard Eastern winters and suffered recurrent sinus infections. Taking antibiotics had become routine.

After a sterling East Coast education, Stephanie ultimately ended up dropping out in the seventies, becoming absorbed in the counterculture and living on a shoestring. She worked outside in her garden from sunup to sundown, smoking marijuana nearly every day and occasionally ingesting psychedelics. "I was trying to live a more peaceful life, and in some ways it was a good time. But there was no control over depression. I experienced bouts of anxiety that seemed never to go away. I always had stomach problems. By the time I was an adult my stomach was trashed."

When Stephanie reentered the "establishment" her problems continued. "I had lived a relatively healthy lifestyle, eating whole, organic foods. But I didn't realize what I was doing to myself by skipping meals. I rarely sat down and ate a meal slowly. I didn't chew my food. I ate too fast. I got colds and flu more often and stayed sick longer." Stephanie continued to suffer a range of gastrointestinal problems, including esophageal reflux, indigestion, diarrhea, constipation and bowel spasms.

Although Stephanie was plagued with a host of health problems, our focus will be on her gastroesophageal reflux disease (GERD), better known as heartburn—a burning sensation under the breastbone that can radiate toward the throat. More than sixty million people in the United States alone—males and females of all ages, including up to 25 percent of pregnant women—suffer from GERD daily.

The physiology of esophageal reflux is fairly simple. As you chew food, enzymes within the saliva act upon it to begin the digestive process. You swallow and the food passes down into the esophagus, a muscular tube connecting the mouth to the stomach. The human stomach is a muscular, elastic, pear-shaped bag lying crosswise in the upper abdominal cavity, beneath the diaphragm. At the entrance to the stomach is a high-tension ring-shaped area called the lower esophageal sphincter, which maintains constriction to prevent the stomach's corrosive digestive juices (measuring 0.9 to 1.75 on the pH scale) from escaping into the esophagus. The pH scale, ranging from 0 to 14, is a measure of the acidity or alkalinity of a solution. For example, a hyperconcentrated solution of sulfuric acid, which is extremely acidic, would measure very low; water, which is neutral, measures 7; sodium hydroxide (lye), which is extremely alkaline, measures 14 within the pH range. The stomach's digestive juices are so powerful that if you were to drop a nail into a beaker full of digestive juices, that nail would melt down within a few hours; if you were to drink digestive juices, your mouth and esophagus would immediately erupt in burning blisters. The stomach lining, however, is protected from this low pH (highly acidic) environment by a barrier consisting of a tight layer of mucosal cells that secrete a gel-like mucus coating.

Food is churned around in the digestive juices by the muscular action of the stomach and is reduced to a semiliquid state. Then it passes through the pyloric sphincter—a ringlike muscle that relaxes, leading to the duodenum, the first section of the small intestine. In the presence of esophageal reflux—when the stomach compresses and the pressure in the stomach builds up—if the lower esophageal sphincter is too weak, the contents of the stomach (foodstuffs and the digestive juices) can backwash into the esophagus, which does not have the stomach's protective layer of mucosal cells. Repeated exposure to digestive juices can cause the lining of the esophagus to erode, become inflamed and even develop scattered ulcerations.

Stephanie had an added problem. "My food doesn't move very quickly out of my stomach, and sometimes after I've eaten, I have a burning sensation in my esophagus, which is stomach acid wanting to come up." Peristalsis is the organized, rhythmic movement that is intended to move foodstuffs from the mouth through the digestive system—a muscular passageway with various compartments. At a sports event, when you see a stadium of people doing the wave, it is like looking at a giant digestive tract from the inside. It is likely that Stephanie's sensation of food moving sluggishly was a result of weak peristalsis. In serious cases of gastric reflux, peristalsis can actually reverse direction, carrying the stomach contents all the way up to the mouth, which Stephanie also experienced.

Stephanie tolerated her gastrointestinal problems and chalked them up as part of life. When she finally did seek medical attention in her fifties, she was given what she referred to as a "garbage-can diagnosis of irritable bowel syndrome." Two years into her lingering illness, her asthmatic condition compelled her to seek medical attention, which included a pulmonary workup. Some individuals experience bronchial irritation when the stomach contents aspirate into the bronchial airways. Stephanie's bronchial irritation was triggered in part by esophageal spasms. Because the bronchial tree is anatomically positioned very close to the esophagus, when the esophagus is constantly irritated and goes into spasms, this can trigger the bronchus to spasm. "My doctor found nothing physically wrong with me," Stephanie said.

Stephanie had shunned Western pharmaceuticals her entire adult life, choosing to read and study about herbs. Reluctantly, she turned to "one of the big hot industries" that have sprung up to capitalize on the landslide of chronic conditions plaguing Americans. She took all of the over-the-counter acid reflux medications, as well as prescription Zantac, Tagamet and Prilosec. Because the presence of acid in the esophagus is considered to be the cause of heartburn, the treatment focus is either to neutralize acid or to block the production of stomach acid with medications—many referred to as $H_2$ blockers—that inhibit the activity of histamine cells that are involved in acid production. It is believed that when $H_2$ cells are blocked, acid production diminishes.

After nine months on Prilosec, Stephanie saw no improvement. Finally, her doctor felt he had the answer: a newly discovered bacterial infection called *H. pylori* to which ulcers and acid conditions can often be attributed. Stephanie agreed to take a high dose of tetracycline and Flagyl. "Those are two of the most obnoxious antibiotics," she said. "So after a ten-day course of antibiotics, whatever was left of my immune system was just wiped out." Stephanie was deathly ill, with horrible pain in her esophagus and stomach. Her lips and mouth were on fire, her tongue an angry red from acid reflux.

At this point, a gastrointestinal specialist took Stephanie's complaint seriously. Up to 20 percent of patients diagnosed with GERD go on to develop complications such as esophageal ulcerations from chronic esophageal acid exposure and inflammation. Prolonged irritation of esophageal tissue by gastric reflux can actually change the cell makeup of the lining of the esophagus, leading to a potentially precancerous condition called Barrett's esophagus. There is a 10 percent chance of Barrett's esophagus progressing to esophageal carcinoma (it is the leading cause of esophageal cancer). The specialist examined Stephanie and ran the gamut of tests, including an endoscopy—taking a look down her esophagus with a flexible scope and snipping biopsies. "Everything was just perfect in there," Stephanie said dryly.

Although heartburn can be triggered by behaviors that lead to diminished lower esophageal sphincter pressure—such as lying down, bending over or lifting heavy objects; eating certain foods such as chocolate, acidic foods, alcohol, caffeine or peppermint; and taking certain medications such as anti-inflammatories, narcotics, tricyclic antidepressants or calcium channel blockers—Stephanie did not kid herself. "I knew anxiety was causing my esophageal reflux. Fear in and of itself is one of the worst motivators in the world. And what it does to the body is unbelievable." Though Stephanie had never had manic episodes, she had been diagnosed as bipolar (manic-depressive) at the onset of her illness, and suffered cycles of panic, depression and anxiety. In that regard, she shared a dark legacy with her paternal grandparents. Her grandmother was schizophrenic, and her grandfather was manic-depressive. Her father, who had served as a model of anxiety, also had manic-depressive illness and had once said, "You didn't grow in a very good garden." For Stephanie, this was bittersweet consolation.

For seventeen years of Stephanie's childhood the act of eating was associated with heightened levels of stress and anxiety. In effect, she had become conditioned. The classic study of conditioning was conducted by Russian physiologist and experimental psychologist Ivan Petrovich Pavlov, who discovered the conditioned response. Pavlov began by ringing a bell (conditioned stimulus) and presenting his dogs with food. At first the dogs salivated at the sight and scent of the food (unconditioned response). But after a number of trials the dogs salivated as soon as the bell had been rung (conditioned response) even without the presentation of food. It took a very short time for Pavlov to detect the conditioning of his dogs to the bell. Yet Stephanie went through *seventeen years* of reinforced conditioning with her parents' nightly battles at the dinner table. To her, eating is associated with stress and anxiety. Fifty years later, she may be sitting with her husband eating in a calm state, but on an unconscious level, that bell of Pavlov's dogs is still ringing. Because Stephanie had consciously sought to reverse this conditioning, when she married Morris she felt safe enough to allow herself to fall apart so she could begin the process of re-conditioning.

At the end of a fruitless two-year search through Western medicine, seeking a cure, Stephanie went to see Dr. Han, who took a completely different approach in treating Stephanie's esophageal reflux.

Western medicine is primarily focused on stomach acid and ways to block it with $H_2$ blockers, or to neutralize it with over-the-counter agents such as Pepto-Bismol. However, stomach acid production and regulation is a complex process. One of the basic mechanisms of your body is to monitor how much acid is in your stomach. When the acid drops below a normal level, your brain releases hormones that trigger the cascade of events leading to increased production of acid. When acid production gets too high, the signal is fed back to the control center, which reduces the hormones and acid production subsides. By neutralizing or blocking the production of stomach acid, you are interfering with the body's own regulating mechanisms. When you neutralize or block acid production, your brain is going to get a signal that says, "Aha! I don't have enough stomach acid. I must make some more." In the long run, instead of reducing stomach acid, there is the risk that the body will continue to make more and more acid. Therefore, the more you take the $H_2$ blockers or neutralizing agents, the more likely it is that you will have to continue to take them.

In Chinese medicine the problem of acid reflux is never a problem in and of the stomach itself; rather, it involves a pattern of relationships among three critical Energetic systems: Stomach, Spleen and Liver. The interaction or interplay of these three systems provides Energy movement and circulation that is critical for the process of digestion. Normally, Stomach Energy descends and Spleen Energy ascends. In Chinese medicine, Spleen Energy represents most of the digestive functions performed by the intestines and colon. The dynamic of Spleen Energy is to extract the nutrients, then transport and distribute these nutrients throughout the body by ascending upward and outward (imagine the gentle flow of a lawn sprinkler). Liver Energy is pivotal in regulating and directing the traffic of Energy flow, ensuring that what should flow upward goes up and that what should flow downward goes down.

Imbalances within Stomach, Liver or Spleen Energy can result in gastrointestinal problems. The circulations of the descending Stomach Energy and the ascending Spleen Energy are mutually dependent on each other. Often when Stomach Energy is going in the wrong direction (backing up), you will suffer gastric reflux, nausea and vomiting. When Stomach Energy backs up, Spleen Energy tends to go in the wrong direction as well (down instead of up and outward), and you will have symptoms of gas, bloating, diarrhea and, if left untreated, likely malnutrition. This can be referred to as rebellious Stomach Qi.

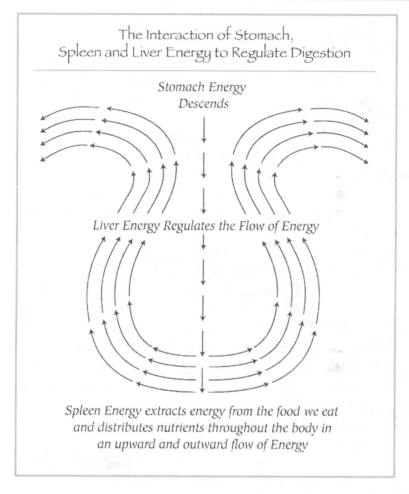

The Interaction of Stomach,
Spleen and Liver Energy to Regulate Digestion

Stomach Energy
Descends

Liver Energy Regulates the Flow of Energy

Spleen Energy extracts energy from the food we eat
and distributes nutrients throughout the body in
an upward and outward flow of Energy

*Figure 20*

In Western medicine esophageal reflux is one diagnosis, and people who suffer from it are pretty much treated the same way—by focusing on neutralizing or suppressing the production of acid. In Chinese medicine, the treatment for esophageal reflux does not focus solely on suppressing or neutralizing stomach acid. In fact, you can even use acid to treat acid. One of the methods Chinese medicine uses is the paradoxical approach of prescribing Sour herbs to treat gastric reflux. Putting Sour herbs into an already "sour" stomach signals the brain not to produce any more acid.

From a Chinese point of view the symptom of esophageal reflux presents a complex situation. Within this diagnosis, there are at least ten different types that can be differentiated, each with a unique Energetic pattern of imbalances.

Treatment takes the form of a multitargeted approach, in which these many imbalances are addressed. In addition, each patient's particular condition must also be taken into consideration. In Western medicine it does not matter, for example, if you are a male or female, if you are strong or weak, if you tend to be hot or cold, work inside or outdoors, or if you tend to be calm or emotional. Chinese medicine factors in *all* of a person's individual conditions when formulating a diagnosis and treatment plan.

Defining one's type and unique condition ensures that the treatment plan will optimally agree with the patient's constitution. In Stephanie's case, one of the two major obstacles to curing her esophageal reflux was that her damaged esophageal lining could not heal because of continued exposure to the caustic contents of her stomach. The second factor was her stress.

One of the most important functions of Liver Energy is to regulate emotions. Among all the Energetic systems, Liver Energy is the most sensitive to the effects of stress. When Liver Energy is affected by stress, its ability to regulate or direct the traffic of Energy flow within the body is compromised. If Stephanie's stress is not resolved, the problem of esophageal reflux will keep recurring. It is important for her to get at the root of her stress and to manage her anxiety as best she can. Herbal treatments can aid in treating Stephanie's stress. If she does not manage her stress, Liver Energy will not be able to regulate the upward and downward flow of Stomach and Spleen Energy. These factors often make esophageal reflux a chronic condition.

Collaboration with Western medical diagnostic techniques can make a significant difference in the formulation of a Chinese herbal treatment plan. For example, if biopsy results from an endoscopy indicate precancerous changes, certain herbs will be selected to address this precancerous state and prevent the evolution to cancer. If a test for *H. pylori* is positive, Western medicine has antibiotics to treat this condition, but these medications can be harsh on the stomach. Using herbs to treat *H. pylori* is a gentler yet equally effective treatment.

Stephanie's formula included Bletilla, a primary herb that melts at body temperature, thereby creating a gel-like coating of the upper gastrointestinal (GI) tract. This insulates the damaged lining (or ulcerations) from the constant erosion and/or irritation of stomach acids, bile and digestive enzymes, allowing these tissues to heal. It also improves microcirculation in the mucosal membrane of the upper GI tract, arrests bleeding and aids in the generation of new tissue, reduces inflammation and pain, and soothes discomforts such as burning, sour feeling and bloating. Corydalis acts as a secondary herb to control pain and discomfort by promoting energy and blood circulation. Notoginseng, another secondary herb, assists Bletilla in repairing the destroyed lining of the GI tract by stimulating growth of new tissue. Notoginseng is also known for its superb ability to both promote circulation and arrest bleeding. Pearl powder is a secondary herb that has an extraordinary ability to heal membranes. Pearl powder is calming and soothing, which helps the patient cope with stress. Peony, Licorice, Bamboo shavings and Ginger were added to regulate peristalsis (so that it would function normally), and additional herbs were added to address her anxiety.

Stephanie had digestive problems as a result of weakened Spleen Energy, so she could not handle a strong herbal formula. Dr. Han prescribed granulated herbs. Another reason Dr. Han chose this particular process is that an herbal decoction from dried herbs would immediately wash down into the stomach. Granulated herbs can be dissolved in warm water to create a creamy consistency. Dr. Han instructed Stephanie to drink this creamy herbal mixture thirty minutes prior to a meal to coat her esophagus and stomach. This multilevel approach would coat her tissues to allow healing.

An important aspect of Chinese diagnosis is examining a patient's tongue. At Stephanie's first visit, Dr. Han saw on Stephanie's tongue that her problems were old and deeply rooted. This came as a relief to Stephanie. "I knew that it would take some time for me to heal and that I'd never be as pristine as I was when I was born. It's just the way it is. And it took about three months before I got any results from the granulated formula. But it felt good. I love the taste of the herbs. They don't taste like medicine—they taste like earth. It's not a bad taste. I was so relieved that something worked—three months didn't seem like a long time, compared to the years I suffered in pain and discomfort."

Although Stephanie claims that herbs are the only treatment that ever worked for her, she deserves the credit. If she had not stuck with the herbal treatment program, she would not have seen the benefits. Stephanie's story demonstrates that in some cases healing takes patience. Stephanie's case of GERD was severe. In the vast majority of cases the inflamed lining of the esophagus can improve markedly within a couple of weeks. Small ulcerations can be healed in about a month.

The home that Stephanie has made with Morris mirrors her creativity, with an upright piano along one wall, a sewing machine set up on the dining room table and jars of herbs and spices lining the kitchen shelves. "When I went through that two-year period of illness I felt that my whole career was a sham—how could I be a therapist helping others if I was that sick? But it certainly has been a gift in many ways. As time went on I began to see that I could be a lot more help to other people. There is nothing more humbling than getting that sick and recovering. I imagine that anyone who has ever been seriously ill and recovered has discovered some compassion and humility."

Stephanie's patience with her healing process combined with the individualized approach of Chinese medicine restored her to a more functional state. As for her gastric reflux, she said, "I'd probably have to live a monastic life in order for it not to be a problem. But Chinese herbs have made it possible for me to live a more normal life." Including dancing with Morris.

## Individualized Program for GERD

Symptoms and indications of rebellious stomach Qi/GERD

- ◆ You suffer from chronic heartburn that may be exacerbated by eating, bending over or lying down.
- ◆ You experience regurgitation, characterized by an occasional sour or bitter taste—less common than heartburn, but may be brought on by the same factors.
- ◆ You experience difficulty in swallowing or a constricted feeling in the esophagus.
- ◆ You feel pain or irritation, a sense of pressure or tightness, sometimes sharp pain upon swallowing, which can radiate to your neck.
- ◆ You have a chronic sore throat, bronchial irritation—coughing and abnormal phlegm—or asthmatic activities.

Ways to treat rebellious stomach Qi to correct or prevent GERD

*Take Extra Steps to Manage Stress:* If you feel you have tried everything to manage your stress and you are still stressed out, it may be time to seek professional help to resolve your emotional issues. In addition, make a habit of listening to positive visualization tapes.

*Quit Smoking:* Smoking irritates the esophagus, which aggravates GERD. See page 150 for more on nicotine and for guidelines to help you quit the habit.

*Modify Your Diet:* From the point of view of Chinese medicine, everything we take into our bodies—air, food and experiences—generates Qi (energy). Thus, to obtain balance it is necessary to make healthy choices regarding the quality of air you breathe, the circumstances you involve yourself in—and especially what you eat and ingest. In Chinese medicine, food has an Energetic dimension and should be agreeable with a person's specific condition as much as possible.

- Foods should be generally soft and light, easy to digest.
- Cold foods (both in physical and Energetic temperatures) such as raw vegetables should be avoided (except for people with Stomach Heat). From the Chinese medicine point of view, just as an individual's constitution can be divided into Yin and Yang (Cold and Hot), Energy from food can also be classified as Yin and Yang (Cold and Hot). Yin foods are Cooling, calming and passive. Yang foods are Warming, stimulating and active. In addition, there are foods that can balance or support each individual Energetic system. Please see chapter 20 for more on the Energetic temperature of foods and your individual constitution.
- Avoid or reduce consumption of foods that reduce esophageal sphincter pressure. Alcohol, coffee, garlic, chocolate, fried foods and sugar contribute to esophageal reflux by allowing partially digested food to escape from the stomach into the esophagus.
- Avoid or reduce the consumption of Energetically Cold or Hot (spicy) foods that can cause direct mucosal irritation such as spicy foods, citrus fruits and tomatoes. Coffee and soft drinks can create hyperacidity when taken with meals.
- Avoid eating heavy meals or overeating.
- Avoid processed foods containing chemicals, preservatives or hormones.
- In Chinese medicine, food and medicine are integrated. The following foods may be helpful and can be found in your Oriental market or online at ancientherbsmodernmedicine.com. Chapter 21 provides medicinal recipes to help treat GERD.

*Foods That Help to Coat the Stomach*

Cream of sweet rice *(a glutinous rice similar to white rice, but sticky and slightly sweet)*

Kudzu starch *(used in place of cornstarch)*
Lotus root starch *(use in blended drinks or stir-fries)*
Potatoes *(preferably in soup)*

*Foods That Help to Promote Esophageal Motility*

Bamboo fluid and shoots *(can be used in stir-fries or tea)*
Cinnamon
Dried tangerine peel *(as a flavoring agent or in tea)*
Ginger *(use in stir-fries or tea)*
Loquat fruit *(can be used in desserts or eaten alone)*

*Foods That Help to Strengthen Digestive Energy*

Chinese dates *(similar to European dates)*
Chinese yams *(similar to American yams but not as sweet)*
Hyacinth bean *(medium-sized white bean, very good for
    digestion—prepare as you would any other bean)*
Licorice *(use for flavoring in desserts)*
Pearl barley *(whole grain)*
Poria mushroom *(a bland mushroom that can be used in soup or
    eaten with rice)*
Rice and sweet rice *(see recipe on page 329)*

*Foods That Are Cooling and Help to Nourish Stomach Yin*

Mung beans *(small green bean, Cooling and detoxifying in
    nature—prepare as any other bean)*
Dandelion greens *(in stir-fries or salads)*
Asparagus
White wood ear mushroom *(Chinese use these mushrooms to
    make dessert, porridge, soup or stir fry)*
Lotus root *(see recipe on page 329)*
Lotus seed *(use in pudding or sweet porridge)*
Lily bulbs *(fresh bulbs can be stir-fried, dried can be rehydrated and
    used in porridge or dessert)*
Soft tofu *(use in stir-fries, soup)*

*Foods That Are Warming and Help Invigorate Energy Flow to the Stomach*

| | |
|---|---|
| Basil | Garlic *(small amounts)* |
| Cardamom | Ginger |
| Clove | Green onion |
| Fennel | Turmeric |

*Foods That Help Reduce Indigestion*

Daikon radish *(can be cooked or used raw in a salad)*
Dried tangerine peels *(use as flavoring)*

*Foods That Help Reduce Pain*

Sichuan pepper *(seasoning)*
Galangal *(Thai ginger)*
Ginger
Turmeric

*Avoid Eating on the Run:* Your autonomic or unconscious nervous system, which regulates the actions of your intestines, is divided into the sympathetic and the parasympathetic nervous systems. During the day, when you are awake, responding to stress, eating and running, you are predominantly in the sympathetic state. When you are in a sympathetic state, peristalsis (the organized, rhythmic muscular contractions of the digestive tract that move food from the mouth through the digestive system) is slowed down. When you eat while in this state, your digestive system cannot function properly. Slow down when you are eating. Never eat at your desk. Walk around slowly, breathing deeply, for a few minutes after meals to allow your autonomic nervous system to shift into a parasympathetic mode, which will get peristalsis moving more effectively.

***Do Not Go to Bed Within Three Hours After Eating a Full Meal:*** Eat smaller, more frequent meals. Elevate your head and upper body six inches when sleeping or lying down, but do not lie down right after a meal, as this may cause the contents of your stomach to back up into your esophagus.

*Lose Weight If You Are Overweight:* Increased abdominal pressure from extra pounds increases the pressure on your esophagus and contributes to GERD. Avoid tight-fitting clothes and belts.

Nurturing a balanced lifestyle will result in healthy weight loss. Eating a balanced diet of real, whole foods can eliminate cravings. Weight loss is discussed further in chapter 19.

*Chinese Herbs and Western Supplements:* Avoid taking antacids on a long-term basis. The excess calcium carbonate in antacids can make your stomach too alkaline, which can actually stimulate more acid production.

Western digestive supplements can be purchased in a health food store. Routinely, before each meal, take one to three (depending on the size of your meal) enzyme capsules containing a combined total of 500 to 1,500 milligrams of the digestive enzymes lipase, amylase and protease.

Routinely, after each meal, take 600 to 1,200 milligrams of betaine hydrochloride, depending on the size of your meal. If you feel a warm, burning sensation in your stomach when taking betaine hydrochloride, drink an eight-ounce glass of water and discontinue use.

Routinely, three times a day, after meals, take 300 milligrams chewable deglycyrrhinated licorice root. Licorice root accelerates the actions of the cells that provide a protective coating of the lining of the stomach.

You can also take Chinese herbal formulas and Western supplements specifically formulated to treat GERD. Within the Western diagnosis of GERD, at least ten types can be differentiated in Chinese medicine, each with a unique Energetic pattern of imbalances. You can find patent formulas to treat each type at your local Chinese herbal clinic or online at ancientherbsmodernmedicine. com. While it is always optimal to consult a Chinese doctor and prepare herbal decoctions of formulas created specifically for you, patent formulas may be used to fill in the gap between the times when you can consult a doctor, or if a doctor is not available in your area.

# 7

## Chinese Herbal Formulas You Can Take for Chronic or Recurrent Illnesses

*Acne, eczema, herpes, psoriasis, irritable bowel syndrome*

By the number of television commercials advertising relief for chronic illnesses, it is painfully evident that Americans are not feeling as well as they would like to. Most people have discovered that over-the-counter remedies offer temporary, marginal relief at best. Some, like Stephanie in the previous chapter, have failed to get relief from Western prescription drugs. Discussing every chronic illness would fill an entire book, so only a few common conditions are covered here.

## Supporting Your Immune System

Medicinal mushrooms such as Reishi, Maitake, Zhu Ling, Yun Zhi, Shiitake, Enokitake, Himematsutake and Dong Chong Xia Cao (Cordyceps) have been shown both in studies and in use for thousands of years to be potent medicine to enhance and support immune function. Mushrooms produce several medicinal compounds, most notably polysaccharides, which are large, long-chained sugar molecules (carbohydrates). These polysaccharides appear to induce a pronounced immune response by increasing the number and activity of killer T and NK (natural killer) lymphocytes, which are normal, healthy immune surveillance cells that eliminate foreign cells (such as cancer). People with severe and chronic diseases have been shown to have abnormally low levels of NK cells. Low levels of NK cells are associated with many chronic viral infections such as AIDS, Epstein-Barr and hepatitis.

Immune modulators allow your immune system to be calmed if it is over-active and strengthened if it is underactive. If you are suffering from a health problem, or you simply want to stay healthy, you can take an immune modu-lating formula separately or in addition to your daily multivitamin/mineral supplement and the Chinese/Western formulas specific to your condition(s).

## Super Green Food

You can also benefit from regularly drinking vegetable juice or super green food (sea algae). Green food will provide your body with phytonutrients (nutri-ents derived from plants), plant enzymes and probiotic cultures (live organisms that benefit the digestive tract and help in the absorption of nutrients) to nour-ish your cells as well as the electrolytes necessary to replace those lost through stress. Chlorella, spirulina and red, blue, green and brown algae infuse your body with nutrients and antioxidants. Sea algae contain bioflavonoids, which are crystalline compounds found in plants that are responsible for their deep colors. They possess antiviral, antibiotic, anticarcinogenic, anti-inflammatory, antioxidant and antihistamine properties. You can make a protein drink in a blender using eight ounces of water, one-half cup crushed ice, one scoop protein powder, a small piece of fruit, one tablespoon of flaxseed oil and one scoop of super green food.

You can purchase immune-modulating formulas, Chinese patent herbal formulas to treat chronic and recurrent conditions, Western supplements and super green food online at ancientherbsmodernmedicine.com. While it is al-ways optimal to consult a Chinese doctor and to prepare herbal decoctions of formulas created specifically for you, patent formulas may be used to fill in the gap between the times when you can consult a doctor, or if a doctor is not avail-able in your area.

## Your Individualized Program

Chronic and recurrent conditions, while not life-threatening, dampen the joy of existence. One of the primary philosophies of Chinese medicine—that every person is an individual—is never so true as when it comes to formatting a health program. Taking Chinese herbal formulas and nutritional supplements is not a substitute for making lifestyle changes. You will experience the best re-sults on a health program that is well rounded and balanced. The best approach is to find a lifestyle that you personally can live with. Making compromises in some areas and being stronger in others allows you room to find a lifestyle that nurtures and supports your particular needs and desires.

The following is the foundation program upon which you can build an integrated Chinese and Western health program that is specific to your concerns. Before you start any program, consult your Western and Chinese doctors to make sure that you have a correct diagnosis of your condition. Discuss with your doctors which Western medical treatments are right for you. Ask your doctors to follow you through any lifestyle, dietary or herbal and nutritional supplement changes you make.

* Eat a balanced diet of real, whole foods to keep your immune system healthy. See chapter 19.
* Manage your stress. See chapters 10 and 16.
* Eliminate toxins from your diet and environment. See chapter 11.
* Take a daily multiple vitamin-mineral supplement that includes Chinese herbs.
* Get regular moderate exercise, incorporating breathing and meditation. See chapter 16.
* Recognize that you are a spiritual being on a human path. See chapter 16.

If you are suffering from a chronic or recurrent illness, find a health care professional who can test you for food allergies or dysbiosis, which is an imbalance of the healthy and unhealthy bacteria and yeast in the gut that may be exacerbating your chronic condition. See page 431 for a laboratory that can refer you to a health care provider in your area who does these types of tests. If you test positive for either of these factors, your health care professional can treat you on an individual basis.

## Acne

Acne is a disorder that can take on various forms, such as blackheads, whiteheads, pustules and cysts. The face is almost always involved, but lesions can also often be found on the chest and back. Most cases of acne are caused by increased production of sebum, obstruction of the follicle and/or inflammation.

In Chinese medicine, acne is considered primarily a Heat and Damp excess in the skin. The Energetic systems involved are Lung and Liver.

Ways to treat acne

*Modify Your Diet:* Eating too much sugar results in high insulin levels, which stimulates testosterone and causes acne. Avoid sugar and reduce your carbohydrate consumption. Avoid spicy foods. Avoid processed, fried foods and hydrogenated oils, which contribute to Internal Toxins.

Drink water to flush toxins from your system. Maintain regularity of bowel movements. Further detoxify by following the vegetable juice detox program on pages 291–296.

*Avoid Dehydrating Skin Products:* Dehydrating face scrubs or products stimulate your body's natural reaction to produce more oil. Treat your skin gently.

*Chinese Herbs and Western Supplements:* You can use Chinese medicinal herbs in recipes to treat acne. See chapter 21 for recipes. You can also take Chinese herbal formulas and Western supplements specifically formulated to treat acne. Formulas can be found online at ancientherbsmodernmedicine.com.

## Eczema

Eczema (or dermatitis) is a pattern of skin inflammation with clinical features of redness, itching, scaling and vesicles in varying combinations. Most commonly, eczema presents as lesions, which can be dry or wet, flaky and often hyperpigmented. They are found in patches in the areas of the elbows, knees, wrists and ankles and around the eyes. Extreme temperatures, sweating, irritating clothing and harsh soaps are known to exacerbate the disease.

In Chinese medicine, Wind, Heat and Damp—or any combination of the three—are usually the cause of eczema. The Energetic systems involved are Lung, Stomach, Liver and Spleen.

Ways to treat eczema

*Reduce or Quit Using Stimulants:* Nicotine, alcohol, chocolate and herbal stimulants such as Ma Huang aggravate and contribute to eczema outbreaks.

*Reduce Stress:* Increase cardiovascular exercises such as walking or Qigong. Breathing exercises such as Qigong breathing (see page 242) are important to stress reduction.

*Modify Your Diet:* Lower or eliminate intake of dairy, fried foods, sugar, processed foods (especially white sugar and white flour products), shellfish, caffeine and spicy foods. Eliminate gluten foods (anything made of wheat) for six weeks to see if there is any improvement, then slowly reintroduce these foods. Research has shown that virtually all skin disorders improve with the elimination of wheat and dairy.

Drink fresh vegetable juices (see pages 291–296) and use sea vegetables (super green food, see page 104) in blender drinks to nourish your skin (via the Blood and Liver), to provide essential iodine and to provide antioxidants to boost your immune system (via the Lung Meridian). Increase foods that nourish Blood and clear Damp and Heat (see chart on pages 310–326). Also, take essential fatty acid supplements such as cold pressed flaxseed oil.

Green tea is Energetically Cooling and therefore can be beneficial to drink in moderation.

*Avoid Aggravating Detergents:* Attempt to discern which laundry detergents, bubble baths, soaps and shampoos have irritating effects and eliminate them. Replace with natural self-care products found in your health food store.

*Maintain Regularity:* Colon cleansing through detoxifications, along with increased fiber intake (fruit, whole grains and vegetables), helps your skin via the Large Intestine Meridian.

*Bathe in Sea Salt, or Swim in the Ocean:* Although it is best to keep eczema dry, wading or swimming briefly in nonpolluted ocean water—which is saline—can be beneficial. Or you can add sea salt to your bath. After bathing, gently and thoroughly pat skin dry. Expose your skin to one half hour of early morning sunshine.

*Chinese Herbs and Western Supplements:* Twice daily with breakfast and dinner, take 50 milligrams zinc picolinate; once a day with breakfast, take 100 milligrams B complex with 500 milligrams pantothenic acid and 400 IU of vitamin E.

You can use Chinese medicinal herbs in recipes to treat eczema. See chapter 21 for recipes. You can also take Chinese herbal formulas and Western supplements specifically formulated to treat eczema. Formulas can be found online at ancientherbsmodernmedicine.com.

## Herpes

A herpes outbreak results when your immune system becomes lax and cannot suppress the herpes virus. Itching, tingling, burning and painful skin lesions break out on the skin. Symptoms of tingling often occur a week or so prior to the lesions first being observed. The lesions usually evolve over a four- to ten-day period.

Herpes infection is classified in Chinese medicine as a combination of the External Causes Heat, Damp and Toxins. The frequency and intensity of symptoms depends upon the strength and balance of the Liver, Kidney and Spleen Energetic systems.

Ways to treat herpes

Follow the guidelines for eczema. In addition, try the following strategies.

*Take Extra Steps to Manage Stress:* Prolonged high levels of the stress hormone cortisol suppresses the immune system, which releases the herpes virus from the restraints of your immune system. Anything you can do to reduce stress will help stop herpes outbreaks. See chapter 16 for more on stress reduction.

*Modify Your Diet:* Avoid sugar, caffeine and excessive alcohol as well as chocolate, nuts and oats, which contain the amino acid arginine, known to aggravate herpes. Avoid shellfish, mushrooms and lamb during the acute phase.

*Chinese Herbs and Western Supplements:* If you are not having a herpes outbreak, take 500 milligrams lysine with breakfast for prevention.

If you are having a herpes outbreak, take 1,000 milligrams lysine with breakfast, lunch and dinner.

See chapter 21 for recipes. You can also take Chinese herbal formulas and Western supplements specifically formulated to treat herpes. Formulas can be found online at ancientherbsmodernmedicine.com.

## Psoriasis

Psoriasis is most commonly seen as a patch of well-defined skin lesions of white to silver scaling with a reddened base. These patches most often occur on the scalp, outside surface of the elbows, knees and pubic area.

In Chinese medicine, psoriasis is generally divided into two categories: excess and deficiency. Heat and Toxin in Blood during the early stage and Blood stagnation in later stages is usually seen in the excess type. Yin or Blood deficiency, leading to undernourishment of the affected area, is commonly seen in the deficient type.

## Ways to treat psoriasis

Follow the guidelines for eczema and herpes. In addition, you can use Chinese medicinal herbs in recipes to treat psoriasis. See chapter 21 for recipes. You can take Chinese herbal formulas and Western supplements specifically formulated to treat psoriasis. Formulas can be found online at ancientherbs modernmedicine.com.

# Chronic Diarrhea

Diarrhea is in itself a sign of underlying pathology, and it is important for individuals who experience chronic diarrhea to pursue a clear diagnosis as to its cause.

The formula offered here for chronic diarrhea is primarily designed for nonspecific diarrhea (meaning that obvious causes have been ruled out). From a Chinese medicine perspective, this type is usually due to Qi or Yang deficiency of the Spleen or Kidney Energetic systems.

## Ways to treat chronic diarrhea

*Check Medications:* Look at the labels of any drugs you are taking to make sure that diarrhea is not a side effect. Be cautious that you are not taking too much magnesium or vitamin C, both of which can cause loose bowels. Increase your fluid intake to compensate for the loss of fluids and to prevent dehydration.

*Modify Your Diet:* Following the BRAT diet—bananas, rice, applesauce and tea—can help stop diarrhea. Avoid foods that are cold in temperature and Energetically Cold. See pages 310–326 for the Energetic properties of foods.

*Chinese Herbs and Western Supplements:* If you notice mucus or undigested food in your stool, you can take the digestive formulas on page 102.

You can use Chinese medicinal herbs in recipes to treat diarrhea. See chapter 21 for recipes. You can also take Chinese herbal formulas and Western supplements specifically formulated to treat chronic diarrhea. Formulas can be found online at ancientherbsmodernmedicine.com.

# 8

## The Gray Zone of Health

*If you are in the "gray zone" of health, your body's
defense can be strengthened with Chinese herbs before
you develop chronic or recurrent illnesses such as
colds, flu, bronchitis or headaches*

Nara Shikibu grew up as a sickly kid who was weaned on antibiotics. Five additional years on tetracycline as a teenager left her feeling run down and wasted. "I fell apart at eighteen. I couldn't keep anything down. I was only able to eat some rice with butter and clear broth," Nara said. "On top of that, I had horrible allergies. I seemed to catch everything that went around and become even sicker, and it would take me a long time to feel better." Over a seven-year period, Nara saw nearly a dozen doctors. She had "all the tests," and nothing came back positive other than a mildly elevated candida level.

Nara got married and tried going to school and working. Even as a very young woman she did not have the stamina to devote time to her marriage, work and study. She ended up divorced and struggling to get up every day and go to work. "The doctors didn't know what to do with me and finally started saying my problems were all in my head."

In 1995 when she was twenty-five, several friends suggested Nara try Chinese herbs. "They told me, 'You won't believe what you'll get out of this.' I went in already trusting in the process, thinking that Chinese medicine has proven to be helpful for others, so it might help me too. When I saw Dr. Han, he immediately saw what was wrong with me. After everything I had been through, it was hugely gratifying to have someone say, 'I can see it on your tongue, I can feel it in your pulses.' "

Nara's condition was representative of an increasing number of people in the West. She was in the gray zone of health—not suffering from a specific illness that could be diagnosed by Western medicine, yet not well.

Western medicine looks at factors that can be objectively measured by a lab test, EKG or X ray, for example. Nara did not have any definitive signs, so it was not possible to diagnose her illness. Without a definitive diagnosis, Western medical treatment is often limited. When one is in the gray zone of health, it is possible to fall through the cracks of the health care system.

From a Chinese medicine point of view, Nara's imbalances were clear from her symptoms. Chinese medicine recognizes that symptoms tend to appear during the early stages of an illness, before the crisis sets in. Disease does not just happen. It is a process, starting as a minor imbalance, gradually developing or worsening when not treated. "Healing is about life, not just disease," said Maoshing Ni, Lic. Ac., D.O.M., Ph.D., known as Dr. Mao, who is the cofounder of the Tao of Wellness clinic and Yo San University of Traditional Chinese Medicine in Los Angeles, California. "Disease is a symptom of life out of balance. Chinese medicine is the healing of *life*. In Chinese medicine, we have a saying from the classics: 'A superior physician treats an illness before it even begins. A mediocre physician treats a condition as it's developing. An inferior physician treats a patient after an illness has occurred.' That would put us all in the inferior category! But prevention is so important. Problems are easier to deal with when they are small."

Nara's imbalance was a combination of deficiency and stagnation. This is one of the most common patterns of imbalances seen in the West. Yet there was also a certain uniqueness to her situation. Both her deficiency and stagnation were extreme. Her internal Energy was depleted. This was seen in her weakened Kidney and Spleen Energies. Her Kidney and Spleen deficiencies were mostly Yang deficiencies, which are not commonly seen types of imbalances in the West.

Stagnation can happen at various levels. Imagine your body's Energy system as a tree. The most superficial level of stagnation would be at the level of leaves. A deeper stagnation would involve the twigs, then the branches, trunks, major roots, smaller roots and ultimately the fine, capillary-like end roots. Nara's stagnation was at the level of the root, involving Qi, Dampness and Blood as well as Liver, Lungs, Spleen and Large and Small Intestine Energies.

Nara's Yin and Yang disharmony was complicated. Because of the Yang deficiency she felt cold all the time. Energetically Cold foods, or foods of cold temperature, exacerbated her digestive problems and fatigue. However, her tongue was coated with a thick yellow moss indicating internal Heat resulting from the long-term accumulation of stagnation. Deficiency and stagnation are opposite Energetically. Deficiency is a weakness—a state of lack of Vital Substance. Dampness is an excess or abnormal accumulation of External Causes. Yet at a deeper level they are related.

Your body's Energetic systems need to be harmonized and balanced, and there is a dynamic to this Energy pattern—a constant movement and free flow of the Energy, which delivers the nutrients—the Essence of Qi—to the body. At the same time, this Energy removes the waste and toxins, preventing and freeing your body from stagnation. One of the basic functions of the body's Energetic systems is to maintain this dynamic movement of Energy flow. Kidney Energy provides the most important source of power for the movement. It is the push behind the movement. Heart Energy assists the Kidney Energy. The Lung Energy helps to distribute the Energy flow that carries the nutrients. The Spleen Energy sustains the other Energy systems by supplying constant nourishment from food. The Liver Energy regulates the movements by directing the Energy "traffic."

When Kidney and Spleen Energy become deficient, the body's ability to maintain Energy circulation is compromised. This leads to a reduction of the nourishment delivered throughout the body as well as a gradual accumulation of toxins and metabolic wastes that are normally cycled out of the body by the Energy circulation. The stagnation then becomes a causal factor in further impeding the Energy flow.

The challenge in designing a treatment plan for Nara was that the herbs for Tonifying or strengthening her deficiencies could potentially fortify and deepen her stagnation. Herbs that disperse or clear stagnation could weaken or even damage her already deficient Qi. Her Yang deficiency required Warming herbs, yet Warming herbs could easily aggravate the internal Heat, whereas Cold herbs, although helpful in clearing Heat, could damage her already weakened Yang Energy. There was a fine line of balance to maintain and a very small margin of error to work with.

Think of your body as a container that is normally filled with Qi and other Vital Substances. When Energy deficiencies occur, your container becomes half empty. To correct (fill) this imbalance seems simple. You would merely fill the container with "good stuff"—vitality and Qi. However, in Nara's situation it was much more complex. Because of the stagnation caused by many years of antibiotics her container was not only half empty but also filled with "bad stuff" that first needed to be taken out. The priority is usually given to the cleanup first so that room can be made within the container for the "good stuff" to be put in later.

The Centers for Disease Control estimates that one half of the 235 million doses of antibiotics prescribed each year are unnecessary. Like Nara, many people who are suffering from the gray zone of ill health turn to their doctors for help and are sometimes given round after round of antibiotics. Often, antibiotics are prescribed for colds and flu, but since antibiotics combat bacteria, they are useless against such illnesses, which are viral infections.

Taking antibiotics to fight a bacterial infection is like fighting an enemy with only one highly trained, technologically powerful soldier. The vast majority of the time antibiotics are effective in disabling the invading bacteria. Your body, while weakened, is still able to eliminate the small amount of remaining bacteria from its system. However, should the bacteria defeat the soldier, the battle can easily be lost. Even if antibiotics do win, they do nothing to strengthen your body or your immune system. Also, antibiotics often possess a single active agent, and invading organisms oftentimes need only minimal mutation to become resistant to this agent. Because of the long-term overuse of antibiotics, more virulent and antibiotic-resistant bacteria are developing. As a result, pharmaceutical companies are constantly scurrying to develop newer and more potent antibiotics to try and stay ahead of bacterial resistance.

From a Chinese medicine perspective, antibiotics are Energetically Cold and Bitter in nature, and tend to aggravate existing Dampness. Bitter flavor generally has clearing and Drying effects. When overused, Cold and Bitter Energy can easily damage Yang or turn into a Dry Energy and damage underlying Yin.

Antibiotics often irritate and weaken the digestive system and lead to decreased vitality and a weakened immune system. Herbs can be used for common infectious conditions to supplement antibiotics, to reduce side effects or as an alternative to antibiotics if a patient does not respond to antibiotic treatment. Although antibiotics are an important method of treatment for dangerous bacterial infections, there are many instances when the use of herbal medicine would be more advantageous. Many herbs are capable of strengthening and supporting the immune system and have antimicrobial properties. These herbs fight the microorganisms that cause disease.

In addition to antibiotics, because of her discomfort and pain, Nara took anti-inflammatories (aspirin or related medicines), which irritated her already sensitive stomach. She was also prescribed Diflucan, an antifungal medication, which is highly toxic to the liver. Dampness is essentially an abnormal accumulation of moisture, which in nature is already Wet and Cold. Adding to her system these medications, which carry with them even more Cold and Dampness, worsened her condition.

What further complicated Nara's situation was the fact that the good and bad were so enmeshed that ridding the container of the bad meant running a risk of further depleting her already weakened Qi. The first step was to separate out the good from the bad. When the stagnation had nothing to cling to, it would be much easier to eliminate. After the cleanup, her container could be filled back up with "good stuff." This would be accomplished by strengthening her Spleen and Kidney Energy.

"Dr. Han went about trying to devise teas that would help me. It took quite a while," Nara said. "We used to joke that I was one of his most difficult patients. My stomach was so sensitive that I couldn't tolerate a lot of herbs he would have wanted to use."

Herbs need to be digested in order to work. Nara's condition was so severe initially that she was unable to digest even the mildest of herbs prescribed, just as she was unable to digest a normal diet of food. Nara required herbs to strengthen her digestive system, but she did not have enough digestive Energy to digest the needed herbs. Hence a catch-22. That is why, when treating people with extremely weak digestive systems, progress is so slow to come about. The herbalist, in a sense, has to inch his or her way along with the patient in order not to overload an already weakened digestive system. As one of Dr. Han's teachers, Dr. Yue Meizhong, physician to Chairman Mao, so aptly put it, "When you need to attack a disease, attack with the force of a tidal wave. But, when patience is required, go slowly as the old woman needlepointing under the table lamp."

After many unsuccessful trials of herbal combinations, Dr. Han used a treatment referred to as herbal transdermal ionization—a concentrated herbal pack applied to her abdomen—to deliver herbal properties transdermally, bypassing her sensitive digestive system. (See page 147 for more on herbal transdermal ionization.) "Right away I felt a little better," Nara said. "Then we spent a year and a half trying different herbal formulas and seeing what worked. Even though my healing didn't take phenomenal leaps, at least I saw a bit of improvement. And that was encouraging. I figured that if I was going to find real recovery back to good health, it wasn't going to come in leaps, it was going to come in slow increments—like a steady climb. And that's what it really turned out to be."

Nara prepared an herbal decoction five days a week for five years. She then began to feel healthy enough to taper off. "It became part of living," she said. "Get up in the morning, make the special tea and drink it. I go back to the clinic for herbs about once a month now. My stomach is still susceptible to stress, and if I don't eat particularly well I'll feel it. But I can eat normal food now. If I start to feel some discomfort, I'll drink tea for a little while to clean out my system. I get fewer flus and colds than other people seem to. When I feel something coming on I'll get an herbal formula and I don't end up getting what's going around in the office. Overall I've got a normal energy level now, so I can lead a normal life. I feel good so I can enjoy life. The herbs turned my health around. It was such a simple thing. It's just tea. But it restored what the antibiotics had done to my body, so my body could be healthy and take care of itself."

## Chinese Medicine Is Designed to Treat Disease as It Evolves

Western medicine tends to focus on a single factor of illness, and then tailors the treatment intervention accordingly. For example, Western medicine will treat a cold. If the person develops pneumonia, the doctor will then treat the pneumonia. If the pneumonia then evolves into the even more serious condition of septic shock, the doctor will aggressively treat the septicemia.

When you go to your doctor, he or she sees only what is happening with you at that period in time. In reality, the disease process began well before you went to the doctor and will end well afterward.

Chinese medicine endeavors to anticipate the development of disease so that one can take steps ahead of time to prevent disease from occurring and avoid complications. It also treats illness at every stage of its evolution. If you have a cold that develops into pneumonia, Western medicine calls this a complication of your disease. In Chinese medicine, if you have a cold that develops into pneumonia, it is considered a different component of the same disease. In other words, these conditions evolve from one another, and they are treated as *different stages* of the *same disease process*. Chinese doctors are trained to take the necessary steps to intervene before a complication occurs. The Chinese doctor will treat a cold and will also provide intervention and support to prevent the evolution of the cold into pneumonia as well as the necessary herbs to treat these complications should they occur.

In Chinese medicine, the objective of the diagnosis is not just to identify the cause (virus or bacteria) but rather to assess the strength of the Cause versus the strength of your Qi.

In the treatment of infectious disease, Chinese medicine views the evolution of the disease in several different stages or levels. The following diagnostic and treatment system, designed to deal with fever-causing infections, identifies four distinct levels:

### First level: Wei (Defense Qi)

Wei is the protective energy that circulates at the very surface of your body. Wei level is the first protective barrier against the Cause. When the Cause confronts Wei, you experience mild malaise, mild sore throat and nasal congestion. At this level, the Cause is not yet very strong and the Qi is strong and intact.

### Second level: Qi

Once the Wei level is breached (or pierced) by the Cause, it reaches Qi, which is the next level. Qi-level involvement is experienced as high fever, chills and pronounced perspiration and thirst. Your body and immune system are actively fighting and resisting the invading Cause. In other words, both the Cause and your Qi are strong.

### Third level: Ying

When the Cause pierces your Qi it enters the Ying level, which is evident in the development of pneumonia, endocarditis and myocarditis, to name a few problems. At this level the Qi begins to be overwhelmed, or worn down, by the Cause.

### Fourth level: Xue (Blood)

If the treatment fails to stop the disease progression at this point, it will culminate in the Xue (pronounced *shh-why*) level, the last or final level, which is critical and potentially fatal. Often, the earmark of the Xue level is the presence of multiorgan failure. The patient's blood coagulation factors are exhausted, which results in internal coagulation and extensive bleeding simultaneously. At this stage, Qi has become depleted.

Are you suffering from Spleen and Kidney Yang Energy deficiencies—the gray zone of health?

- You have a Cold constitution (see chapter 20 to determine your Energetic constitution).
- You have a sensitive digestive tract and have loose stools.
- You have decreased appetite along with a feeling of bloating after eating.
- You suffer from chronic candida.
- You have low endurance and stamina.
- Your body tends to retain fluid or your ankles tend to become swollen.
- You have a weak lower back and knees.
- During cold and flu season you frequently catch these illnesses.
- Colds and flu linger.
- Your sex drive decreases during the winter.
- You tend to have a lot of mucus buildup.

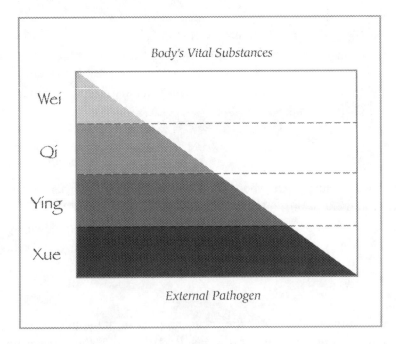

*Figure 21*

*The white area represents your Vital Substances. The shaded areas represent External Causes in your system. As the illness descends from Wei to Xue, your body experiences a diminishing amount of Vital Substances and an increasing amount of External Causes.*

There are a number of ways to strengthen Spleen, Kidney and Lung Energies to treat the gray zone of health.

*Avoid Overtaxing Your System:* Get regular rest—at least eight hours of sleep every night. Take rest periods and/or naps during the day. Avoid overexercising. Excessive exercise increases the stress hormone cortisol, which weakens your immune system. Ideal exercises for you are Qigong, Tai Chi, yoga and walking. Moderate exercise allows you to strengthen and repair the body so that you go forward without setbacks. Moderation and discipline are the key to preserving and cultivating your Kidney and Spleen Energies.

*Limit Caffeine Intake:* Caffeine is a stimulant that increases the stress hormone cortisol, which weakens your immune system. Limit caffeine intake to one cup of coffee in the morning; quit if you can. See pages 148–150 for more on caffeine and guidelines to help you quit the habit.

*Quit Smoking:* Nicotine is an External Cause that contributes to the gray zone of health. See pages 150–151 for more on nicotine and for guidelines to help you quit the habit.

*See a Health Care Professional:* The goal in seeing a health care professional is to strengthen your body's defenses to optimize the function and decrease the toxin load of every system in your body and to keep your intestines as healthy as possible to optimize the absorption of nutrients.

* Have your adrenal hormones tested, as depleted adrenals (often reflect Kidney Energy deficiency) are a major contributing factor in lowered immunity. See chapter 10 for restoring adrenal function.
* Have your amino acid levels tested. If your body is not breaking down the proteins you eat into amino acids, this can exacerbate fatigue and symptoms of depression. Amino acid supplementation can boost your energy as well as supply your body with the necessary precursors to neurotransmitters.
* Stool, hair and blood tests can determine if you have (1) high levels of accumulated heavy metals in your system, (2) sensitivities to foods or (3) dysbiosis, which is an imbalance of the healthy and unhealthy bacteria and yeast in the gut, any of which may be weakening your immune system and draining your energy.

See page 431 for a laboratory that can refer you to a health care provider in your area who does these types of tests. If you test positive for any of these factors, your health care provider can treat you on an individual basis.

*Modify Your Diet*: Dairy products and fried foods create Phlegm, an Intermediate Cause, and are best avoided or limited if you are in the gray zone of health. Avoid sugar, including too much fresh fruit, which is Cooling, or refrigerated or iced foods and drinks. Cooling foods weaken Spleen Energy.

Soups with protein such as legumes, organic meats and poultry are Warming and boost Spleen Energy. Eat Yang (Warming) foods that will warm your Yin (Cold) constitution, such as congees (see pages 327–328 for recipes). When you eat raw vegetables, which are Cooling foods, have a cup of hot ginger tea too. Drink herbal teas with Warming spices such as cinnamon, cayenne, ginger and cloves. Pages 310–326 provide lists of the Energetic properties of foods that you can use as a guideline. Chapter 21 provides medicinal recipes to treat the gray zone of health.

*Chinese Herbs and Western Supplements*: If you do not currently have a cold or flu, for prevention take 250 milligrams vitamin C, with breakfast and dinner.

When you do have a cold or flu take 1,000 milligrams vitamin C with breakfast and dinner—if this causes loose bowels, reduce amount.

You can also take Chinese herbal formulas and Western supplements specifically formulated to treat the gray zone of health including colds and flu. Formulas can be found online at ancientherbsmodernmedicine.com.

*Flu Prevention*: Along with lifestyle changes, nutritional supplements and Chinese herbs, you may choose to have a flu shot during flu season. Flu shots can provide relatively good protection (85 percent efficacy) against influenza infections, yet their effectiveness is limited and depends on the following factors:

◆ *Accurate coverage.* It is not always easy to predict which subtypes of viral strains are likely to cause the epidemic for the next flu season. The flu virus is highly mutable and constantly creates new strains by self-modifying its gene sequences. Some changes are gradual through a series of minor mutations, and some are sudden and drastic through major mutations. The prediction can sometimes be off. Part of the difficulty in guesstimating is that the forecast has to be made eight to ten months ahead of time to allow enough time for pharmaceutical companies to manufacture the vaccine.

- *Sufficient coverage.* There are over six thousand different flu viral gene sequences identified and stored currently in the data bank of Los Alamos National Laboratory. As transcontinental travel becomes increasingly easier and more accessible, the traditional pattern of one dominant strain of virus per type per year is changing as well. Especially for the areas such as coastal regions of the United States and Western Europe, there can be multiple strains of the flu virus going around in any given year. Yet the flu shot usually contains the vaccination for only two or three major types of viral strains. In other words, it will provide protection most of the time for two or three viral strains if the prediction is right on but will not shield you against other strains that are going around at the same time.

- *Individual differences.* A flu shot apparently works much better for young and healthy individuals (nearly 100 percent efficacy) than it does for older or chronically ill individuals. Sometimes even with the vaccination, these people will often require additional support, such as immune-enhancing and antiviral herbs.

- *Chinese medicine can play a significant role in the prevention and treatment of the flu.* Certain Chinese herbs have antibacterial properties, others have antiviral properties and others can stimulate or strengthen your immune system. When applied to a petri dish cultured with the bacteria causing pneumonia, well-known Chinese herbal formulas designed for upper respiratory infection showed no effect. However, when a few drops of blood are added to the petri dish and formula, the bacteria will begin to die off. This demonstrates the fact that herbal formulas do not cure but rather strengthen your body, in particular your immune system, to assist your body in healing from illness.

Antiviral properties are unique to Chinese herbs. In Western medicine, aside from a few recently developed drugs that are somewhat effective in treating chronic viral infections, there really are no medications available in the treatment of acute viral infections. That is why Chinese medicine is preferable for the treatment of most viral infections. Even for severe viral conditions, such as encephalitis and meningitis, specific herbs have been shown to be very effective in counteracting the viral cause.

As far back as 1962, Chinese researchers began studying the effectiveness of herbs against acute viral infection. In a study of 1,150 patients suffering from cold and flu symptoms including fever, chills, headache, sore throat and fatigue—

characterized by Chinese medicine as Wind and Heat—the average length of time to full recovery when taking Chinese herbs was 2.7 days, down from the recovery period of 4 to 7 days when treated with Western over-the-counter medications. Many Chinese patent herbal remedies are well tested, and most have at least several hundred years of history.

# 9

## Mental Illness, Anxiety and Depression

*Chinese medicine believes that the mind and body are
intimately entwined and interactive*

Over the past two decades Western psychiatry has evolved from the stereotype of a bespectacled, bearded middle-aged man in a cardigan sweater sitting behind the head of his reclining patient to face-to-face medically based assessment and diagnosis. With remarkable breakthroughs in understanding how brain chemistry functions, Western medicine is now armed with numerous medications that can effectively treat a range of psychiatric disorders.

## The Open-Box Versus Sealed-Box Approach

Compared to the much more scientific orientation of other medical specialties, the field of psychiatry remains a blend of art and science. In Western medicine the body has become an open box. In fact, the Western approach began with gross anatomy by opening the box of the human body to find out what was inside—organs, blood, bones. As medical technologies evolved, those boxes were opened to find other boxes—cells, molecular structures and on down. This analytical approach has allowed scientists to discover the cures for many diseases. Western medicine takes the position that the whole cannot be understood until the components that make up the whole are analyzed and understood. In treating a health problem, Western medicine looks for the cause. In looking for the cause, many boxes must be opened.

Over the past twenty years there has been a tremendous improvement in the quality and effectiveness of the medications utilized to treat a variety of psychiatric disorders. However, given the ethical prohibitions against removing the top of people's skulls to do research on the brain, the inner workings of the brain have remained a sealed box—a mystery. Recently with the advent of MRIs and PET scans Western medicine has begun to acquire a rudimentary understanding of the inner workings of the brain. However, for the most part, the brain still remains a closed box. When a person is suffering from a mental illness, X rays, blood tests or even spinal taps will not show any meaningful, supportive information.

The Chinese medical approach is a sealed-box approach. Unlike Western medicine, Chinese medicine does not attempt to open the box (the human body). If a person is depressed, the Chinese doctor asks questions about the person's symptoms, then prescribes herbs and observes how these symptoms change. Say a person is suffering from a particular type of depression. Considering that this type of depression has afflicted people for a couple of thousands of years, a wealth of knowledge has accumulated over generations and generations and Chinese doctors have this wealth of knowledge to draw from. This accumulation of knowledge is referred to as empirical evidence—in other words, it is derived from observation and experimentation.

Psychiatry is much like Chinese medicine in that the psychiatric field relies on symptoms and outward appearances and manifestations to make the best scientific/experiential judgment regarding a diagnosis as well as the first best guess as to what medication and dosage to prescribe. The patient is then observed and monitored over several days, weeks and months—in a fashion very similar to Chinese medicine.

## The Human as a Whole

The philosophy of wholeness is at the very heart of Chinese medicine. The whole is in constant motion and involves many factors simultaneously. No part can be accurately studied without its dynamic connection to the whole.

Everything that happens inside a body is reflected outwardly. For example, you can look into a person's eyes and see what is going on in their Liver. The Liver Energetic system is considered to be a regulator of Energy flow, circulation and emotions. That is what it means to be holistic. Your body is wired by Qi, so every part is related to some other part. You do not have to cut into the body to know what is going on internally.

Think about the way Western medicine diagnosed scurvy. Descriptions of scurvy are found in ancient writings and clear accounts are found in records of medieval crusades. For hundreds of years on ships where fruits and vegetables were not supplied, men suffered and died of scurvy. In the 1500s French explorer Jacques Cartier observed as Huran Indian healers cured his dying men with white pine tea. Nearly two centuries later, this account, along with the empirical evidence of hundreds of years, inspired Scottish naval surgeon James Lind to perform experiments that demonstrated the link between citrus and scurvy. British ships began taking limes on board—and the sailors subsequently earned the moniker limeys. Like this story of the discovery of the connection between scurvy and citrus fruit (vitamin C), Chinese medicine has several thousand years of empirical knowledge from which to cull information about herbs and their effects and benefits.

## Chinese Medicine Does Not Make Distinctions Between the Mind and the Body

Chinese medicine revolves around the philosophy that the mind and body are intimately entwined and interactive. In Chinese medicine Internal Causes—Anger, Joy, Sadness, Grief, Pensiveness (anxiety or obsessiveness), Fear and Fright—influence your body's Energetic systems. These emotions are neither good nor bad in themselves, but when they are excessive or out of control, they can lead to imbalances (illness). For example, anger is toxic to Liver Energy, causing stagnation and leading to depressive or anxious tendencies. Lack of Joy weakens Heart Energy, which drains joie de vivre—the vitality for life—and can lead to a feeling of isolation and alienation from humanity. Sadness and Grief weaken Lung Energy, which interferes with the reception of Qi, resulting in depression. Pensiveness knots up Spleen Energy, resulting in loss of appetite and a propensity toward eating disorders and chronic anxiety. Fear and Fright damage Kidney Energy, resulting in anxiety, arrested development and insomnia, and can lead to addictions. When Internal Causes dominate we tend to make poor choices in life, either through neglecting aspects of our body, mind or life or through choosing toxic or injurious substances or activities to self-medicate or to temporarily escape. Therefore, the disorders typically considered to be psychiatric in nature can be treated by rebalancing and harmonizing the appropriate Energetic system(s).

## Integrating Chinese and Western Medicines to Treat Mental Illness

Many of the prescription medications currently used in the treatment of mental disorders are far less likely to cause intolerable side effects compared to those used as recently as five or ten years ago. Even so, side effects are the primary reason mentally ill patients discontinue their medications or take less than the prescribed dose. In an attempt to help people deal with medication side effects, many physicians prescribe additional medication(s), which can leave patients with a whole new set of side effects.

The use of integrative medicine has been proven to hold great promise in providing the mentally ill with much more effective health care. Just as the integration of psychotherapy and psychopharmacology (treating mental disorders with prescription medications) has shown greater effectiveness than either intervention used alone, the use of specific prescription medications along with the use of specific Chinese herbs has also been found to provide improved effect. Moreover, it has been found that patients have greater compliance when these two approaches are integrated.

A second obstacle to accessing mental health care is the cost of ongoing treatment. The use of certain Chinese herbs can help counteract the side effects of many psychiatric medications. Oftentimes, the cost of these herbs can be significantly less than the prescription Western medications also designed to counteract side effects. By making the total cost of care less expensive, while still effectively treating side effects, overall compliance and efficacy are likely to improve.

Although cost and medication side effects are indeed two primary obstacles faced by the mentally ill, these problems can pale in comparison to the social stigma of mental illness. Fear of stigmatization often prevents people from accessing necessary care and treatment. This social stigma includes fear of being found out by your employer, family members and friends. Some occupations exclude those who have been or are being treated for mental illness, whether it be something as common as depression and anxiety or more severe conditions such as schizophrenia.

## Panic Attacks

Panic attacks are becoming increasingly common in our stressful world. There is a big difference between an appropriate fight-or-flight response and panic attack. The fight-or-flight stress response is an appropriate physiological response to a perceived danger. A panic attack is the same response, but it occurs in the absence of any identifiable danger or threat. A panic attack is a sudden onset of intense apprehension, fearfulness or terror, often associated with feelings of impending doom. During a panic attack one may suffer shortness of breath, palpitations, chest pain or discomfort and choking or smothering sensations, accompanied by the fear of going crazy or losing control.

Think of a TV set that is constantly scanning the room waiting for a signal from the remote. We can describe the TV as being in standby mode. Unconsciously, we are constantly scanning our environment (being vigilant) for any potential threat. When you click the remote, the TV set turns on. Likewise, the adrenals are programmed to respond to danger signals by secreting the stress hormones necessary for the body to mobilize for fight or flight. We hear an explosion and turn sharply to see and assess the perceived danger. Most of the time, we will say, "Oh, a car backfired." Some individuals, however, do not have the capacity to respond to an assessment of no true danger and readjust back to a standby mode. Their adrenal glands secrete large amounts of adrenaline inappropriately, resulting in a panic attack.

More recently people suffering from panic attacks have been prescribed medications such as Paxil, Prozac and Zoloft, which are selective serotonin reuptake inhibitors (SSRIs) that increase serotonin levels in the brain. Serotonin is the most widely found neurotransmitter—a chemical that carries messages between cells—within the central nervous system. Low levels of serotonin can create depression, panic attacks, obsessive-compulsive disorder, eating disorders and sleep disorders, to name a few problems. In treating panic attacks, increased serotonin levels calm the hot centers of the brain thereby returning the output signals to the adrenal glands back to normal. Other medications such as clonidine and guanfacine work by blocking signals between various centers within the brain so that the ultimate output signal to the adrenal glands returns to a normal range and stress hormones are not secreted inappropriately.

From a Chinese medicine perspective, panic attacks are caused by imbalance in certain aspects of Kidney and Liver Energies. Kidney Energy has a particularly strong association with the feeling of centeredness, emotional stability and self-confidence. When Kidney Energy is compromised, the individual will be susceptible to fear and panic. Liver Energy plays an important role in regulating emotions. Imbalances of Liver Energy can create over- as well as underregulation of emotions. Overregulated Liver Energy can result in aggression, anger and anxiety attacks, a hyperactivity of emotions. Underregulated Liver

Energy can result in depression, withdrawal and isolation. The interactions between Liver and Kidney Energies are supportive of each other. Kidney Energy nourishes Liver Energy, and Liver Energy regulates Kidney Energy. When one system is out of balance, over time it will affect the other system as well. Sometimes due to this mutually supportive relationship between the systems, the imbalances can develop into a vicious cycle.

Severely mentally ill people are best put under close supervision to protect themselves and others. In these cases, Western medicine is equipped to provide specific drugs and a controlled institutional setting. Yet, controlling or stabilizing mentally ill people is quite a different matter from healing them, and that is why an integrative approach to mental illness would produce gentler results and fewer side effects than drugs. Chinese medicine has accumulated much experience in treating so-called mental illnesses, ranging from depression, anxiety disorder and cognitive dysfunction to even schizophrenia. The effect is often reliable yet gentler and well sustained, especially for mild and moderate cases. Its effectiveness is rooted in Chinese medicine's recognition that mental illness is not purely mental *but involves a person's whole being.*

## Ways to Address Internal Causes to Treat Mental Illness, Anxiety and Depression

Catalogue your symptoms and be your own advocate

Almost all of us can relate to experiencing temporary periods of depression. And some of us would go so far as to admit that we had periods of our lives in which we experienced obsession, whether it be over a girlfriend or a boyfriend, a new car, overeating or undereating or something else. Emotional fluctuations are a normal part of a human's makeup. As the stress in our day-to-day lives increases, it is not unexpected to see emotional ups and downs increase.

Depression is usually accompanied by a certain degree of anxiety. Certain emotionally uplifting medications used to treat depression may raise anxiety levels. Conversely, medications that are intended to sedate and reduce anxiety often send the patient deeper into depression. Some medications cause people to lose touch with their emotions and feel a lack of motivation and inspiration. For these and other reasons, many people cannot tolerate pharmaceuticals used to treat depression and anxiety.

Western medicine focuses on correcting underlying biochemical abnormalities. Consequently there is a risk of overcorrection. Because of their regulating

## Descriptions of emotions that may help you define your problems

### Depression

| | | |
|---|---|---|
| Angry | Disillusioned | Not myself |
| Bitter | Fatigued | Pessimistic |
| Brokenhearted | Foggy-headed | Regretful |
| Cynical | Gloomy | Resentful |
| Defeated | Hopeless | Sad |
| Despondent | In a funk | Sorrowful |
| Disappointed | Joyless | Unhappy |
| Discouraged | Miserable | Worried |

### Anxiety

| | | |
|---|---|---|
| Agitated | Feeling dread | Restless |
| Being jittery | Fretting | Stressed |
| Being in mortal | Having the creeps | Tense |
| terror | Irritated | Troubled |
| Concerned | Nervous | Uneasy |
| Discontent | Obsessing | |
| Disgruntled | Quarrelsome | |

properties, however, herbs can reduce depression without aggravating anxiety and still keep a person emotionally centered. Depression and anxiety disorders can be well treated by Chinese medicine alone, especially for mild and moderate cases. The effect is often comparable to that of Western medicine. The basic approach is to harmonize and balance certain aspects of the major Energetic systems such as Liver, Kidney, Heart and Spleen, and sometimes certain minor Energetic systems such as Gall Bladder.

Many people do not understand how to recognize and catalogue their symptoms. Sometimes people have learned to live with a symptom, other times their symptoms may be dismissed as irrelevant or insignificant.

Our society uses words such as *anxiety* and *depression* to explain a wide gamut of emotional experiences. Depression to one may be a whole different experience than it is to another. People who are sad, who are severely disappointed, who have low energy, who worry, who obsess, who are anticipating a significant challenge like taking a test, will all describe themselves as anxious. A psychiatrist's job is to tease out of the patient as clearly as possible the true feeling being experienced.

As the majority of people with psychiatric challenges will likely go to their primary-care physician rather than to a psychiatrist, the more accurately you can describe your problems, issues and symptoms, the more able your primary-care doctor will be to treat you effectively. Before you go to your doctor, write down all of your questions, and do not let the doctor leave the room until they are answered. Write down or tape-record the doctor's answers so that after you leave you can review and absorb everything the doctor said.

## Develop meaningful relationships

A very important aspect in healing from mental illness from both a Western and Chinese medicine perspective is to establish meaningful relationships. Such relationships breathe Vital Energy (Qi) into your life and remove stagnation, helping you to heal. The support provided by these relationships can be very important in providing the strong foundation for improving your condition. To prevent severe isolation from developing, contact with at least one other person every day is crucial, whether it be family or friends.

You can find meaningful relationships by following your interests. Joining a Qigong, yoga, Tai Chi, spiritual/religious or meditation group is one way of being around other people in a positive environment.

## Focus on your spiritual outlet

From an Eastern perspective, our thoughts, desires and actions reflect the degree of whatever it is we are stuck on. Meditation is a way of reflecting on the motivations behind our actions. Usually our motivations are based on some perception of a need that we feel will relieve whatever it is we are suffering from. In meditation emotional wounds from the past that unconsciously shape and motivate our thoughts, desires and actions can be experienced directly and the unconscious grip loosened. Meditating in a group is particularly comforting and can provide the security and safety you feel lacking in your life. See chapter 16 for more on meditation and healing Energy.

Emphasize movement in your life

Movement and breathing therapies such as yoga, Tai Chi and Qigong consciously combine mind and body to induce a relaxation state that can purify the emotional residue of painful feelings.

Deep breathing exercises break up stagnation. It can be as simple as just taking deep breaths throughout the day, or as involved as participating in a Qigong class with others. The Chinese practice of Qigong combines graceful physical movements with mental concentration. This practice balances your body's Energy along the Meridians. Health is restored when your body's Qi is flowing and rebalanced. See chapter 16 for more on Qigong and healing Energy.

Take on life's challenges

Another important aspect in getting your Vital Energy moving is to take on life challenges, no matter how big or small, in such a way as to try not to be overwhelmed. This may mean taking challenges one day, one part of a day, one hour or maybe even just one minute at a time. Allow yourself to grow into challenges; rather than "eating the elephant all at once and choking on it, eat one small piece at a time," as an old Chinese saying goes.

See a health care professional to be tested for food allergies or dysbiosis

A health care professional can test you for food allergies or dysbiosis, which is an imbalance of the healthy and unhealthy bacteria and yeast in the gut that may be inhibiting the absorption of nutrients or otherwise stressing your body, which would inhibit the optimum production of neurotransmitters.

Blood tests can determine amino acid levels. Amino acids build proteins, which build brain chemicals (neurotransmitters) that are important for mental health. If you are lacking in amino acids, you can take free-form amino acid complex, which provides readily absorbable amino acids (see page 132). See page 431 for a laboratory that can refer you to a health care provider in your area who does these types of tests. If you test positive for any of these factors, your health care professional can treat you on an individual basis.

Modify your diet

Eating sugar causes blood sugar imbalances that ultimately imbalance your brain chemicals. Eating a balanced diet of real, whole foods, including protein with every meal and snack, will keep your blood sugar levels balanced and will help stabilize your brain neurotransmitters.

Eat foods that have beneficial effects on depression and anxiety or panic. See pages 151–155 for guidelines on raising serotonin levels. Pages 338–339 provide a medicinal recipe to alleviate the anxiety associated with mental and emotional illness.

## Chinese herbs and Western supplements

The Western treatment of the vast majority of mood and anxiety disorders consists of medications that increase neurotransmitters such as serotonin, dopamine and gamma-aminobutyric acid (GABA). When these medications are used appropriately, most people experience significant improvement in their symptoms of depression or anxiety. Severe cases of depression, anxiety and panic disorders require the evaluation of a psychiatrist and an appropriate prescription medication. However, mild cases of mood problems and anxiety can be treated with naturally occurring herbs, amino acids and other nutritional supplements. These do not require a doctor's prescription and can produce a similar increase in neurotransmitter levels in the brain, thereby improving your condition. 5H-GABA and GABA are amino acids that bind to the same receptors as the minor tranquilizer Valium—but they are non-addictive and can effectively alleviate panic attacks. 5H-GABA is a more usable form than GABA.

Routinely, at bedtime, on an empty stomach take 100 milligrams 5-H GABA. If you do not feel the calming effects after one night, increase to 200 milligrams. Or take 500 milligrams GABA. If you do not feel the calming effects after one night, increase to 750 milligrams.

Routinely, thirty to forty-five minutes before breakfast and dinner take 1,000 milligrams free-form amino acid complex.

To ensure your body is absorbing all the nutrients in the food you eat, routinely, before each meal take the digestive formulas on page 102.

You can take Chinese herbal formulas and Western supplements specifically formulated to treat depression and anxiety. To order formulas log on to ancient herbsmodernmedicine.com.

# PART THREE

## Modern Plagues

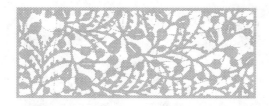

# 10

## Adrenal Burnout/ Kidney Energy Deficiency

*Combining Chinese and Western medicines to*
*rebalance your stressed-out body*

On January 6, 1996, a blizzard ripped across the eastern seaboard, bringing the New York area to a crawl. Twenty years earlier, Dimitri Stojanov had entered the country illegally from Russia with little education and few words of English. He landed a job on the production line in a defense company. In a mercurial rise to a senior management position, by age forty Dimitri had achieved his white-collar American dream, with citizenship, a prestigious job with a penthouse office, a luxurious home in a nice neighborhood, a loving wife and three children. Now, with the expressways reduced to parking lots, Dimitri's normal three-hour round trip commute from his home to the factory was taking him over seven hours. But he was used to hardship and sacrifice and was not going to let nature stand in his way. He did have one nagging worry, however. Inexplicably, although he could still function, he was plagued with a numb sensation over half of his body.

Around that time Dimitri was flying back and forth regularly to the West Coast on business. On his first trip, he heard about Dr. Han and went to see him. Dimitri explained his concern about the numbness he was experiencing. He admitted he was taking a megadose of Xanax. He said he had given up his lunch break to go to the gym to work out, but his waistline was still spreading. He either could not sleep or would drag himself home from work and be dead to the world. Dr. Han began by prescribing herbs to help Dimitri reduce the dose of Xanax he was taking. After two weeks, Dr. Han was able to reduce Dimitri's medication by 25 percent but could not lower the dosage any further without Dimitri suffering acute anxiety. The numbness had not resolved. In fact, Dimitri was not seeing any real improvement in any area of his health. The herbs Dr. Han prescribed went into him like a handful of sand into the ocean, with hardly a ripple.

On a subsequent trip to the West Coast, Dimitri began to open up to Dr. Han. "During the Cold War there were a lot of opportunities in my company for advancement," he said. "When the Cold War ended, government orders slowed down. My workforce was reduced from twelve hundred to eight hundred people, but I was still expected to keep up a certain quota." In addition, Dimitri had been called upon by the board of directors, who had learned that one of their vice presidents was involved in money laundering—an activity that directly involved his division. "I knew about the vice president's racket. The board members promised that my testimony against him would be kept a secret. So I went along. But the man I testified against had enough control in the company so that the board wasn't able to squeeze him out of the company. He found out that I had testified against him and started verbally terrorizing me. After two weeks of this, half of my body went numb."

Dimitri was an extremely driven individual who worked six days a week. He was determined not to show signs of weakness. He made no friends at work and would spend his entire workday focused on his responsibilities. He described his stomach as "being tied in knots" for as long as he could remember. He had not had a natural bowel movement in two years. He drank coffee from the moment he woke up until shortly before going to bed. He kept a two-pound can of sugar on his desk to add to his coffee, and replenished this supply every week. On his drive home, he would stop once or twice at a convenience store to refill his coffee mug so that he would not fall asleep while driving. After listening to his story, it was clear to Dr. Han that Dimitri was worn down by stress. He bluntly told Dimitri that it was a miracle that he had not dropped dead from a heart attack.

## Stress from a Western Point of View

As the world seems to spin out of control, modern medicine has been compelled to examine the effects of stress on human health. The overwhelming consensus is that stress kills. Although we are all familiar with the immediate unpleasant effects of stress, the most dangerous and insidious effects of chronic stress are cumulative.

Stress is derived from the concept in physics of an outside force having an impact on a given body. The human body has set levels that all its systems are designed to return to in an attempt to keep the body's processes in a state of status quo. This state is referred to as homeostasis. The body's adaptive responses to stress are an attempt to return from what the body perceives as an abnormal state, back to homeostasis. When you exercise, your body generates heat due to muscle contraction and the use of energy. In an effort to return to its homeostatic 98.6 degrees your body will begin to sweat; the evaporative cooling of perspiration ultimately brings your temperature down. Likewise, when you are cold, your body starts to shiver; these muscle movements release heat in an attempt to return to homeostasis. Or, when you are walking at higher altitude than you are accustomed to, your respiratory rate will increase in an attempt to maintain your body's homeostatic level of oxygen and carbon dioxide. All warm-blooded animals possess this innate drive to maintain homeostasis.

Understanding the body's drive to maintain homeostasis, it is easy to understand why *any* change is perceived as stress. To the body, it makes little if any difference whether your stressors are good or bad. Normal everyday life activity and events cause stress. Stress cannot be avoided; the only way to be truly free from stress is to be dead.

Since the systems of the body are interconnected, the impact of chronic stress is so complex that a full explanation would take an entire book. For simplicity's sake, the focus here will be on your endocrine adrenal glands. Your two adrenal glands are small triangular organs perched above each kidney. Stress hormones are secreted from your adrenal glands in response to acute and chronic physical and emotional stress. Stress hormones influence nearly every bodily function. Every excitatory situation will result in an initial adrenaline rush from the adrenal medulla to help your body deal with the stressful situation. If stress is chronic, the hormones cortisol and dihydroepiandrosterone (DHEA) are next secreted from the adrenal cortex to help your body function in the long term.

*Functions of Adrenaline*

Causes immediate, emergency response *(fight-or-flight)*
Accelerates heart rate
Increases breathing
Raises blood pressure
Increases metabolic rate
Intensifies blood flow to muscles, brain and lungs
Sharpens mental focus

*Functions of Cortisol*

> Maintains blood pressure and fluid balance
> Diminishes inflammation
> Directs many other systems of your body to operate effectively
> Regulates immune responses

*Functions of DHEA*

> Decreases recovery time from exercise
> Decreases the risk of cardiovascular disease
> Increases the production of human growth hormone
> Improves your immune response
> Increases energy and fat burning

Constant demands on your adrenal glands to secrete stress hormones results in a diminishing of their functional abilities. Police cars get driven twenty-two hours a day. If they are not regularly maintained and repaired, within six months their gas mileage starts to diminish. A private citizen's car might not begin to show a change in gas mileage for several years. Like the police car, your adrenal glands cannot be driven day and night past their ability to rejuvenate and repair. Without rest and maintenance their reserves will diminish and the overall functioning of your adrenal glands and stress hormone secretion will gradually falter. Adrenal fatigue affects all the interconnected systems of the body. These systems include your entire endocrine system, your neurological system and your immune system to name a few—thus the progression from stress to illness.

## Adrenal Burnout Is the Equivalent of Depleted Kidney Energy

All five major Energetic systems are involved in stress response, particularly Kidney, Liver and Heart Energetic systems, which are associated with the fluctuations of emotions when an individual is under physical and psychological stress. Chinese medicine intentionally does not distinguish between the physical and psychological aspects of our bodies.

Stress on the body weakens and exhausts Kidney Energy. Kidney Energy regulates your body's ability to deal with stress and provides vitality while supporting all the other systems. Kidney Energy maintains structural integrity and

## Kidney Energy Is So Essential That It Is Often Considered the Base of Life Force

You are born → *Kidney Energy is generated*
You grow into an adult → *Kidney Energy develops*
You reach full maturity → *Kidney Energy peaks*
You begin to age → *Kidney Energy declines*
You die → *Kidney Energy is extinguished*

function of the bones and joints. It is closely associated with some of the most important cognitive functions such as memory, information processing, focus and concentration. It is particularly associated with emotions such as fear and courage.

Early Kidney Energy decline is much more prevalent in Western cultures. The difference is due to Lifestyle Factors, which are a Non-Internal, Non-External Cause in Chinese medicine. What makes the Western culture unique is the hidden stress—the kind of stress that permeates day-to-day life and the basic fabric of this culture. It is always in the background, as a constant reminder of the things one is expected to accomplish, of demands and consequences.

When stress is extreme and prolonged, the constant demands on your adrenal glands to secrete stress hormones will cause them to tire. Adrenal fatigue negatively affects all the interconnected systems of the body, including your endocrine, neurological and immune systems, to name a few. When you suffer from adrenal burnout you begin to suffer from chronic illnesses.

From Dr. Han's many years of consultations with Americans he has come to understand that many people who appear to be successful are actually only a few short steps from major financial crisis. From a Chinese perspective Americans tend toward overdoing, whether it is work or enjoyment. There is a lack of moderation, discipline and balance that wears on Kidney Energy so that it declines much faster and earlier than it is supposed to. The majority of people in the West, even those who are considered healthy, have a weakened Kidney pulse.

*Factors That Deplete Kidney Energy*

* Overwork
* Overplay

- Chronic worry
- Use of stimulants
- Lack of proper nutrition
- Exposure to and ingesting toxins

*Symptoms of Kidney Energy Deficiency/Adrenal Burnout*

- Achy and weak muscles
- Any discomfort for which you have sought medical attention, but after extensive testing all results come back unable to indicate anything wrong
- Bowel habit changes—ill-formed stool, feeling of incomplete elimination, persistent constipation, loose stool or diarrhea—for no apparent reason
- Burning, watery, itchy eyes
- Difficulty focusing
- Dragging feeling
- Emotional fluctuations or mood swings for no reason
- Exhaustion upon awakening even if you have slept
- Feeling easily out of breath
- Feeling of low-grade fever, but fever is not indicated on a thermometer
- Fitful or restless sleep with nightmares, intense or "busy" dreams
- Frequent urinary tract infections, vaginal infections, abnormal vaginal discharge
- Heart palpitations
- Lack of cognitive clarity—feeling of foggy-headedness
- Lack of sense of well-being
- Lapses of short-term memory—difficulty in retrieving people's names, a familiar phone number or your social security number, for example
- Light-headedness or feeling faint
- Night sweats or spontaneous sweating for no apparent reason
- Prone to colds, flu, other types of upper respiratory infections, recurrent sinus or middle-ear infections
- Tongue becomes unusually coated or develops fissures or cracks on the surface
- Vague digestive discomfort—feeling that food is "just sitting there" or "not going away"
- Wishing you could take a nap during the day

# Recovering from Adrenal Burnout/Depleted Kidney Energy

The fundamental way of preserving and cultivating Kidney Energy is through maintaining a lifestyle of moderation and discipline. In Chinese medicine there are two distinct preventative approaches. First is the prevention of the development of disease, and second is the prevention of already existing illness from evolving or escalating into an even more serious disease. In addition to taking herbs, lifestyle changes are imperative in restoring adrenal function and rebalancing your Energetic systems.

## Ways to Strengthen Your Heart, Liver and Kidney Energies and Resolve Adrenal Burnout

### Observe moderation and discipline in diet, work, play and exercise

The American culture has become excessive in many, if not all, aspects of life. Overconsumption of food is the norm—the average meal served at a restaurant has been shown to be two to three times the recommended amount for a serving. People are overworked and overextended financially. Some are too sedentary, others are addicted to extreme sports and exercise. Then there are those who play—too much sex, alcohol, drugs and partying depletes Kidney Energy and creates an imbalance of Liver Energy. Even on vacation people cannot relax, running from one tour to the next, from one flight to another. They return home feeling more exhausted than before they left. It is only when an individual is able to achieve and maintain moderation throughout his or her life that the need for medical intervention or support can be effectively minimized.

### Get enough rest and sleep

Your autonomic nervous system is divided into the sympathetic and the parasympathetic nervous systems. You can think of your sympathetic mode as the Yang and your parasympathetic as the Yin of your nervous system. Like Yin and Yang, there is a dynamic relationship between the sympathetic and parasympathetic mode. Your sympathetic and parasympathetic nervous systems are constantly adjusting—just like Yin and Yang—in an attempt to keep your body in balance. Your autonomic nervous system is constantly adjusting and accommodating the processes within your body and all of your external input such as food, drink, environment and stimuli. Just like Yin and Yang, there is never perfect balance, as the sympathetic mode and the parasympathetic mode each have a purpose and are beneficial to your body when appropriately set into action.

During the day you are predominantly in the sympathetic state as you go about your life, eating, working, living. Internally your body is reacting to and facilitating metabolic processes and stimulating your adrenal glands to increase output of stress hormones whenever you are stressed. The sympathetic mode creates acids as by-products of metabolic processes, which tend to make your system more acidic.

At night, your parasympathetic mode counteracts the physiological effects of the sympathetic nervous system by stimulating digestive secretions, slowing your heart, constricting your pupils and dilating blood vessels. It also brings your body from an acidic state back to a more neutral pH. Your body's homeostatic mechanisms strive to maintain an extremely narrow range of pH—very close to neutral—which requires a skillful balancing act. Your body needs an ebb (Yin) and flow (Yang) rhythm like night and day. Nighttime is the appropriate time for your body to flow into a parasympathetic mode to balance the day's accumulated acidity. This is known as the alkaline tide. The alkaline tide is important because the biochemical processes within your body depend on a specific pH balance. When your body remains too acidic for too long, numerous metabolic processes are shut down. The cellular flow is slowed, interrupted or stalled and your cells collect toxins. If this imbalance is not resolved, it can ultimately damage your system on a cellular level, accelerating the disease and aging processes. Malnutrition, stress, sleep deprivation, drugs, stimulants (including sugar) and exposure to toxic substances are all factors that keep your body in a sympathetic state.

At night our autonomic nervous system is supposed to move from a sympathetic state of breaking down (acidic) to a parasympathetic state of building up (alkalinizing). But most of us stay up far past sunset and intentionally cut back on sleep to catch up on work or other activities. By doing so, we create a heightened state of sympathetic dominance (adrenal excess) that prevents or delays the shift into the parasympathetic mode necessary to sleep, digest food, absorb nutrients and repair.

One of the most common factors that lead to depleted Kidney Energy is sleep deprivation. If you are not sleeping deeply for six to eight hours a night because you have difficulty falling asleep or maintaining sleep, or if you awaken too early in the morning, or if your sleep is fitful, you are suffering from insomnia.

Insomnia is the inability to fall asleep or to remain asleep restfully through the night, or the tendency to awaken too early. From a Western point of view, insomnia in itself is not a disease, but rather a symptom of another problem, such as stress, anxiety, too much caffeine, chronic pain, depression, gastroesophageal reflux, medication side effects, muscle spasms or hormonal fluctuations, to name some factors.

*The Stages of Sleep:* Sleep is divided into two major categories based on brain activity and EEG (electroencephalogram) wave patterns: nonrapid eye movement (NREM) sleep and rapid eye movement (REM) sleep. NREM sleep is divided into four stages. Stage one of NREM sleep is a short transitional period between being awake and being asleep. It is considered to be one of the least restorative stages of sleep. In stage two NREM sleep, the individual has less voluntary muscle tone than in stage one. The greatest proportion of time asleep is spent in stage two. Stages three and four—characterized by slow-wave EEG patterns called delta waves—are deeper and more restorative stages of sleep than stages one and two. Periods of slow-wave or delta sleep are associated with vital restorative brain processes, such as neurotransmitter replenishment, cellular repair, cerebral metabolism, neuroendocrine release and resynchronization of circadian rhythms.

REM sleep is defined by characteristic rapid eye movements. The brain wave pattern of REM sleep includes low-wattage, relatively fast-frequency EEG waves. REM sleep is associated with dreaming, rapid oculomotor (eye) movements and loss of muscle tone of voluntary muscle groups. Most REM sleep occurs during the last third of the night, shortly before awakening. During REM sleep, the brain is very active metabolically, with high blood flow and blood sugar utilization. The brain wave activity pattern during REM sleep actually looks similar on an EEG to that of being awake.

Western medical treatment for insomnia includes medications to aid in sleep. None of these medications provides a long-term answer, and they can lead to tolerance and/or addiction. However, in the cases of transient, short-term problems with insomnia in an individual who otherwise does not suffer from sleep difficulties, these medications can be rather safe and effective in temporarily resolving sleep problems until the issue that is causing insomnia is resolved or becomes less unsettling. In recent years more people have begun to find relief from insomnia by using over-the-counter herbs, amino acids and hormones.

Serotonin is the primary neurotransmitter involved in the wake/sleep cycle. Tryptophan is the building block of serotonin. Having a snack high in tryptophan, such as warm milk, cottage cheese with banana, peanut or almond butter, plain yogurt with nuts, or sliced turkey before bed can help you sleep. See pages 154–155 for sleep formulas.

*Chinese Medicine's Approach to Insomnia*: From a Chinese medicine perspective, there are many ways to treat insomnia. Usually, it attempts to harmonize and balance Heart, Liver, Kidney and Spleen Energies—depending upon what the specific diagnosis calls for. Acupuncture is commonly and effectively used to treat insomnia. The same acupuncture points that can be needled to interact with the central nervous system to reduce pain also participate in the regulation of sleep-wake cycles. Acupuncture can induce alpha waves, thereby promoting REM sleep. With electroacupuncture, electric stimulation patterns can be synchronized with the alpha waves. Acupuncture is also an excellent way to assist the patient in relaxing, which will of course also help improve the ability to fall asleep. Compared to the use of medications to help induce sleep, which act primarily upon the central nervous system, acupuncture is able to help induce sleep by affecting both the central and peripheral nervous systems. Oftentimes, once the muscles are well relaxed, via the effects of the peripheral nervous system, the central nervous system follows suit.

Consult with a health care professional to resolve your health issues

A health care professional can assess your adrenal hormones and prescribe replacement hormones if indicated—see chapters 17 and 19 for more on hormone replacement.

Have your amino acid levels tested. If your body is not breaking down the proteins you eat into amino acids, this can exacerbate fatigue and symptoms of depression. Amino acid supplementation can boost your energy as well as supply your body with the necessary precursors to neurotransmitters.

Stool, hair and blood tests can determine if you have (1) high levels of accumulated heavy metals in your system, (2) sensitivities to foods or (3) dysbiosis, which is an imbalance of the healthy and unhealthy bacteria and yeast in the gut, any of which may be weakening your immune system and draining your energy.

See page 431 for a laboratory that can refer you to a health care provider in your area who does these types of tests. If you test positive for any of these factors, your health care professional can treat you on an individual basis.

## See a health care professional to help resolve back pain

Back pain often accompanies adrenal burnout/Kidney Energy deficiency. Back pain affects an estimated 80 percent of all people at some time of their lives and is the leading cause of disability for people under the age of forty-five. Chronic back pain is defined as pain lasting more than six months or recurring every three months for at least three years. Because an exact diagnosis is often impossible to establish, as many as 85 percent of patients with back pain will never receive a definitive diagnosis. Western medicine has a limited number of interventions for back pain. For example, after the acute phase of back pain—which is usually two to four weeks—people are encouraged to begin an exercise program with strength and endurance exercises. For overweight individuals with chronic back pain, weight loss is recommended. Complete cure of chronic back pain is usually considered an unrealistic expectation.

Western medicine approaches the treatment of back pain from the outside inward. Back pain is considered a localized musculoskeletal and/or mechanical disorder. Chinese medicine approaches treatment from the inside outward, as it recognizes the interplay of internal Energetic systems. For example, in many situations, weakened Kidney Energy leads to vulnerability of one's back. People with deficient Kidney Energy have a tendency to develop premature degenerative back problems. One of the important functions of Kidney Energy is to support the function and structural integrity of the bones. Through strengthening Kidney Energy the back can also be strengthened. For example, the treatment of osteoporosis and rheumatoid arthritis is often approached by fortifying Kidney Energy.

In treating the most common types of back pain, herbs and acupuncture are often utilized in combination to treat the Energy deficiencies. Acupuncture is utilized to alleviate the pain during the acute flare-up and herbs are then used more often to address the root causes. Back muscles can be strengthened and stabilized by supporting the underlying Energetic systems. The three Energy systems intimately involved in back pain are Kidney Energy, associated with bones; Spleen Energy, associated with muscles; and Liver Energy, associated with tendons and ligaments. By addressing all three of these Energy systems and bringing them into balance, Chinese medicine can effectively treat and help strengthen your entire system.

Moxabustion, explained on page 58, a combined herbal and heat therapy treatment directed at specific acupuncture points, is often used to treat chronic back pain. Also, acupressure can be effective in treating back pain, particularly for those patients with anxiety about needles used in acupuncture. Acupressure has been found to be particularly effective in treating people with muscle spasms.

## Gua Sha (cupping)

Cupping is perhaps one of the oldest forms of treatment in Chinese medicine, even predating acupuncture. Cupping can be used to stimulate the circulation of Qi and to "draw out" stagnation causing muscle spasms, tension, pain and lack of range of motion. Cupping uses bell-shaped cups in varying sizes, from the size of an espresso cup to the size of a wineglass. Cups are made of glass, rubber, bamboo, plastic or ceramic. The most commonly used are glass cups. Traditionally, fire is used to create a vacuum inside the cup. One method is to light an alcohol/herb-saturated cotton ball and place it into the cup. The burning herbs create a vacuum within the cup that sucks the cup tightly onto your skin. At the same time, the herb particles will be dispersed by the heat created. These particles move rapidly and are absorbed by the increased circulation in the skin beneath the cup. The heat (fire) cupping method requires skill and should be attempted only by a well-trained and experienced practitioner.

The modern vacuum cups have a pump to create the vacuum, which is more controllable. An electric pump is used to evacuate air within the cup. Sometimes the practitioner applies a thin layer of oil, herbal cream or aloe vera to your skin prior to treatment, which allows the cups to be moved during treatment to cover a wider area. During the treatment the skin beneath the cup will turn light red to purple and even almost black. Every five to ten minutes the cups are lifted or slid from one area to another. After the cups are removed the deepened skin color will gradually diminish over twenty-four hours to a few days. After a cupping treatment you are "open" to outside exposure. For that reason it is advised that you:

- Do not drink alcohol for twenty-four hours.
- Do not drink cold or iced liquids for twenty-four hours.
- Keep the treated areas lightly covered and warm for twenty-four hours.

Herbal Transdermal Ionization (HTI)

The newest treatment for back pain includes the use of an ultramicrowave or infared heat lamp along with topical herbs. The technique is designed to promote circulation and relax muscles as well as help the topical herbs to penetrate deeply into the affected muscles. Another method is known as herbal transdermal ionization treatment (HTI). HTI is an effective way of concentrating and delivering the herbs deep into the affected sites by converting the herbs into electrically charged particles in an electric field, then, through polarity, forcing the herbal particles with the same electric charge as the electrode to penetrate deeply into the body. As a basic law of physics, electrically charged particles are drawn toward each other if they have opposite polarity (charges), and like charges will repel each other. During a treatment the herbal soaked pad is placed between the patient's body and an electrode. By applying electricity to the electrode it will push (repel or drive) the herbal particles with the same charge as the electrode into the patient's body.

## See a health care professional to help resolve constipation

By brutally driving himself, Dimitri had suppressed peristalsis—the natural rhythm of the digestive tract that pushes food along the various stages of digestion—which meant that he could not have a bowel movement without the use of laxatives or even enemas. Dr. Han prescribed a potent herb to increase peristalsis. While 10 percent of the dose of this herb would have sent most people running to the bathroom all night long, the herb had no effect on Dimitri whatsoever.

In Chinese medicine constipation is not ideally treated with laxatives, since one's body can easily become dependent upon them. Optimal treatment for constipation focuses on restoring normal peristalsis. Unlike Western medicine, Chinese medicine distinguishes between various types of constipation based on the underlying causes. The type of constipation will direct the choice of appropriate herbs and herbal formula.

Constipation can be due to deficiency or excess (stagnation), each requiring different measures of treatment according to the diagnostic principles of Chinese medicine. Within a deficiency there are distinctions of Qi, Blood, Yin, Yang, Jing or Fluid deficiency or a combination of these. Excess (stagnation) can be due to Heat, Cold, Blood, Dampness, Dryness, Food or a combination of these. The deficiency and stagnation can appear simultaneously in some situations. The herbs need to be selected and put together carefully and each patient's uniqueness needs to be addressed and well targeted.

## Modify your diet

Burned-out individuals are often lacking in electrolytes. Electrolytes are elements required by your cells to regulate the electrical charge across cell membranes. Having a protein drink with super green food every day will provide your body with the electrolytes necessary to replace those lost through stress. See page 104 for more on super green food. Chapter 21 provides medicinal recipes to strengthen Kidney Energy and restore adrenal function.

## Engage in practices that integrate mind, body, breathing and meditation

Meditative practices buffer the damaging effects of stress. See chapter 16 for more on meditation.

## Quit caffeine

Dimitri's numbness—the problem that initially caused him to seek treatment—was due to blockage of Energy circulation partly from deficient Kidney Energy. It was also partly due to deeply rooted stagnation, the result of Liver Energy imbalance and long-term overuse of stimulants, sugar and refined white flour products such as cake, cookies, pasta, bagels and pretzels.

From a Chinese medicine point of view, everything we take into our bodies—air, food, liquid and experiences—generates Qi. Thus, to obtain balance, we must make healthy choices regarding the quality of air we breathe, the circumstances we involve ourselves in and especially what we eat and ingest.

As Dimitri's energy level had decreased over the years, he had begun drinking large amounts of coffee to stay alert, and when he started taking Xanax he had to pound even more coffee to counteract the medication's sedating effect. He began his day with coffee and continued drinking pot after pot all day with so much sugar that when he finished a cup of coffee there was an inch of syrup at the bottom. He had even taken to stopping at 7-Eleven on the way home from work to tank up on more coffee. Although we all experience a lift from coffee, according to Chinese medicine caffeine does not generate Energy, it merely borrows it. Caffeine drains your Kidney Energy, just like taking out a withdrawal from your bank account. If you do not put a deposit in your system, it will become depleted little by little.

True energy is not a nervous energy but a sense of feeling confident, substantial and calm. The American culture associates calmness with tiredness and equates energy with being highly stimulated. "When I discuss quitting coffee and other stimulants with my patients, many are afraid that their energy is going to crash," said Maoshing Ni, Lic. Ac., D.O.M., Ph.D., cofounder of the Tao of Wellness clinic and Yo San University of Traditional Chinese Medicine in Los Angeles, California. "In the Chinese culture, calm has a wonderful connotation. It means that your head is clear; you are sharp and in control and you can manage your energy properly. In the Eastern culture we sip green tea. The tea is a calming, soothing, contemplative beverage. You sit and think and clear your head. Americans are a coffee-gulping culture. You gulp coffee because you are always on the go, go, go. Caffeine stimulates the brain that there is danger, which results in the release of adrenaline from the adrenal glands. Drinking coffee turns on your survival mode. While the rush is pleasurable, your adrenal glands are also telling your immune system to gear up because you are going to fight or run to survive, and you may be injured and need help along the way. Consuming caffeine results in a sharp blood sugar drop, which is why you feel cravings soon after your high wears off. It is also highly addictive and depletes your adrenal glands and immune system. There are herbs that can build up your system—not in a stimulant way, but rather with solid strong Energy. When one feels that type of Energy, it is very different from the false energy that comes from drinking coffee or using stimulants."

Pages 151–155 provide suggestions for ways to boost serotonin levels to help you quit caffeine. Wean from caffeine slowly. Schedule your allotted amounts of caffeine on your calendar. Week one, decrease by one-half cup per day. Week two, decrease by one cup per day. Continue until you are down to one-half cup per day. If you want to quit drinking coffee and other caffeinated beverages but enjoy the ritual of your morning or afternoon drink, you have several options:

◆ *Green tea* is known for its anticarcinogenic effects. While it is not advisable for people who do not consume caffeine to begin drinking green tea, which contains caffeine, if you are a caffeine drinker, green tea is an excellent alternative. See pages 187–188 for more on green tea.

◆ *Yerba maté* is a South American herbal drink known as the "drink of the gods." It has been revered by the South American Guarani Indians for centuries for promoting health, vitality and longevity. The gauchos (cowboys) of the high plains traditionally drank yerba maté throughout the day while doing their strenuous work. Analysis shows there are 100 milligrams of caffeine in a seven-ounce cup of yerba maté, in contrast to 115 to 175 milligrams of caffeine in a seven-ounce cup of coffee. A report published by the *Review of Natural Products* states that yerba maté contains vitamins A, C and most of the B vitamins as well as several minerals including potassium, calcium, magnesium, iron and iodine, in addition to fifteen amino acids.

◆ *Teeccino* (pronounced *tea-chee-no*) is a caffeine-free herbal "coffee" made from roasted carob, barley, chicory root, figs, almonds, dates, extract of Mexican vanilla and natural flavors. Teeccino contains potassium, an electrolyte. It comes in original, vanilla nut, chocolate mint, almond amaretto, hazelnut, mocha and java flavors. A simple formula for quitting coffee: Begin blending 1 part Teeccino with 3 parts coffee grounds. Gradually increase the Teeccino and decrease the coffee grounds. This process is best undertaken very slowly to allow your body to adjust to lesser amounts of caffeine. You can find product information online at ancientherbsmodern medicine.com.

◆ *Decaffeinated coffee* is not caffeine free. Most decaffeinated coffees are processed using chemicals and contain methylene chloride, which is carcinogenic. Swiss water processing removes some—but not all—caffeine from coffee using water rather than chemicals.

## Quit Nicotine

Nicotine is an External Cause. Nicotine tobacco products are proven to cause vascular disease and cancer. Although stimulants give you a lift, according to Chinese medicine stimulants such as tobacco products do not generate new Energy; they merely borrow and consume Energy. Stimulants tap into your Kidney Energy reserve. As a result, in the long run, you end up with an empty tank.

Patches, chewing gum and other products containing nicotine are promoted to help people kick the nicotine habit but can be addicting themselves. While not as deadly as tobacco products, these substances are nevertheless toxic to the human body. You may choose to take the prescription drug Zyban (bupropion) as part of your quitting-smoking program. Zyban is a nicotine-free pill that has helped many quit smoking—even those who have smoked ten years or more. Zyban is believed to mimic nicotine's effects on the brain by boosting levels of the chemical messengers dopamine and norepinephrine. Zyban must be prescribed by a doctor.

When considering whether to use Zyban, consider the following:

- The most common side effects are dry mouth and insomnia.
- There is a dose-dependent risk of seizure. Do not use Zyban if you have had a seizure disorder.
- If you have severe liver disease, your doctor may advise you to use a less frequent dose.
- Do not use Zyban if you are taking Wellbutrin.
- Do not use Zyban if you have ever had bulimia or anorexia nervosa.
- Do not use Zyban if you are taking or recently have taken a monomine oxidase inhibitor.

## Quit herbal stimulants such as Ma Huang

The herb Ma Huang contains ephedra, a substance that has adrenaline-like properties. Ma Huang is an ingredient in many over-the-counter diet, sports and performance-enhancing supplements. Ephedra extracted from Ma Huang (which is often used to treat asthma) has a strong stimulating property—so strong that it is banned in international athletic competition. Ephedra is one of the first herbs taught in Chinese medical school. Dr. Han's teacher Song Tian Bing taught his class, "Ma Huang has Energy like a wild untamed horse, so you never want to relinquish control. Don't ever forget when you use Ma Huang that you saddle it so that you have the reins."

In Chinese medicine Ma Huang is considered to have a strong tendency to exhaust Kidney Energy and is never to be used for people who already have preexisting weakness. It is only to be used for a very brief period of time, usually only for *a few days,* and the patient's Kidney Energy must be protected at the same time. *Do not take herbal stimulants unless monitored by an experienced Chinese practitioner.*

## Focus on boosting your neurotransmitters naturally before turning to antidepressants

Given the incredibly hectic lifestyles and pressures of today's Western culture, the levels of stress and accompanying anxiety experienced by most individuals are much greater than in generations past. Our culture is suffering en masse from diminished brain neurotransmitters that are necessary for feelings of well-being.

To respond to this need, Western medicine has developed a vast array of antidepressents such as the tricyclics Elavil, Sinequan and Pamelor. More recently an entire new line of antidepressants, the selective serotonin reuptake inhibitors (SSRIs), have arrived on the scene—Prozac, Zoloft, Paxil, Luvox and Celexa. Antidepressants can make the difference between misery and a sense of well-being, thus providing a bridge that allows individuals to address the problems that led to depression.

Although SSRIs have very few and rare significant side effects and are often very effective in helping treat depression, they do not treat the underlying problems of stress or anxiety. To address anxiety, there are the so-called minor tranquilizers such as the benzodiazepines Valium, Xanax, Ativan, Tranxene and Klonopin. Benzodiazepines are the leading prescribed minor tranquilizers for the treatment of stress and anxiety. Dimitri's Western doctor had prescribed Xanax, but it had not completely eased Dimitri's anxiety. For someone like Dimitri, with his chronic anxiety, for Xanax to be effective he would have to be taking the pills like M&Ms. Although for the most part effective, benzodiazepines are highly addictive, both psychologically and physiologically. They are not meant to be taken daily or over the long term. If taken regularly, dependency increases and efficacy decreases. The negative impact of addiction to tranquilizers on a person's work and family often leads to even greater levels of stress and anxiety.

Since Western medicine has been unable to develop another class of medications that are as effective in treating stress and anxiety as the benzodiazepines but do not have the addictive quality, some enlightened Western doctors have begun incorporating nonmedical techniques into their treatment plans to combat anxiety. Biofeedback has been found to be effective in some cases. Biofeedback is the monitoring of physiological functions such as blood pressure and muscle tension. The person is allowed to visually or audibly sense the fluctuations in signals. This enables the person to fully appreciate what is happening in his or her body and attempt to control—through strict mental focus—the fluctuations of physiological functions such as breathing, pulse and blood pressure. Biofeedback sessions often help people alter their reactions to stressful events and situations. The downside of biofeedback is that routine training sessions with a specialist in the field are often required.

People suffering from significant levels of stress and anxiety can benefit from Chinese herbs. There are many well-tested and proven Chinese herbal formulations effective in treating anxiety without side effects, including no physical or psychological dependency. In many ways these herbal formulations may be safer and more effective.

The following guidelines can boost your neurotransmitters and strengthen your Kidney Energy, which will subdue cravings and the physical need for stimulants.

- Eat a balanced diet, including protein at every meal. Eating more frequent meals will help to stabilize your blood sugar and keep your neurotransmitters at a healthy level, which will help reduce cravings for stimulants.
- Have regular acupuncture treatments before and after quitting stimulants to help reduce cravings. Auricular (ear) acupuncture is often used to ease withdrawal symptoms. Ask your acupuncturist for "seeds." Some acupuncturists use the actual seed of the Wang Bu Liu Xing plant (Vaccaria), while others prefer to use stainless-steel beads. Seeds are attached to surgical tape and adhered to certain specific acupuncture points on the ear. When you feel anxious, stressed or experience cravings from withdrawal from cigarettes, sugar, caffeine or other stimulants, stimulating the seeds with the tips of your fingers can provide relief. The seeds can stay in place for as long as a week before being replaced.
- Eliminate white sugar and white flour products from your diet.
- Stop eating processed and junk foods, which contain unhealthy chemicals.
- Learn deep breathing techniques. See ancientherbsmodernmedicine.com for books and tapes that can help you develop breathing practices.
- Pray or meditate.
- Instead of drinking coffee, switch to organic green tea, which has half the caffeine of coffee—or quit altogether.
- Drink Sleep Tea, developed by Lincoln Hospital in New York City to ease withdrawal symptoms. It contains chamomile, peppermint, catnip, skullcap, hops and yarrow. Sleep Tea is available at your health food store.
- Practice positive thinking and visualization. See ancientherbsmodernmedicine.com for recommendations for books and tapes to help you learn these positive techniques.
- Exercise moderately and regularly to recharge, clear your mind, have fun and boost dopamine levels in your brain.
- Get a good dose of sunshine every day.

## Vitamin B$_6$, the amino acid tryptophan and the minerals calcium and magnesium are necessary for serotonin production

| Vitamin B$_6$ | Tryptophan | Calcium | Magnesium |
|---|---|---|---|
| Brown rice | Almonds | Asparagus | Almonds |
| Chicken | Cottage cheese | Brewer's yeast | Apples |
| Corn | Peanuts (peanut butter) | Broccoli | Avocados |
| Eggs | | Cabbage | Brewer's yeast |
| Green leafy vegetables | Shellfish | Dairy foods | Brown rice |
| | Soy foods (tofu, tempeh, miso) | Dandelion greens | Cod |
| Legumes | | Dulse | Flounder |
| Meat | Tuna | Filberts | Green leafy vegetables |
| Nuts | Turkey | Green leafy vegetables | |
| Peas | | | Halibut |
| Poultry | | Kale | Salmon |
| Salmon | | Kelp | Sesame seeds |
| Shrimp | | Mustard greens | Shrimp |
| Soybeans | | Oats | |
| Spinach | | Parsley | |
| Sunflower seeds | | Salmon (with bones) | |
| | | Sardines | |
| | | Seafood | |
| | | Sesame seeds | |
| | | Tofu | |
| | | Tuna | |
| | | Turnip greens | |

◆ If you are quitting smoking, focus on healing from nicotine. Take an extra amount of antioxidants to help your lungs heal from smoking. Three times a day, with meals, take 20 milligrams coQ$_{10}$ and 100 milligrams alpha-lipoic acid.

◆ To boost neurotransmitters to help quit addictions (and also to help with insomnia), twice a day, on an empty stomach thirty minutes before breakfast and lunch, take 100 milligrams 5-HTP. Before bedtime take 100 milligrams of 5-HTP, with a small amount of carbohydrates, such as a few raisins. If you do not see any improvement within two weeks, increase the dose, but do not exceed 1,000 milligrams. Take with 25 milligrams vitamin $B_6$ and 100 milligrams magnesium.

## Chinese herbs and Western supplements

If you are extremely fatigued and suspect you are suffering from adrenal burnout, a simple blood or saliva test can check your cortisol and DHEA levels. If your cortisol is too high, you can take 100 milligrams of phosphatidylserine (available in health food stores) three times a day, with breakfast, lunch and dinner, to help lower cortisol levels.

If you have been under chronic stress and are over forty, your adrenal glands may have decreased DHEA production. DHEA is a hormone that balances cortisol. It improves immunity, stimulates fat burning and improves energy. DHEA is reported to promote longevity, reduce chronic fatigue and suppress autoimmune diseases. DHEA must be taken in physiologic doses, which is an amount that would be normal for your body to produce on its own. Pharmacological doses—above what a human body would normally make on its own—could have serious side effects. *DHEA must be taken under the supervision of a doctor.*

Holy Basil is an Ayurvedic herb considered sacred by many Indians. Pharmacological studies have demonstrated that Holy Basil is a powerful antistress herb with blood sugar–balancing properties. If you have been under prolonged stress, take 800 milligrams of Holy Basil twice a day, with breakfast and dinner.

If you suffer from digestive discomfort such as bloating, gas, constipation or diarrhea, before each meal take the digestive formulas on page 102.

You can take Chinese herbal formulas or Western supplements specifically formulated to treat symptoms of adrenal burnout such as addictions, insomnia, chronic back pain, constipation, anxiety and depression. You can buy herbal formulas online at ancientherbsmodernmedicine.com.

# 11

## Environmentally Related Illnesses

*Allergies/asthma, autoimmune conditions and*
*chronic fatigue are the diseases of our age*

July 11, 1990. The sky had darkened with ash as a firestorm swept the seaside community of Santa Barbara. The air was dry and hot, making it difficult to breathe. Despite the temperature outside, forty-one-year-old Heather Daniels had her heater turned up to the highest setting. She shivered in a cocoon of blankets, her hands and feet icy cold. Heather's environmentally related illnesses had frustrated her doctors and had made her a virtual prisoner in her home for three long years. For eight years she had not worked in her profession as a piano teacher. Electrician's tape sealed the cracks around her windows. Her house had been stripped clean of carpeting and otherwise dismantled to remove any detectable synthetic materials. Even with these precautions, Heather was acutely sensitive and fragile. She had recently undergone oral laser surgery, which had left a nasty burn in the back of her throat. The trauma had triggered a bad spell, and Heather lay, head wrapped in a towel, exhausted from two days and two nights of nonstop hiccuping.

Heather is an attractive, dark-haired woman with an exuberance that defies the years she endured illness, isolation and financial ruin. In 2001, at fifty-two, her face was remarkably free of lines. She laughed readily and seemed eager to put her ordeal behind her. "In 1987, when I was thirty-eight, my housemate put in new carpet and repainted the house while I was away on vacation. I went into a toxic shock within a few minutes of coming back to the house. I never recovered from that episode, but experienced an acute shift in my health and became highly allergic. After that I lost everything. I almost lost my life."

## Our Changing Environment

Thousands of years ago, the External Causes Chinese medical doctors dealt with were bacteria, viruses and parasites. In today's world we have eradicated many plagues with immunizations. We can prevent bacteria from multiplying through the use of antibiotics, sanitation, refrigeration and food preservatives. Ancient Chinese medical doctors could not have foreseen the terrible consequences the introduction of modern External Toxins such as industrial chemicals, solvents, heavy metals, hormones, pesticides and herbicides would have on the environment and food chain. At the same time, Chinese medicine is designed to take any disharmonious factors into consideration, including alterations in the environment.

Heather Daniels's illnesses had a direct relationship with our now toxic environment. What made this situation worse is that Heather was born with a sensitive constitution. Repeated exposure to environmental toxins further sensitized her system until it was on overload. Her immune system became overreactive as a result. Heather developed what is known as environmental sensitivities, also known as multiple chemical sensitivities. This type of sensitivity is often triggered by a catastrophic exposure such as Heather's chemical poisoning. The person becomes acutely sensitive and reactive to many things in the environment, and this sensitivity can be further exacerbated by added trauma such as, in Heather's case, the laser burn. There are people like Heather who are born with allergic constitutions who react strongly to typical allergens such as pollen and dust, as well as to everything else from perfume to gasoline. Because our environment is now permeated with substances that have never before been part of the environment and food chain, these more sensitive individuals are developing environmental sensitivities.

## Chinese Medicine Views the Human Body as an Integral Part of Its Surroundings

Chinese medicine understands that your body constantly interacts with and reacts to the environment. This interaction and reaction create a cascade of physical, physiological and psychological changes. At the same time, the changes that occur are also determined by your unique constitution. For example, some people can tolerate the heat of the desert; others will become distressed in that environment. Some people remain balanced in humid conditions, while others become imbalanced. Some people can tolerate certain toxins, while others are gravely affected by them.

Chinese medicine considers much more than seasons and geographical locations. Ancient Chinese practitioners recognized that humans have varying constitutions and react differently to varying factors. For this reason, Chinese medicine evolved to take all of the factors of one's environment into consideration. As a part of the whole, many other things in addition to seasons and geographical locations are taken into account when a practitioner evaluates and diagnoses a patient. Every recognizable factor that impacts the human body is considered. Some of the relevant factors are your age, your gender, what type of work you do, where you live, your diet, your stress level and *all* the aspects of your environment—including your reactions to your geographical location and the seasons.

Office workers tend to show different symptoms than construction workers who are outdoors much of the time. People of varying work environments also respond to treatments differently. Women, men, children and adults are treated differently. Some Chinese doctors even pay attention to the time of the day that your treatment is administered because of your body's biochemical and biological rhythms.

## Allergies

When Dr. Han made a house call and found Heather disabled by hiccups he treated her with acupuncture and stopped the hiccuping. He asked Heather many questions about herself, her lifestyle, history and environment. Because Heather reacted negatively to many foods, Dr. Han knew that she would also be sensitive to herbs. He worked out a formula that would support and desensitize her immune system without triggering an allergic reaction.

Allergies are acquired abnormal immune responses to antigens such as pollen, food, drugs and, increasingly, environmental toxins. For the majority of people, allergy symptoms are seasonal. A stretch of sunny days followed by wind will usually stir up airborne allergens. The most common symptoms of airborne allergies are nasal congestion, runny nose, sneezing spells, irritation or itchy eyes and stuffy ears. Severe allergies can result in recurring sinus infections and affect an individual's concentration and cognitive clarity. The drainage associated with an overtaxed immune system can cause chronic irritation, hoarseness and sore throat. Sinus discharge can drain into the stomach and cause upset stomach, or can drain into the bronchi and create a cough. Airborne allergens or food allergies can also trigger asthma attacks.

Food allergies commonly cause a wide range of problems. Some people, like Heather, experience an allergic reaction to certain foods and the toxins in food and suffer headaches, chronic fatigue and attention problems. There are four types of allergic reactions, which run the gamut from life threatening to relatively mild. Type I involves immediate, violent reactions, such as to a penicillin shot, bee sting or shellfish. With Type I allergies, chances are that you will have to avoid that substance for the rest of your life. Eighty percent of all allergies are Type IV, which involves a milder reaction and is often delayed anywhere from two hours or two days. Type II and III are somewhere in between.

## Systematic desensitization from food allergies

The logical approach to dealing with food allergies is to avoid the allergen. However, in some cases people begin to avoid some foods, then others and then others and their body becomes increasingly sensitive. Eventually the person is left with an extremely confined selection of foods from which to choose. If you suffer from Type IV food allergies, systematic desensitization is a way to actively address your allergies instead of passively avoiding them. Begin by asking your Western doctor for a blood test to determine what foods you are allergic to and the level of your intolerance.

*If your allergic reactions to foods are mild to moderate:* The antibodies to the foods that you are allergic to will usually subside if you completely avoid those foods for three to six months. At the end of this period of abstinence, introduce a small amount of one food. Three months later, introduce a larger amount of that food, gradually increasing the amount of food you can eat until you feel that you have reached your allergic threshold. It is important to rotate the food in this process and eat it no more than once every three days. Repeat this process with all the foods on your allergy list.

*If your allergic reactions to foods are severe:* Consult a physician to ascertain whether or not the desensitization process would be appropriate for you.

Whether your allergic reaction to foods is mild or moderate, in time, and with patience, you should be able to tolerate and even enjoy most of the foods on your list without suffering an allergic reaction. It is important to note that this method is effective only with real food and not processed foods or junk food. Everyone, including those without food sensitivities, would benefit from avoiding these products.

If you are extremely sensitive or debilitated, like Heather, this method may not be the best choice for you. Heather was afraid to try the systematic desensitization method. Instead, she started with a simple herbal formula that she could tolerate, and gradually built up to a stronger formula. As her system desensitized, her immune system became stable and she was able to eat more foods. Heather's recovery using Chinese herbs was long. "Dr. Han had to be very careful with my herbs," Heather said. "In the beginning I was reacting to just about everything in my environment. But I never had a bad reaction to the herbs. I took them regularly for over two years. Still, I can't say much about that time because I was very ill. I wasn't able to talk or think clearly."

On a regular herbal treatment program, Heather's immune system slowly began to recover and to protect her from sensitivities to foods and to the environment. One year later, she felt strong enough to teach piano one day a week, progressing to two days a week. Her herbal formula was redesigned weekly for the next several years. Heather is now back to teaching piano full time.

If you are suffering from food allergies, discuss both approaches with your Western and Chinese doctors to determine which approach is right for you.

## Chronic Fatigue

Jan Koorwinder was the type of woman who never sat still. An immigrant from the Netherlands, she embraced the hectic pace of the United States. She raised three children and made a warm and welcoming home for her family. At the same time, she took care of herself. She jogged and led an otherwise active lifestyle. She was fifty-seven years old when she began to notice an unusual shift in her energy level. The fatigue continued for several months until it became debilitating. "I have always been a very, very energetic person," Jan said. "Before I got sick I could do anything! Suddenly I began to experience a laundry list of problems. The most debilitating was that I felt intensely tired. In the morning, even after a good night's rest, just to lift a finger felt like too much trouble. It got to the point that, mentally, I was not there anymore. There were times I was reading and when I finished I simply didn't have the faintest idea what I had read. My husband and children would talk to me and I'd look at them, and I do understand English, but what they were saying did not penetrate at all. I was like a zombie and began to fear that I had Alzheimer's disease."

Jan also began to suffer from infections and a chronic earache. Other elusive symptoms plagued her. "My bones felt painful," she said. "I would go to the doctor again, and find that there was nothing wrong. My impression was that they thought I was a complaining woman who didn't have anything else to do with my time. I eventually found a doctor who ran a number of tests but found nothing."

Through two years of doctor shopping Jan understood that there are conditions that Western medicine does not readily recognize. Depression often accompanies chronic fatigue. However, Jan's story is also an example of how the mind influences the body. During her illness, even when she held no hope of a medical cure, she held on to the belief that she would someday feel better again. "I strongly believe that maintaining a positive attitude is half of the battle," she said. "If you think that you are deathly sick, you become sicker and sicker and more and more miserable. But if you are optimistic, then you have won half of the battle."

Jan's problem, chronic fatigue syndrome, is a condition that has foiled Western medicine and wreaked havoc in millions of people's lives, yet many go untreated. Many people in Jan's situation are truly sick but are often dismissed as neurotics and referred to a psychiatrist. After a two-year-long search for an answer within the Western medical community, Jan began looking for alternative remedies.

## Chinese Tonic Herbs

Chronic fatigue is often diagnosed by Chinese medicine as deficiencies in any or all of the Five Major Energetic Systems, so the treatment plan revolves around strengthening those systems affected. Within the repertoire of Chinese herbology are tonic herbs, which are a unique group of herbs. The properties of tonic herbs cannot be found in any other herbology system in the world. Tonic herbs possess strengthening properties. Rather than stimulating or transferring already existing Energy, tonic herbs actually generate new Energy. Therefore tonic herbs can be used to treat any sort of weakness or deficiency condition that requires production of Qi. Tonic herbs are designed to strengthen the body, including the immune system, hematological (blood) system, endocrine system and nervous system. By definition, tonic herbs correct deficiencies and replenish what is lacking in the body. These herbs are unique in treating chronic fatigue and other conditions such as immune system deficiency, adrenal burnout, weak digestive system, low libido and chronic back pain.

"From the time I started taking the herbs, I can only say I went upward," Jan said. "It was amazing. Within a couple of months I was back to my old self. When I go in to see Dr. Han, he adjusts the herbs absolutely perfectly to my complaints. If I am very tired or my head feels like a cotton ball, he throws a little more twigs or leaves or pieces of bark in the tea and it works. I am in good shape now. If staying healthy means I have to take these herbs the rest of my life, then that's what I will do."

In cases when an illness cannot be clearly defined and diagnosed, the treatment choices can be severely limited in Western medicine. In Chinese medicine, the objective is to recognize all the signs and symptoms and utilize this information to develop an appropriate treatment protocol. If symptoms are present, a person can always be treated with Chinese medicine.

## Autoimmune Diseases

Forty-nine-year-old Lance Mayamoto grew up on a farm near Omaha, Nebraska. "When I was growing up, we used to spray 2,4,5-T to kill brush—which is the active ingredient in what the military called Agent Orange," Lance said. "We also used paraquat—a toxic herbicide chemical formula—by the gallon. We used gasoline as a degreasing cleaning solvent. I worked in electromechanical types of jobs and used carbon tetrachloride that was left over after it was outlawed, then trichloroethane, until it was outlawed. Later I used methylethylketone, acetone and lacquer thinner as solvents. I never used gloves or a mask. I didn't know that chemicals could affect my health, and in fact I was upset when they were outlawed, because it made my work harder."

Autoimmune processes seem to be linked to certain genetic traits triggered by factors such as viral infections, chronic stress, environmental toxins and hormones, especially estrogen and xenohormones. Xenohormones (xenoestrogens or xenobiotics) are foreign compounds and/or chemical toxins that mimic the effects of hormones in the body. Xenohormones are present in man-made chemicals such as chlorofluorocarbons, herbicides and pesticides and in industrial by-products from plastics, paper and the incineration of hazardous wastes.

In 1967, Lance's mother, at age forty-nine, was diagnosed with scleroderma, an autoimmune condition which causes hardening of the skin and certain organs, including the gastrointestinal tract, lungs, heart and kidneys. The course of the disease was quick and she died within one year. In 1982, at age thirty-five, Lance began to suffer from migraine headaches. By 1986 other symptoms followed—numbness on the left side of his body, extreme fatigue, limb weakness and joint pain, which progressively escalated until the pain consumed his entire body. "I went to doctor after doctor, and each prescribed pain medication. I had CAT scans, MRIs and blood tests, and my doctors could not find a cause. So I lived with the pain."

In 1995, Lance moved from Oregon to Utah. For the next five years he continued to see doctor after doctor as his condition worsened. A neurologist diagnosed him with a rare autoimmune condition called vasculitis, which causes the immune system to attack the vascular system.

Twenty years ago, the word *autoimmune* was not the household word it is today. In the twenty-first century, autoimmune conditions such as thyroiditis, lupus, Crohn's disease, rheumatoid arthritis, insulin-dependent diabetes, multiple sclerosis, Graves' disease, myasthenia gravis, interstitial cystitis and Sjögren's syndrome are an increasing problem. Many diseases not previously well understood in Western medicine have been found to be autoimmune problems. Autoimmune conditions occur when the immune system begins to react more aggressively than is appropriate. The first sign might be that you get a raging reaction to bug bites or poison oak, while someone with a healthy immune system would experience only minor itchiness. If your immune system reacts even more aggressively, it can lose the ability to distinguish between normal, healthy cells and destructive foreign invaders. Your immune system begins attacking your own healthy cells. When this occurs you have an autoimmune condition.

Autoimmune conditions have risen dramatically with the rise in environmental toxins and stress. As we become more technologically advanced and our lifestyle is further separated from the traditional, natural way of life, we will likely see an increasing amount of these problems. The chemical revolution of the past fifty years has produced thousands of man-made chemicals that have not been tested for their effect on the public's health and safety. On March 21, 2001, the Centers for Disease Control released a report documenting the dangerous levels of toxic chemicals that are accumulating in the bodies of average people. High levels of mercury were noted. Women of childbearing age are regularly exposed to a class of chemicals known as phthalates, which are used in plastic products, cosmetics and personal-care products, and which are clearly linked with developmental defects in animals. Extremely high levels of pesticides were detected in 10 percent of those tested.

Because the earth is steeped in poisons, allergies, asthma, chronic fatigue and autoimmune conditions will likely continue to rise. Highly toxic (and now banned) chemical substances were used liberally on the farm and in the work-place where Lance grew up. Both he and his mother developed autoimmune conditions.

"I am third-generation Japanese," Lance said. "My family was Christian, but my family on my grandmother's side was Samurai, and she taught me the Samurai tradition. Being strong and ignoring pain was part of the culture. When I grew up, I pursued the martial arts, which are the warring arts." Because of this conditioning Lance had always been able to mentally control his response to pain. But after nearly twenty years the severity of his migraines and total body pain had worn him down.

When the narcotic analgesic Demerol did not help, Lance began a protocol of low-dose antidepressants in an attempt to control his pain. Tricyclic antidepressants have been available for the treatment of depression and pain syndromes for decades. Because this class of medication alters the level of neurotransmitters in specific areas of the brain, they have been found to be effective in managing certain types of pain syndromes by altering the brain's interpretation of pain impulses.

He began taking the anti-inflammatories ibuprofen and naproxen. When these medications did not effectively control the inflammation, he was prescribed prednisone. Prednisone is a synthetic steroid, similar to cortisone, that has been prescribed for some autoimmune diseases to suppress the immune system. Because steroids are typically administered in pharmacological doses—often over and above what your adrenal glands would typically produce—the treatment often introduces a host of other problems. When Lance tapered off prednisone as directed, the pain was worse than before beginning treatment. His doctor put him back on one 10-milligram pill a day, then two. Lance was on prednisone for six months and started to experience some of the typical side effects of daily steroid use such as weight gain.

Eventually, even when taking prednisone, the attacks of pain and weakness returned as bad as ever. Lance decided to again taper off the prednisone but suffered extreme depression as a side effect. "At that point, I did not think I would live until I could retire at age fifty-five. I had developed bowel problems and stomach problems in addition to the migraines, body pain, numbness and weakness. I felt that death would be a welcome relief from the twenty-plus years of pain I had gone through. My plan was to fight on until I could retire so that my wife would receive my retirement benefits. I felt it was just a matter of time before I was finished."

In April 2001, Lance's brother came out to Utah on business. "My brother told me about his wife's experience with Chinese herbs," Lance said. "His wife had had a brain tumor. Although she had had surgery, she was having seizures and her Western doctors couldn't stop them. When she started taking herbs her seizures stopped. My brother took herbs for things like colds and was impressed with Chinese medicine. He started bugging me to go to Dr. Han. I thought it really couldn't hurt. I was flying out to California for a business trip anyway, so I took the opportunity to see Dr. Han."

Dr. Han is experienced in treating difficult autoimmune conditions. He immediately recognized the urgency of creating an herbal formula that would modulate Lance's immune system. The immune system is not a single biological function but a complex system that involves many actions. If your immune system becomes fatigued, it can be tired and wired at the same time. For example, your immune system might be too fatigued to defend against foreign invaders, so you will come down with colds, flu and other infections, but at the same time the wired aspect of your immune system causes it to turn on healthy tissues, resulting in an autoimmune condition. This example allows you to see that a fatigued and overreactive immune system cannot be effectively treated by simply suppressing the immune system. In the case of autoimmune conditions, Chinese herbal formulas can support the weakness and tune down the hyperactivity at the same time. Chinese medicine takes a completely different approach to autoimmune conditions. Most important, Chinese medicine does not suppress the immune system, but rather strives to balance it.

"I was on my second week in my efforts to wean myself off the steroids," Lance said. "When I started the herbs, I felt better than I had felt in a long time. Before, when I weaned off steroids the pain level was intolerable. I couldn't sleep or work. Since I started the herbs, there are periods during the day when I actually feel pain free." He also started on patent herbs to control his stomach pain and migraine headaches. "I've used Tagamet, Zantac and Prevacid for twelve years to control stomach pain. Dr. Han gave me some patent pills that look like BBs. From the day I got started taking them I have not taken any other medications, and I have not had any stomach problems, my incidence of headaches has gone way down and my use of headache medication is almost zero."

Because of Lance's illness, he had to come to terms with the fact that he was not in control of his life. "There is a dichotomy between my cultural belief, which says to be strong and self-reliant, and my religious belief as a member of the Church of Jesus Christ of Latter-day Saints, which says not to trust in the 'arm of the flesh.' I always had enough determination and tenacity to work through everything, until the final years of my illness. When I became unable to do a lot of things, it was a humbling process. Prayer has always been a big part of my life. I learned that prayer is not just having a two-way communication with God; it is a conduit of power. I prayed, and members of my church prayed for me. In the early history of the Mormons, they used faith, mild foods and herbs. I have done all three. I believe that Chinese herbs are part of the answers to those prayers."

One year after starting Chinese herbs, Lance calls his recovery "miraculous." "I recently did some concrete work at my house and spent hours manually digging up a pipe. Before, I wouldn't have been able to do it without extreme pain. But now, I was only mildly sore afterward. I'm sleeping better. I have fewer headaches. Everything has improved. I'm off the painkillers entirely, and I'm calmer. I haven't been able to do push-ups in years, but I can do push-ups with one hand now." Although Lance experiences ups and downs in his recovery, his condition is relatively stable. He continues to take herbs regularly.

More people are flocking to doctors with symptoms similar to those experienced by Heather, Jan and Lance. These people characteristically suffer from a conglomerate of serious problems traditionally considered independent of one another, such as chronic fatigue, immune weakness, hypersensitivities or allergies, chronic viral or candida infection. These are the illnesses of our new age. Western-managed care often refers to those people as "heavy utilizers." Western medical doctors are trained to consider anyone with more than six symptoms to be a psychiatric case, which is why many people with environmentally related illnesses end up being told their problems are "in their heads" and are referred to psychiatrists.

From a Chinese medicine point of view, all symptoms are considered legitimate. Chinese medicine understands that environmentally related illnesses are complex—the profound deficiencies and the pronounced stagnation are tightly entangled. These types of illnesses are stubborn and chronic and present a significant challenge to heal.

## Ways to Treat External Toxins/ Environmentally Related Illnesses

Consult with a health care professional

If you are ill, you need to see a health care professional to work with you and follow your healing progress.

Have your adrenal hormones tested, as depleted adrenals are a major contributing factor in lowered immunity.

Have your amino acid levels tested. If your body is not breaking down the proteins you eat into amino acids, this can result in decreased neurotransmitter production, which will result in fatigue and symptoms of depression. Amino acid supplementation can boost your energy as well as supply your body with the necessary precursors to neurotransmitters.

Stool, hair and blood tests can determine if you have (1) high levels of accumulated heavy metals in your system, (2) sensitivities to foods or (3) dysbiosis, which is an imbalance of the healthy and unhealthy bacteria and yeast in the gut, any of which may be weakening your immune system and draining your energy.

See page 431 for a laboratory that can refer you to a health care provider in your area who does these types of tests. If you test positive for any of these factors, your health care practitioner can treat you on an individual basis.

## Protect yourself from further chemical exposure

Environmentally related illnesses can result from overexposure to External Toxins. External Toxins influence the Energy systems differently depending on each individual and his or her situation. External Toxins come from air, water and food. Become an active participant in your health by learning as much as you can about the chemicals in our environment and actively avoiding exposure. To protect yourself, David Steinman, a nationally recognized authority on environmental toxins and author of numerous books on the subject, advises:

- Avoid exposure to home and garden pesticides.
- Use biodegradable, toxic-chemical-free, environmentally safe products.
- Avoid electropollution. Electropollution is the stray electromagnetic radiation propagated through the atmosphere. That most harmful to humans usually comes from broadcast towers, radar installations, microwave appliances and the magnetic fields surrounding electrical appliances and power lines.
- Avoid chemical solvents.
- Use toothpaste without fluoride and avoid drinking fluoridated tap water. Studies on animals have shown that fluoride may contribute to the development of cancer, and recent government tests have demonstrated that fluoride appears to be carcinogenic.

◆ Exercise to remove toxins and strengthen the immune system.
◆ Take antioxidant vitamins and minerals.
◆ Avoid heavy-metal exposure such as 1) lead in tap water—drink bottled water, 2) mercury in dental fillings—have fillings removed by an expert in this procedure and/or opt for composites rather than amalgams; mercury in fish such as shark and swordfish, 3) cadmium in plastics, stabilizers, pigments, animal products and vegetables—use environmentally safe self-care products and eat organically grown meats and produce, 4) aluminum exposure—do not cook with aluminum foil and pots. (Note: these are only some of the heavy metals you can be exposed to in the environment. See page 432 for David Steinman's books for further reading on this subject.)

### Modify your diet

Americans have come full circle from the excitement about and dependence upon processed foods that began in the forties to a growing understanding that the human body needs and thrives on a consistent diet of real, whole foods. More people are turning away from a diet consisting of overly processed or adulterated foods that come from a factory and moving toward a diet consisting of foods that could, in theory, be picked, gathered, milked, hunted or fished.

Food is medicine. There is a long tradition in China whereby food is used as a means of treatment or of correcting certain imbalances. In fact, there is a rather significant overlap in Chinese herbology between food and medicine. There are a large number of herbs that can be consumed as a food and still provide strong medicinal effects. In China there are restaurants that specialize in cooking dishes that taste good, promote wellness and also treat a certain imbalance or illness. Each restaurant has an herbalist who recommends certain dishes to customers. In chapter 21 you will find medicinal recipes that have been created especially to treat a specific condition(s)—they use real, whole foods that are delicious, nutritious and medicinal.

Malnutrition in this country is primarily a result of the processing of foods. Much of the processing actually depletes the food source of its vital minerals, vitamins and other nutritional aspects. If you suffer from brittle nails, constipation, cravings, dry and thinning hair, scaly and itchy skin, infertility, insomnia, mood swings, depression or weight gain, chances are you may be suffering from some degree of malnutrition and are Energetically imbalanced. David Steinman advises:

* Eat certified organic meats, dairy, vegetables, fruits and nuts.
* Avoid processed or chemically adulterated foods.
* Avoid genetically engineered foods.
* Avoid irradiated foods.

Over-the-counter and prescription medications for allergies work by blocking histamine receptors. Flavonoids prevent the release of histamines. Fruit and vegetable juices contain bioflavonoids, which are a crystalline compound found in plants that is responsible for the deep colors. They possess antiviral, anticarcinogenic, anti-inflammatory, antioxidant and antihistamine properties. Drinking vegetable juice can prevent allergic reactions. See pages 291–295 for more on vegetable juicing.

Many chronic fatigue syndrome (CFS) or chronic fatigue immune dysfunction syndrome (CIDS) patients feel worse after drinking fresh vegetable juices because they are Kidney and/or Spleen Yang deficient. Energetically Cold foods such as raw vegetable juices are too Yin and Damp for these types. Some of these patients also have systemic candida, which is a Cold and Damp disharmony, and juicing can aggravate this disharmony. On the other hand, juicing can be a powerful means for these patients to get a tremendous amount of nutrients and for them to cleanse their systems of certain toxins. Because CFS and CIDS are not singular imbalances in Chinese medicine, the only way for a CFS or CIDS patient to use juicing safely and effectively is to have a customized juicing program for his or her condition—just as with everything else in Chinese medicine. Dr. Han often creates a cleansing program with different juicing formulas to target the imbalance or disharmony of different Energetic systems based precisely on the diagnosis. For example, there are juicing formulas for Liver cleansing, Heart cleansing, Spleen cleansing, Lung cleansing and Kidney cleansing. Each can be used alone or in combination with other cleansings. For patients with Yang deficiency or Damp stagnation, juicing formulations must be carefully balanced to minimize the Cold or Damp nature of the juice. At the same time, an herbal formula will be designed to support the patient's Qi and counteract the Cold and Dampness from the juice. Under Dr. Han's close supervision, patients with conditions inherently incompatible with juicing can drink reduced doses for ten days or less. *If you are suffering from CFS or CIDS, do not attempt a juice cleansing unless closely supervised by a doctor of Chinese medicine or an herbologist who is experienced in treating CFS or CIDS.*

## Quit caffeine, nicotine or other stimulant chemicals

Seven hundred volatile substances have been identified in coffee, including more than two hundred acids, alcohol, aromatic compounds, carbonyl compounds, esters, hydrocarbons, heterocyclic compounds and terpenoids. Nonvolatile substances in coffee include caffeine and other purines, glycosides, lipids, melanoidins, caffeic acid and chlorogenic acid. Coffee often contains pesticide residues and other contaminants such as nitrosamines, solvents and mycotoxins. The chemical decaffeination process leaves decaffeinated coffee tainted with methylene chloride, which is carcinogenic (Swiss water processing removes some of the caffeine from coffee using nontoxic means and is therefore a safer choice).

In addition, it is a well-known fact that burning food can create carcinogens, and coffee beans are often burned in the roasting process. The numerous acids in coffee contribute to gastrointestinal distress. Caffeine depletes your body of calcium, potassium, iron and trace minerals.

Many soft drinks contain harmful chemicals, especially diet sodas containing aspartame. Aspartame has been linked to breast cancer, brain cancer, seizures, neurobehavioral symptoms, headaches, blurred vision, depression, nausea, insomnia, danger to a developing fetus, memory loss, hyperactivity, muscle and joint pain, fatigue, ringing in the ears, diarrhea and loss of control of limbs (symptoms similar to multiple sclerosis). See pages 148–155 for guidelines to restore neurotransmitters to help quit caffeine, nicotine and other stimulants.

## Detox on a regular basis

If you are suffering from an environmentally related illness, practicing regular detoxification can help to break up stagnation and get your Qi moving to speed your recovery. Since detoxification can be hard on the body, if you are seriously ill, do not attempt detoxification on your own. You must be supervised closely by a health care practitioner. If you are not suffering from a particular illness, our toxic environment makes it important to practice regular detoxification. See pages 291–296 for more on detoxification.

## Drink plenty of clean water

In addition to detoxifying your system, there are daily detox precautions you can take, such as drinking eight to ten eight-ounce glasses of pure water every day. The Environmental Protection Agency (EPA) estimates that one in five Americans consumes tap water that violates EPA safety standards under the

Clean Water Act. Studies have identified more than 2,110 contaminants in the nation's water supplies. Because it is expensive to treat your entire incoming water supply, it is most efficient to treat water at points of use, such as at cooking and drinking sources. There are two basic processes to clean water: filtration and purification. Some systems combine both methods. Begin by testing your water so that you know what issues to address. Buy a system that addresses those problems. Water testing and purification systems can be found online at ancientherbsmodernmedicine.com.

## Have your environment tested for mold

The presence of mold in your environment can be a factor contributing to your environmentally related illness. The presence of mold in the environment is generally considered by Chinese medicine as a form of Dampness or Toxins. You can test your home and office for mold contaminants. For information on where to buy mold-testing kits log on to ancientherbsmodernmedicine.com.

It is important to find out what kinds of mold are in your environment. Some are more dangerous than others. Testing allows you to identify dangerous molds and the ones that you may be highly allergic to. The level of mold will provide an indication of the contamination. The type of mold will also dictate the seriousness of that contamination. If you test your environment and get a very high reading but you do not know where the excessive moisture is coming from or you are not aware of any structural damage, an on-site inspection by an industrial hygienist could possibly identify the source. There are many professionals who know what to do to identify the problems but not as many who know what to do to prevent the problems in new construction or how to solve the problems in existing structures.

## Keep your indoors free of volatile organic compounds (VOCs)

Cigarette smoke and dust mites are obvious pollutants. Building materials and interior furnishings can emit gaseous volatile organic compounds (VOCs) into the air, many of which can be toxic, including new carpeting, draperies and other fabrics, vinyl tiles and wallpaper, paints, stains and solvents. Products as diverse as spray deodorants, hairspray, air fresheners, bug sprays, appliances, dry-cleaning fluid and office equipment and supplies all emit VOCs. There are too many VOCs to list here. You can purchase air-purification systems that dehumidify, deodorize, kill germs, bacteria and mites and absorb fumes. Also available are desktop units and air-to-air heat exchangers that blow stale air out of your home and pull fresh air in without significant heat or cooling loss. Product information can be found online at ancientherbsmodernmedicine.com.

## Exercise caution when having vaccinations

If you travel out of the country frequently, be aware that there has been much discussion and significant evidence indicating that multiple and frequent vaccinations can indeed trigger significant autoimmune reactions.

## Chinese herbs and Western supplements

If you suffer from any type of environmentally related illness, find a health care practitioner who can give you vitamin B injections or intravenous vitamins such as vitamin C, or a "Meyer's cocktail," which is a combination of calcium, magnesium, vitamin C and vitamin B complex.

Routinely, thirty to forty-five minutes before breakfast and dinner take 1,000 milligrams free-form amino acids.

Routinely, before each meal, take the digestive formulas on page 102.

To prevent allergy attacks, drink Allergy Season Tea—available at health food stores. This tea is made with ginger root, licorice root, peppermint leaf, anise seed, tulsi leaf, gotu kola, skullcap root, cardamom seed, eucalyptus leaf, orange peel, black pepper, clove bud, cinnamon bark, amla extract, angelica root, magnolia flower, peony root and poria mushroom.

When you have an allergy attack take 1,000 milligrams of buffered vitamin C crystals two to three times a day with 500 milligrams quercetin. If you do not see any improvement after one day, increase to 2,000 milligrams vitamin C and 1,000 milligrams quercetin—but do not go above this. If you experience diarrhea, reduce the vitamin C.

Your body cannot detoxify if you are constipated, since the toxins will remain in your intestines and be reabsorbed. If you suffer from constipation, you can take a Chinese herbal formula along with a detoxification formula. Drink eight to twelve eight-ounce glasses of purified or filtered water per day.

You can use Chinese medicinal herbs in recipes to treat the symptoms of environmentally related illnesses. See chapter 21 for recipes. Environmentally sensitive individuals can also benefit from taking Chinese herbal formulas created to prevent illness when traveling. These formulas and Western supplements specifically formulated to treat environmentally related illnesses can be purchased online at ancientherbsmodernmedicine.com.

# 12

## Cancer

*Treating cancer with integrative medicine*

The painful urination did not seem like anything to worry about. Twenty-two-year-old Jamie Ingersol dismissed the symptom as a bladder infection, as she had had similar episodes in the past. In early February 1998 she was treated at a student clinic, but the condition did not resolve. When a clinic doctor performed a pelvic exam, he noticed a mass over her left ovary and referred her to a gynecologist.

After a physical exam and an ultrasound of the area, the gynecologist was not concerned. He explained that Jamie had a dermoid cyst. A dermoid cyst is a fairly rare, nonmalignant cystic tumor created when an unfertilized egg begins to replicate. The cysts often contain elements derived from the cells of a developing embryo, such as hair, teeth and skin. Although benign, the doctor felt the cyst should be surgically removed and that she should wait no longer than six months.

It was one of those perfect southern California days in July 1999 when Jamie recounted her story. Her smile, slightly tentative, belied the depth of trauma she had gone through over the past year and a half. "When the doctor told me about the dermoid cyst, I was frightened of the idea of surgery," she explained. "But I thought that since he didn't seem concerned I really shouldn't worry." Jamie, a second-year student of Chinese medicine, knew there were treatment modalities outside of Western medicine to explore before immediately going ahead with the surgery. She began asking around. "I talked to a woman who had a dermoid cyst who had shrunk it by changing her diet. So I decided to cut out red meat, dairy products, sugar and processed foods. I ate a lot of whole grains, vegetables, tofu and fish."

Four months passed. Every morning Jamie awoke and felt the growing mound with her fingers. She went back to her doctor in late July 1998. The cyst had grown considerably and was now the size of a small grapefruit. The second ultrasound showed fluid accumulation in her abdominal cavity. Again, the doctor did not appear to show significant concern, though he urged her once again to have the cyst surgically removed. He spent a few minutes explaining the surgery.

With the doctor's apparent lack of concern, Jamie was mostly worried about the scar the incision would leave. She had heard about laparoscopic surgery and wanted to check out that option. Her mother went into high gear, making phone calls and inquiries to find another doctor who could perform the laparoscopy. Over the phone, another doctor told her that the presence of fluid surrounding a mass could be a very serious situation. It was the first time the word *cancer* was mentioned. Jamie and her mother were both stunned.

Jamie immediately went to see the second gynecologist. He ordered a C-125 blood test, the commonly used ovarian cancer marker. Jamie's test result showed the C-125 to be significantly elevated. The doctor explained that an elevated level meant that the mass could be cancerous. Jamie was referred to a gynecologic oncologist. Jamie and her parents sat in terrified silence as the oncologist explained that the lab results and the ultrasound indicated that surgery was imperative but that they could not know for sure if she had ovarian cancer until after they operated. Biopsies and the subsequent pathology report would provide a definitive diagnosis. Jamie explained that, even with this sobering discussion, the urgency of her situation did not fully sink in. "It was the end of the semester, and final exams were coming up. It was a lot of memorization—a lot of hard work. I wanted to put the surgery off for two weeks so I could take my finals."

But the surgeon did not want to wait that long. Ovarian cancer is an aggressive cancer with a high degree of malignancy. The abdominal cavity is large and loosely filled with organs that can easily move around to accommodate a growing tumor. By the time the tumor grows to a size that causes discomfort and is subsequently diagnosed, it has usually metastasized. It is one of the few cancers that afflict young women. The five-year survival rate, after aggressive intervention with Western medical treatment, is only 5 percent.

Jamie had only a few days to prepare for major surgery. She went to see Dr. Han because she knew that herbal treatments would be helpful in her situation. She also wanted to know if Dr. Han thought she could put off the surgery.

Jamie's case is an example of how both Chinese and Western medicine can work together in a patient's treatment. Dr. Han had her diagnostic test results from Western medicine. The Western medical diagnosis of an elevated C-125 and fluid surrounding a growing mass in her abdomen presented a definitive picture that carried a great sense of urgency. He advised her to go ahead with the surgery as planned. But because of the clarity of the Western medical diagnosis, Dr. Han was also able to immediately access his knowledge of Chinese herbs to aid in preparing her for that surgery. In addition to her Western medical reports, he used Chinese medical diagnostic methods, which focus on the relationship between cancer and the whole body. Because Dr. Han had seen the results of Jamie's Western diagnostic tests, he had a clear picture of the existence of the malignancy. The result was a treatment plan that was based on the overall picture of the deficiency and stagnation of her Energy.

While a common prescription will include ten to fifteen herbs, because of the severity and complexity of Jamie's condition, Dr. Han used a combination of twenty-three different herbs in creating her formula, which was designed to reduce bleeding during the operation, to promote tissue healing and to strengthen and support her immune system. Almost half of the herbs in her formula had anticancer properties, which would help to contain or suppress the growth of malignant cancer cells.

Jamie was to prepare a pot of herbal tea daily. She would reheat and drink three cups of tea during the day. She was vigilant about preparing and drinking the tea prior to her surgery.

On August 1, six months after she first noticed the mass in her abdomen, Jamie checked into the hospital for surgery. In a radical, three-hour procedure, the surgeon began by draining over a liter of fluid from her abdomen. Cancerous tissue often has the appearance of cottage cheese, which makes it discernible from normal tissue. At first glance, the surgeon must have seen that the cancer had, indeed, metastasized and invaded multiple sites in her abdominal cavity. He removed the grapefruit-sized tumor, along with three-quarters of her right ovary, and a tumor the size of a large egg, as well as a quarter of her left ovary. The entire greater omentum—the sheet of connective tissue that covers the abdominal organs—was implanted with metastasized tumors, and had to be removed. With a laser beam, the surgeon burned off two BB-sized lesions deep in the right lobe of her liver, and peeled off a marble-sized metastasized tumor from her right kidney. The surgeon then excised three quail-egg-sized cancerous implants—two from her abdominal wall and one from her pelvic wall—as well as three marble-sized implants from her sigmoid colon. Ten lymph nodes from her pelvic and abdominal cavities were removed.

Jamie awoke in the recovery room with an incision from her groin to her navel, too drugged and too sick to talk. She was hospitalized for a week. It was a difficult recovery. It was only when she felt strong enough to visit the surgical oncologist's office, two weeks after she went home, that he explained the results of her surgical report and outlined his recommended course of chemotherapy. He had been able to remove the visible cancer tissue during surgery, but given the widespread nature of her cancer, it was all but inevitable that microscopic cancer cells remained throughout Jamie's abdominal cavity. The only way to eradicate those cells was for her to undergo an arduous course of chemotherapy.

During this visit, Jamie's mother appeared more shaken than her daughter. Chemotherapy was something she had not considered. "My parents had supported the surgery, but they were adamantly opposed to chemotherapy and thought it was going to kill me," Jamie said. "They fought it tooth and nail. My mom had been raised with natural foods and didn't even use antibiotics. In many ways, I agreed with her philosophy, but I was also just scared."

Jamie's mother launched into research on natural alternatives to chemotherapy, spending hundreds of dollars on books and talking to everyone she could find who would listen or offer information. Jamie, her two older sisters and her parents would get together to heatedly discuss what Jamie should or should not do regarding further medical treatments. "My mom and dad were totally on the natural side, and one of my sisters was totally fighting for the Western side. My other sister was just trying to figure it out and kind of going in between. And then I'm stuck there listening to all of them. We went through endless hours of discussion."

Jamie's case presented an interesting twist. She was training in Chinese medicine, yet she was not opposed to Western medicine. Her parents were pressuring her to pursue a natural alternative to chemotherapy. Regardless of the sides they chose to defend, the Ingersol family's debate over Western versus natural medical approaches is a microcosm for the debate going on now in the United States. Advocates of each approach have mostly gotten stuck in camps where the other side is viewed with suspicion, even disdain. Once camps get established and battle lines drawn, it is difficult to move from either/or thinking to also/and reasoning.

To the extent that individuals have available to them complementary options, their chances of considering and receiving comprehensive medical treatment are enhanced. But just as Jamie had to negotiate the high-volume discussion within her family, Americans must navigate the biased voices that, for the most part, insist that one approach is the only way. In case after case it can be shown that the use of complementary approaches enhances the treatment, recovery and wellness of patients with a wide range of disorders. Unfortunately, Jamie did not have the luxury of having a complementary team of doctors conferring with one another and advising and reassuring her. She had to go it alone.

One of the approaches Jamie's mother heard about was injecting the patient's blood into a lactating cow that would then produce specific antibodies in her milk. "My mother was presenting these options to me and to everybody else around, like my boyfriend and my sisters, anybody who'd listen to her. We would find holes in every solution, so she was getting really frustrated."

Jamie was more circumspect. "When I originally thought I had a dermoid cyst, I tried dealing with it naturally with diet and so forth, and that didn't work. I didn't want to make the mistake of trying to do just herbs and diet and different things like that and have the cancer spread all over my body. On the other hand, I wanted to make sure Western medicine wasn't overtreating me with chemo when it wasn't really necessary."

She went back to Dr. Han, who she assumed would side with her mother and suggest an herbal alternative to chemotherapy. "I hadn't really discussed Western medicine with Dr. Han before. So I didn't know where he'd be coming from. But you have a certain picture of people who are in alternative medicine, that most of them are against using Western medicine."

It was understandable that Jamie resisted chemotherapy, as it is an invasive and often debilitating treatment protocol. In Dr. Han's opinion, she had very little chance of survival without this treatment. Although Chinese medicine alone has been known to be effective in treating many types of cancers, he did not know of any documented cases of advanced ovarian cancer being cured with Chinese herbal medicine alone. To make sure, he consulted with his mother, Dr. Huiwen Luo, a Western-trained gynecologist and surgical oncologist in practice in China.

Dr. Luo had extensive experience in treating ovarian cancer. In 1966, at the onset of the Cultural Revolution, the then forty-five-year-old Dr. Luo was charged as a "bourgeois counter-revolutionary scholastic authority," stripped of her right to practice medicine and led away to prison. Four years later, she was exiled to western China for "reeducation" through forced labor. She was sent to the remote Hui County, which was inexplicably plagued with a high rate of uterine, ovarian and especially cervical cancers. Dr. Luo requested and was granted the right to return to medical practice because of the dire situation there. Girls as young as twelve years old were dying of cancer. Dr. Luo, in 2001, at seventy-nine years old, remembered clearly how thirty years ago she spear-headed a small but devoted band of doctors in an effort to stave off the slippery slope of death in Hui County. "The total number of patients my team diag-nosed with cancer was in the thousands," Dr. Luo said. The conventional ap-proach for cervical cancer is surgery during the early stage, and for terminal patients, radiation therapy. As a result of inadequate medical services, when vil-lage women developed cancer they would usually not survive. Dr. Luo devel-oped an integrative medical approach that she called comprehensive therapy, which included surgery, chemotherapy, immunotherapy and Chinese herbal medicine.

The first step was to assess each patient's stage of cancer. Uterine cervical cancer is categorized into stage I, II, III and IV depending on the severity. Cate-gorizing stages is valuable in deciding on the type of therapy the patient needs. Stages I and II are generally curable. Stage III and IV cancer are both considered advanced with a guarded prognosis, but stage IV is usually considered terminal. These patients were not good candidates for surgery, as their bodies were sig-nificantly weakened by widespread metastasis and they were not likely to sur-vive surgery. "But I didn't give up on these patients. All of my patients, especially those with advanced stages of cancer and those with extremely weak-ened immune systems, were treated with comprehensive therapy in an effort to improve their conditions and prepare them for surgery."

In addition to chemotherapy, Dr. Luo used immunotherapy and Chinese herbal medicine to bolster patients' immune systems. Immunotherapy is thought to stimulate the immune system to produce large amounts of antibod-ies against cancer cells. Dr. Luo began by taking a sample of cancerous tissue from a patient. She then mixed this tissue with tuberculosis vaccination, which is made of tuberculosis bacteria that has been treated to reduce its ability to cause disease. She injected patients with this preparation. After using extensive herbal therapy, immunotherapy and chemotherapy, many previously inopera-ble patients became operable. In addition to taking herbs before the surgery, Dr. Luo typically asked the patient to take herbs for at least a year postsurgery to aid in recovery and significantly reduce the possibility of recurrence.

Dr. Luo documented the results of her treatment plan in a study involving 120 patients in the third and fourth stages of cervical cancer. With a ten-year survival rate, the survival rate of her patients was 42 percent in stage III patients and 37 percent in stage IV. (For a ten-year survival of ovarian carcinoma that has reached stage III or IV, 5 to 7 percent is considered optimistic.)

When Dr. Han discussed Jamie Ingersol's case with his mother, Dr. Luo, she confirmed that in her fifty years of experience treating gynecological cancers she had rarely seen cases of advanced ovarian cancer successfully treated with Chinese medicine alone. He knew, however, that even with aggressive Western medical intervention, the survival rate was still very low and that the best chance for Jamie would be a combination of Chinese medicine and Western medicine.

There were several crucial reasons to combine these two approaches. It was vital to Jamie's survival that all existing cancer cells in her system be eradicated. The most reliable treatment available was chemotherapy. What often makes chemotherapy a success or failure is how well a patient tolerates the treatment. Chinese medicine can reduce many of the side effects and make it possible for patients to tolerate higher doses of chemotherapy by sensitizing the cancer cells. Herbal treatment can also enhance the therapeutic efficacy of chemotherapy and radiation therapy. The dose of chemotherapy can sometimes be significantly reduced and still attain the targeted therapeutic effect. In the meantime, Chinese herbal medicine can support and strengthen the immune system and give the patient a much better sense of well-being during treatment. Chinese herbal medicine can also help reduce the possibility of the recurrence of cancer.

Discussing her options with Dr. Han gave Jamie the perspective she needed to make her decision. "It felt so good to hear Dr. Han's opinion about chemotherapy," Jamie said. "I felt secure in knowing that he knew about both medicines and that his mother was trained in both Chinese and Western medicine. She didn't just say, 'Oh, do it the Western way because that's all I know' or 'Do the Chinese way because that's all I know.' Since she knew both, she knew what was the best thing to do."

Jamie's mother had accompanied her on her visits with Dr. Han. "She wanted to hear his side of it," Jamie said. "She wanted to be there so she could ask questions and debate with him. She didn't really say anything while we were there, but I thought she felt more reassured when we left his office." In fact, Jamie had made up her mind to go forward with the chemotherapy, but her mother was still not convinced. "I think she felt a little bit better knowing that Dr. Han was in favor of the chemo. But she was still scared about it. There was nothing we could say that would subdue her emotions at all, even to the last minute of my last treatment."

Jamie was living at home and had to deal with the strain of her parents' disapproval of her choice. "It was harder to deal with my family's opposition than it was to deal with the cancer. It was a really difficult time. Even when I was about to get the chemo, I still wasn't one hundred percent behind it. I thought

## Studies Demonstrating the Efficacy of Using Chinese Herbs When Undergoing Western Cancer Treatments

Daizhao, Zhang, and Piwen, Li. "Prevention and Treatment by Chinese Medicine of the Side Effects Due to Chemotherapy and Radiation Therapy in Cancer Treatment."
*Journal of Traditional Chinese Medicine* 35 (August 1994): 498–500.

In China, the use of herbs in conjunction with chemotherapy or radiation therapy has become routine and very much accepted, even by the Western-trained medical community. The complementary use of Chinese herbal medicine and Western medicine in the treatment of cancer has been extensively researched and documented in Chinese literature. In a review of 127 studies published between 1984 and 1994, involving over 11,000 cancer patients with various forms of cancer receiving chemotherapy and/or radiation therapy, Chinese herbs were evaluated for three factors: (1) reducing the toxicity of radiation and chemotherapy, (2) increasing the therapeutic effect of radiation and chemotherapy, and (3) improving the long-term survival rate.

Study patients were treated with herbs along with radiation and/or chemotherapy. Control patients were treated solely with radiation and/or chemotherapy. Three criteria were used to evaluate the success of the treatment: (1) tolerance of chemotherapy so that the patient could complete the course of treatment, (2) the lessening of side effects, and (3) survival rate.

Among the studies examined in the review, a study done by the Oncology Department of Sino-Japan Friendship Hospital, involving 115 cases of various cancers, looking at the chemotherapy patients alone, showed that 88 percent of the study group (receiving herbal treatments) were able to complete chemotherapy, as opposed to only 55 percent of the control group. In a study done by Guanganmen Hospital in Beijing, involving 326 terminal stomach cancer patients, 95 percent of the study

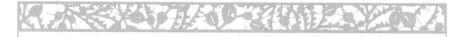

group were able to complete chemotherapy, as opposed to only 75 percent of the control group. Another study in the same hospital involved 115 cases of esophageal cancer. During chemotherapy, 87 percent of the patients in the study group had white blood counts remaining above the required acceptable range and were able to continue treatments, versus 64 percent in the control group. Another study of patients with terminal stomach cancer focused on herbal treatment before and after surgery, chemotherapy and radiation treatments. The results demonstrated that herbs helped to reduce postoperative complications and shortened the duration of the hospital stay.

The combined results of the various studies on cancer treatment and the use of Chinese herbs demonstrated that the study patients using herbal treatment during therapy more than doubled their five-year survival rate. The five-year survival rate tripled for the study patients who continued to receive herbal treatment for six months after chemotherapy or radiation.

that it was what I should do, but it's hard to be one hundred percent behind something that's so intense."

Dr. Glenn E. Miller has counseled many patients in preparation for chemotherapy treatments. The majority of chemotherapy agents are delivered into the bloodstream intravenously. Many believe that the experience in itself will be painful and potentially life threatening. A surprising number of patients have described their fears to Dr. Miller in almost exactly the same words: "The needle is going to go in and I'm going to feel the chemo going in like a burning poison. I'm going to feel it burning through my veins." In reality, because the drug has been hanging on the IV pole in the air-conditioned hospital room and is much colder than the bloodstream, patients end up reporting that the drug actually feels a bit cool as it goes in. There is no sense of the chemo agent coursing through their bodies. Knowing this to be true and easing a patient's fears are two entirely different things. Psychologically, the first treatment is usually the worst because the patient is scared to death of the unknown. In Jamie's case, she had the added stress of the conflict with her family regarding her choice of treatment. To make matters worse, she had not fully recovered from major surgery.

Jamie was scheduled for six chemotherapy treatments, three weeks apart. Her first treatment was on August 31, four weeks after her surgery. Given the severity and widespread nature of her particular cancer, a highly aggressive chemotherapy regimen was required. She was given a combination of carboplatin and Taxol, which are often used for ovarian cancer.

Chemotherapy agents are designed to seek out and destroy rapidly dividing cells by interfering with their division. The human body is in a constant cycle of breaking down and building up as cells die and are replaced by new cells. Through this regenerative cycle, all cells divide to make new cells. Some healthy cells divide more rapidly than others, but in a *controlled* manner. Cancer cells also divide more rapidly than healthy cells, but in an *uncontrolled* manner.

Unfortunately, chemotherapy drugs attack both cancer cells and normal cells indiscriminately, and the more rapidly dividing the cells (both healthy and malignant) the more affected they are by chemotherapeutic agents. Some of the healthy, normal cells in the body that are most affected by chemotherapy agents are located in the bone marrow, the lining of the gastrointestinal tract, the lining of the bladder and the hair follicles.

Bone marrow suppression poses the greatest threat to chemotherapy patients. Bone marrow produces white blood cells, which are vital to the body's natural defense against infection. When the level of white blood cells drops below a certain point, the immune system is weakened and infection can set in; consequently the patient may run a low-grade fever. Bone marrow suppression can also result in anemia, occasionally severe enough to require a blood transfusion.

The mouth and gastrointestinal tract are both lined with a protective layer of rapidly regenerating cells. Because the mouth and gastrointestinal tract are exposed to a variety of potent enzymes and acids excreted to break down food, these cells are the first line of defense, preventing the acids and enzymes from corroding through the underlying layers of tissue. The protective cells are regularly sloughed off and an underlying layer of cells advances to take their place. As these rapidly dividing cells are targeted by chemotherapeutic agents, when enzymes and acids are next released, the protective barrier has been greatly weakened. The acids and enzymes then erode the unprotected tissue. Patients may experience a burning sensation inside the mouth and throat and may develop painful multiple ulcerations inside the mouth, tongue and lips that make it hard to eat or sleep. These ulcerations can occur in the intestinal tract, causing digestive problems such as cramping and diarrhea. Since chemotherapy agents are often filtered through the kidneys and then the bladder—which is protected in the same way by a lining of rapidly dividing cells, which are constantly sloughing off—patients can suffer from cystitis (inflammation of the bladder).

A legitimate, and the most common, fear of those facing chemotherapy is the resulting nausea and vomiting. The human body is magnificently designed so that all of its functions serve a biological purpose. When a poisonous substance is introduced into the body, nausea and vomiting are the body's attempt to expel the toxin. Chemotherapy, essentially a corrosive and poisonous agent, is something the body tries to reject. In fact, vomiting occurs in approximately two-thirds of patients.

Because cells within hair follicles are rapidly dividing, they are also affected by chemotherapy agents. Therefore, most patients receiving chemotherapy drugs will lose most of their hair. The cells that generate the gelatinous material that forms fingernails and toenails are also rapidly producing and targeted by chemotherapy drugs. As a result, the patient's nails will often turn yellow.

In addition, many patients complain of hypersensitivity of the skin, hot flashes, tenderness, even lesions of the palms of the hands and the soles of the feet, making it painful to walk. All of these symptoms add up to profound weakness and fatigue and an overall lack of a sense of well-being. It is important to note, however, that everyone has a different tolerance level. Some people have severe side effects from chemotherapy, others sail through with very little discomfort.

After Jamie's first chemotherapy treatment, she immediately returned to Dr. Han to discuss her side effects, including fatigue, abdominal cramping, diarrhea, low-grade fever and nausea. Jamie's low-grade fever indicated that her white blood cell count had dropped. A key criterion to whether a patient can continue chemotherapy is how quickly the patient's white blood cell count comes back up. Dr. Han increased the potency of her herbal formula to strengthen her immune system, counteract bone marrow suppression and bring her white blood cell count up. He increased the herbs to address her gastrointestinal symptoms.

From then on, during the five-hour chemotherapy treatments, Jamie sipped the herbal medicine. "My doctors knew what I was doing. In fact, I took my herbal tea to the hospital and asked the nurses to heat it up in their microwave. It would stink up the whole floor and I would be sitting there drinking this stuff that looked like mud."

By using Chinese herbs along with her chemotherapy treatments, Jamie Ingersol had a very different experience. "I had a frame of reference because during the first treatment I wasn't really drinking that many herbs. Throughout the rest of the treatments, Dr. Han increased the amount of herbs I used and each treatment got easier. I got sick to my stomach after the first treatment. That was basically my only serious problem through the five months I went through chemo." Between treatments, Jamie's white blood count was monitored. "My white blood cell count was hopping back pretty quickly, and the doctors were happy with that."

The herbal tea did not prevent Jamie's luxurious mane of black hair from falling out. "It started about three weeks after my first chemo. I started cutting it then. I tried different styles as I was losing it. But after a while I could grab a handful and pull out a clump of hair. At that point, I said, 'Okay, let's get rid of it.' One of my sisters shaved my head. She did all these funny patterns on my head with the hair that was there, and it was kind of fun. Luckily, I have a good-shaped head. Everybody complimented me on it, so that was easier."

In October 1998, after three treatments, Jamie's chemotherapy was interrupted by a second surgery, initially intended as an exploratory laparoscopy, which is a less invasive surgical procedure in which a thin fiber-optic tube and probe are used. However, when the surgeon inserted the fiber-optic scope through the small incision, he ran into a honeycomb of scar tissue that prevented exploration. He had no other choice but to make a large incision. The surgeon biopsied Jamie's transverse colon, sigmoid colon, left and right ovaries, left pelvic area and small bowel. He removed approximately two inches of her small bowel, which was densely knotted with adhesions. He rinsed her pelvic organs with saline solution and collected that fluid for lab analysis.

This time Jamie woke up in recovery with a fresh vertical incision running all the way from her groin to two inches above her navel. The good news was that the pathology report showed no recurrence of cancer. After her second surgery, Jamie had three more chemotherapy treatments before she was declared in remission. Her last treatment was January 1999.

## Causes and Treatments for Cancer

"I was in great shape before this happened," Jamie said. "I swam and hiked and did something physical six out of seven days. I ate really well. I don't smoke or drink. I don't know what causes cancer, but I shouldn't have gotten it."

Many people believe that trying to be healthy by eating well, exercising and avoiding the factors we know cause cancer such as smoking and consuming processed foods, should protect us from acquiring diseases, particularly cancer. Reality, however, is harsh. Even when we do all the right things, cancer can still rear its ugly head.

Cancer rates have risen along with the accumulation of toxins in our food and environment. Lorne Feldman, M.D., founder of BIOS—B'shert Integrative Oncology Services—in Los Angeles, integrates Western medicine with complementary medicines in the treatment of cancer. Feldman is a four-time cancer survivor, having survived kidney cancer, non-Hodgkin's lymphoma and two kidney metastases. "I see the causes of cancer being one-third genetic base, one-third toxin exposure from either food or environmental toxins and another third tobacco related," Feldman said. "You can't do anything about your genes— you are born with them—but you can do something about the other exposures. We need to learn how to educate the population on the importance of a healthy lifestyle. My biggest fear is what will happen to our kids' generation who are weaned on fast food. When we grew up there weren't as many trips to fast-food restaurants. Now kids go there every day for lunch. The fast-food industry is currently coming under the same scrutiny as the tobacco industry. People are beginning to understand how fast food contributes to the development of disease and are questioning why it is so prevalent in our society."

The exact cause of cancer has evaded both Chinese and Western medicines. Both systems provide only partial answers. The Chinese medical view sees cancer as a continuous process that begins with a minor imbalance. If the balance of Qi is upset, there will be a slowing down of the Energy flow, which prevents toxins and metabolic waste from being sufficiently removed. This slowing down can evolve into stagnation if it is not corrected. The stagnation can then develop into a blockage of Qi. The blocked energy can become concentrated to form a mass. In the case of cancer, when the mass absorbs certain toxins, it can become malignant. Because of the nature of this process, active intervention can change the course of the development of this imbalance. Chinese medicine pays attention to the relationship between cancer and the entire body, particularly the condition of the immune system. Strengthening the immune system is pivotal in prevention, treatment and improving the quality of the patient's life.

On the other hand, Western medicine is making rapid progress in researching how cancer occurs on a subcellular and molecular level, which is providing a more detailed, clearer picture of the pathology. As a result of this research, more effective drugs are being developed to target cancer cells.

Increasingly, Western scientific research is being done on Chinese herbs.

Memorial Sloan-Kettering in New York and Dana-Farber Cancer Institute in Boston as well as a handful of other prominent cancer centers are now successfully treating a particularly virulent form of leukemia with intravenous arsenic trioxide. This drug is a purified version of a Chinese herbal decoction made from two types of ground rock and toad venom. Another Chinese herbal formula, known as PC SPES, has recently been shown, through multiple testing centers throughout the United States, to be effective in treating prostate cancer as well as lowering the prostate-specific antigen (PSA) level, which is often used as a prostate cancer marker.

As Dr. Luo's work demonstrated, Western and Chinese medicine's very different views of cancer can complement one another by providing a more complete picture of malignancy and a well-rounded treatment program. Cancer treatment is an excellent example of the effectiveness of Chinese herbal medicine in working alongside Western medicine to make certain medical treatments and drugs more effective and to ease Western drug-related side effects. Yet until recently only the brave and pioneering, like Jamie, knew how to access Chinese herbal medicine. Still, her situation was not a true integration of Chinese and Western medicines. In addition to finding herself in the untenable position of having to defend her choice of chemotherapy to her family, it was up to Jamie to seek out and use Chinese herbs on her own. A true integration would have been an active communication and collaboration from doctors on both sides throughout her diagnosis, treatment and recovery.

Today, more and more doctors in both Western and Chinese practices are willing to work together to maximize the benefits of medical treatments. As this becomes the norm, people in Jamie's situation will have a comprehensive and allied medical team that can ameliorate the pressures she went through.

In a second interview, it was apparent that Jamie had come to terms with many of the events surrounding her cancer. Her voice was pleasant and her laugh melodic. Except for regular blood tests, life has returned to normal, and she appears determined to put her ordeal behind her. She refocused her energies on her studies and took the exams she missed the previous summer; she was working as an intern at a Chinese medical clinic. Her hair was growing in beautifully. The short style was flattering, and she smiled as she tugged on it as if to prove that it was there to stay. "If I hadn't gotten cancer, there's a lot of things in my life that I wouldn't have dealt with," Jamie said. "I grew up in a spiritually oriented home. When I got sick, I decided that I could either be positive or I could feel sorry for myself and feel hopeless. I chose to believe that the cancer happened for a reason and that I could make use of the experience and learn from it. I was able to deal with a lot of issues in my life, and I think I am a happier person for it now."

Jamie has never discussed her chemotherapy with her parents. "We don't really talk about it. I think they are glad that it's over, and if I had to go through it again, they would probably still be against it. But if I had to do it all over again, I would do both chemotherapy and herbs. Ultimately, I think the ideal is like in China, where they have hospitals that integrate both Chinese and Western medicines. I had a choice to make. For me, they worked well together."

## Ways to Strengthen Your Immune System

### Focus on your spiritual connection

Focusing on your spiritual connection will assist you in combating the stress that accompanies a serious illness.

- This is an appropriate time to sever any stressful relationships.
- Practices that combine meditation, movement and deep breathing, such as Qigong, Tai Chi and yoga, boost the immune system and provide exercise without draining any of your vitality. See chapter 16 for ways to incorporate breathing and meditative practices.
- Get twenty minutes of sunshine every day to increase neurotransmitters in your brain, which will help you maintain an optimistic attitude.

### Protect yourself from further chemical exposure

Follow guidelines for environmental illnesses on page 167.

### Modify your diet

Eliminate white sugar and refined white flour products, which rapidly turn into sugar in your system. It is known that sugar can accelerate tumor growth.
Follow nutritional guidelines for environmental illnesses on pages 168–169.

### Quit caffeine, nicotine or other stimulant chemicals

Guidelines for quitting caffeine and nicotine can be found on pages 151–155. If you are a coffee drinker and do not want to give up the ritual entirely, you may choose to switch to green tea. Green tea is produced from the tea plant, *Camellia sinensis,* an evergreen shrub. Green tea contains polyphenols (catechins), which have been shown to lower cholesterol and improve lipid metabolism. They also possess anticancer, antioxidant, anti-inflammatory, antibiotic and antimicrobial properties. Considered a strong medicine, green tea has been part of the daily life of the Chinese for over four thousand years.

Other benefits of drinking green tea daily:

- Can act as a bronchodilator in people with asthma
- Prevents high blood pressure
- Protects your heart by lowering cholesterol and improving lipid metabolism—reduces the LDLs (bad cholesterol) and increases HDLs (good cholesterol)
- Reduces the development of bacteria growing in dental plaque
- Kills oral bacteria that cause bad breath
- Scavenges for free radicals that cause cellular damage, which can result in cancer
- Has antibacterial properties
- Slows accelerated aging
- Stimulates the production of saliva and reduces acids formed in the mouth
- Strengthens a weak immune system against common illnesses such as the flu, bronchitis or other infections
- In extract form, can lower blood sugar

Green tea contains caffeine and theophylline, which is a close relative to caffeine and is a stimulant. It is not advisable for non-caffeine drinkers to begin drinking green tea. However, if you are a caffeine drinker, green tea is an excellent alternative. Drink two to three cups of green tea a day instead of coffee. If you are not a coffee drinker, you can take 150 milligrams green tea extract per day, which contains 40 to 60 percent catechins.

Practice regular detoxification

Because detoxification can be hard on the body, you should follow the detoxification program on pages 291–296 with the supervision of your health care professional.

See a health care professional to be tested for food allergies
or dysbiosis

If you have cancer, you need a health care professional to work with you and
follow your healing progress. The goal is to optimize the function and decrease
the toxin load of every system of your body and to keep your intestines as
healthy as possible to optimize the absorption of nutrients.

Have your adrenal hormones tested, as depleted adrenals are a major contributing factor in lowered immunity. If you are extremely fatigued and suspect
you are suffering from adrenal burnout, a simple blood or saliva test can check
your cortisol and DHEA levels. If your cortisol is too high, with breakfast, lunch
and dinner take 100 milligrams phosphatidyleserine to help lower cortisol levels.

If you have been under chronic stress and are over forty, your adrenal glands
may have decreased DHEA production. DHEA is a balancing hormone to cortisol. It improves immunity, stimulates fat burning, improves energy and is reported to improve longevity, treat chronic fatigue and suppress autoimmune
diseases. DHEA must be taken in physiologic doses, which is an amount that
would be normal for your body to produce on its own. Pharmacological doses—
above what a human body would normally make on its own—could have serious side effects. *DHEA must be taken under the supervision of a doctor.*

Have your amino acid levels tested. If your body is not breaking down the
proteins you eat into amino acids, this can exacerbate fatigue and symptoms of
depression. Amino acid supplementation can boost your energy as well as supply your body with the necessary precursors to neurotransmitters. Routinely,
thirty to forty-five minutes before breakfast, lunch and dinner take 1,000 milligrams free-form amino acids.

Stool, hair and blood tests can determine if you have (1) high levels of accumulated heavy metals in your system, (2) sensitivities to foods or (3) dysbiosis,
which is an imbalance of the healthy and unhealthy bacteria and yeast in the gut,
any of which may be weakening your immune system and draining your energy.

See page 431 for a laboratory that can refer you to a health care provider in
your area who does these types of tests. If you test positive for any of these factors, your health care practitioner can treat you on an individual basis.

Modify your diet

The Chinese approach to cancer is to support the body so that it can combat cancer cells. One of the critical factors in the development of cancer is toxins; thus a detoxifying diet is recommended.

It is well documented that people who eat a plant-rich diet suffer lower rates of cancer. Western studies have shown that cruciferous vegetables guard against cancer by stimulating protective enzymes that detoxify and flush carcinogens out of the body and that deeply colored vegetables and fruits contain phytonutrients that provide vital nutrition and antioxidants that neutralize free radicals. Follow the nutritional guidelines for environmental illnesses on page 169. Chapter 21 provides medicinal recipes to treat cancer.

## Do not eat chicken skin

Chicken skin contains xenoestrogens—molecules that exert estrogenic influences on your body—which can stimulate the growth of certain cancers such as ovarian and breast cancer. It also contains an ingredient that accelerates mitosis—a stage of cell division—if that cell is abnormal. Avoid commercial chicken broth, which is processed using chicken skin. Be aware that restaurants often use chicken broth and order accordingly.

*Seaweed*: Most of the members of the seaweed family are excellent for reducing abnormal growths (benign or malignant), such as cancer, cystic tissue and fibroid tumors.

- *Agar.* Vegetarian "gelatin," gels at 100 degrees, sets at room temperature. Cooked with fruit juice and allowed to set, agar makes a delicious dessert.
- *Dulse.* High in iron, lysine and protein. Pleasant and pungent taste.
- *Hiziki.* Known as the "bearer of wealth and beauty," as it nourishes the hair and helps reduce dryness and split ends. Lubricates the intestines to promote elimination and is high in vitamins A and E and calcium (one tablespoon equals the calcium in one glass of milk).
- *Irish moss.* Beneficial to lung problems and reduces obesity. High in minerals. Usually used in tea form instead of with food.
- *Kombu.* The strongest seaweed medicinally. Balances the absorption of minerals, detoxifies, protects against degenerative diseases, aids in weight reduction, aids in recovery from radiation. Softens and shrinks nodules, masses or other abnormal growths.
- *Nori.* Less Cooling than the other seaweeds. High in minerals, vitamin A and the B vitamins.
- *Wakame.* Lowers blood pressure, activates blood circulation. In women, improves ovarian function, thus regulating sex hormones.

Seaweed (except Nori) must be soaked briefly before use (except when using in soup). After soaking, cook the seaweed for about 20 minutes or until tender. Eat seaweed two to three times per week for the greatest benefit.

Some of the health-giving properties of seaweed are:

- Clears Heat and detoxifies poisons
- Benefits the lymph system, thyroid and lungs
- Dissolves phlegm and hard masses
- Lowers cholesterol and body fat
- Provides many minerals for healthy hair, skin and nails
- Binds with toxic metals and eliminates them from your body
- Promotes urination

## Chinese herbs and Western supplements

You can take Chinese herbal formulas and Western supplements specifically formulated for cancer prevention, treatment and to take while undergoing chemotherapy and/or radiation. Formulas can be found online at ancientherbs modernmedicine.com.

# 13

## Hepatitis

*Degenerative and progressive diseases can be
treated with Chinese medicine*

Along an old frontage road to Las Vegas lies a nondescript, drive-by town
with run-down strip malls and gas stations. Here, Rosie Beauregard and her
mother, Brenda, share a trailer in a shadeless and neglected trailer park. The
first impression of Rosie is startling. A platinum blond with surprisingly clear
green eyes, at forty-three her face is childlike and innocent. However, Rosie is
terminally ill.

Rosie is completely dependent on her mother, who helps her out of bed on
the mornings she is able to rise. Rosie is suffering from hepatitis C, cirrhosis of
the liver, pancreatitis, an enlarged spleen and an inflamed gall bladder. She en-
dures chronic and acute abdominal pain, gastric reflux, a constant upset stomach, nausea, inability to keep food down, frequent nosebleeds, hypoglycemic
attacks and chronic constipation. She is carrying twenty pounds of fluid in her
abdominal cavity. Her torso is covered with an inflamed rash.

In 1991, at thirty-five years of age, Rosie was diagnosed with hepatitis C.
Until that time, she had been symptom free. Viral hepatitis is a systemic illness
that causes liver inflammation and liver cell necrosis (cell death). To date, seven
different types of viruses have been identified. According to the World Health
Organization (WHO), an estimated 500 million people worldwide are infected
by hepatitis viruses. In the United States, an estimated 4 to 4.5 million Americans carry the hepatitis C virus, with 150,000 to 180,000 new cases occurring
each year.

In the West, hepatitis C is the single most prevalent cause of liver cirrhosis and liver cancer. About 20 to 30 percent of hepatitis C patients will develop liver cirrhosis. Hepatitis C is the leading cause for liver transplantation in the United States, and liver transplantation is the only and final solution for cirrhosis and liver failure. A vaccine is not anticipated in the near future. Moreover, a vaccine cannot help those individuals who are already afflicted with the disease.

What makes hepatitis C particularly dangerous is its insidious nature. A high rate of individuals infected with the virus do not experience symptoms when they are first infected—or the symptoms are mistaken for the flu. HCV can evolve without symptoms for many years, while it causes permanent liver damage and ultimately liver failure or liver cancer.

Meanwhile, since many infected individuals do not engage in or expose themselves to known risk factors for infection, these individuals have no reason to suspect they are infected and the virus remains undetected and untreated. These individuals form an insidious pool of infection spreading the virus unaware.

Risk factors for hepatitis C include exposure to infected blood and blood products, intravenous drug abuse, unprotected sex with partners who have the virus and travel to endemic areas of hepatitis such as Africa, Asia, India, Mexico, Central and South America and the Middle East, where blood and water supplies are not properly monitored or maintained.

Rosie is not sure how she contracted hepatitis C, but her history reveals high-risk behaviors. "I married at fourteen," Rosie said. "I started drinkin' and doin' the stuff I was not supposed to do. We was livin' in North Carolina and my husband's business was over in the Bahamas. He was bringin' in tons of illegal cargo—coke and heroin." Rosie's husband served two seven-year terms for smuggling narcotics. After his first prison term, Rosie divorced him and remarried. That marriage ended in tragedy. "They blew my husband's brains out," Rosie said. She is not sure who "they" were; her first husband may have played a role. "After my second husband's death, I started drinking real heavily. It was constant, just drink, drink, drink. Then I started using heroin."

Among all reported acute hepatitis cases, about 43 percent are the result of intravenous drug use, including the practice of sharing needles. The risk of infection from a needle stick is approximately 10 percent. Since 1990, when screening for HCV in blood donors began, transfusion-related HCV infection has dropped. About 5 to 6 percent of HCV cases result from transmission from mother to fetus. Infection through sexual contact also occurs at a low rate.

Symptoms of HCV include enlarged and tender liver, jaundice, swollen lymph nodes, anorexia, fatigue, chronic headaches, neuralgic pain in a joint or joints, nausea and vomiting. Other diagnostic clues are clay-colored stools, dark or tea-colored urine, skin lesions and a marked aversion to tobacco smoke.

By March 1996, at age thirty-nine, Rosie was too sick to fend for herself. Her mother flew her from North Carolina and moved her into her trailer in Las Vegas. They began rounds to various doctors searching for a treatment plan that would help Rosie.

Western medicine has developed interferon therapy, which has been shown to be effective in treating 25 to 50 percent of HCV cases. Interferon is a naturally occurring substance that is produced by the immune system against infections. Interferon is synthesized from human cell cultures and administered in a dose that is much higher than naturally occurs in the human body. When synthesized interferon was first developed there were high hopes within the medical community. Recently, interferon has been altered molecularly to enhance the therapeutic effects. Despite the fact that interferon was initially hailed as a miracle drug, the side effects often are severe, including fever, muscle aches, rigors, depression, anxiety, insomnia, hypothyroidism, decrease in white blood cells and platelet count, hair loss, visual disturbances, headaches and weight loss. A significant number of patients relapse after completing the course of treatment. Many individuals cannot tolerate the side effects of interferon therapy and therefore cannot complete a course of treatment. These individuals often find that the cure is worse than the disease. In addition, there are also some individuals who complete a course of interferon therapy and whose blood work shows marked improvement but who continue to feel poorly.

There are a number of factors that exclude a person from interferon therapy, such as ongoing drug or alcohol use, the onset of cirrhosis of the liver or a history of psychiatric problems, particularly depression and suicide attempts. Rosie was excluded because of cirrhosis of the liver. She inquired about a liver transplant but was turned down. Because of the shortage of organs, those who have a history of drug or alcohol abuse or are currently on opiate-based pain killers are not eligible for liver transplants.

Her doctor did prescribe other drugs to treat her symptoms, including morphine in pill form. The drugs did little to alleviate Rosie's suffering or pain. Eight months after she moved in with her mother, upon the recommendation of a friend, Brenda packed Rosie into a car and drove to Santa Barbara to see Dr. Han. At that point, Rosie had been told by her Western doctors that she had only a few months to live.

## Chinese Medicine Does Not Consider Hepatitis to Be Simply a Liver Problem

Hepatitis involves multiple Energy systems. In the acute phase the primary Cause is Dampness. Causes can also involve Heat, some Blood stagnation and an External Toxin. As hepatitis evolves into a more chronic condition, the nature of the imbalance tends to shift from Dampness to Blood stagnation. As the general condition worsens and the immune system is weakened, deficiencies will inevitably set in.

A big part of Rosie's misery was her constant nausea and inability to keep anything down. Imbalanced Liver Energy compromises the liver's ability to regulate the Energetic movement of the digestive system. Rosie's Stomach Energy was backing up, causing her nausea, vomiting and constipation. (See the chart "The Interaction of Stomach, Spleen and Liver Energy to Regulate Digestion" on page 95.) In the meantime, her Spleen Energy was deficient, causing her bloating. Both of these factors interacted to prevent her from absorbing adequate nutrition and depleted her body's immune system's ability to fight her illness. Moreover, Rosie's constipation was so severe that the toxins that were supposed to be discharged from her body were accumulating in her system, putting even more stress on her liver.

Rosie's herbal formula was designed to counteract (suppress or cleanse) the virus and support her immune system, which was near depletion. In Chinese medicine this depleted immune state is often equivalent to Spleen, Liver or Kidney deficiency or a combination. The herbal formula was also designed to reduce the ascites (fluid accumulation in her abdominal cavity) and edema (the swelling in her legs), counteract the progression of the liver cirrhosis and soften her liver. The process of cirrhosis or scarring of the liver is a process of progressive Blood stagnation. Over the next several weeks, Rosie's liver enzymes normalized, her jaundice cleared, most of the fluid accumulation in her abdominal cavity cleared and her energy improved.

A standard prescription for one week consists of one bag of herbs per day. However, Rosie could not afford to continue to consume a bag of tea every day; instead, she stretched out a week's supply over one month. This diluted approach was not giving her the benefits she needed. Brenda and Rosie made several attempts to file claims with Medicare. "Whenever we filed a claim to get some help for the herbs it was denied, so I don't even bother to call our social worker anymore," Rosie said. Without continual, routine use of herbs, Rosie's health began to deteriorate. Her life was reduced to sleeping and watching church programs on TV. "When I die there'll be no more pain," Rosie said. "No more heartache. I'll be able to eat, eat, eat. But I'm scared. I don't want to die."

In the past those who were terminally ill were faced with accepting death as inevitable when they were told by their doctors that there was nothing more they could do. Chinese medicine has much to offer those afflicted with incurable and potentially fatal, chronic, degenerative and progressive diseases. The first step is to support and strengthen a person's innate restorative power so that the body can begin to heal itself.

Rosie was able to obtain financial assistance from a charitable source to resume Chinese herbal therapy. This time, Dr. Han formulated a concentrated herbal enema so that her body could have a better opportunity to absorb some of the herbs. Again she showed marked improvement in a very short period of time.

Rosie and her mother are devout Christians. They believe that Chinese medicine is the answer to their prayers. Throughout her illness, Rosie has remained faithful. "He is always with me, and I put myself in His hands. No matter how sick I get, I will never turn away from God. Chinese herbs were the answer to my prayers."

In the next ten to twenty years, the hepatitis C epidemic is likely to overwhelm the health care system of this country. Chinese herbal therapy can play a major role in the management of hepatitis C as well as other types of hepatitis. The effective rate of hepatitis C treatment by Chinese medicine herbal remedy has been shown in clinical trials to be 67 to 89 percent, with significantly fewer side effects than interferon therapy. Furthermore, it is important to note that Chinese herbal treatment can, to some extent, reverse cirrhotic change, which is considered irreversible by Western medicine.

## When Hepatitis Progresses to Liver Cancer

Art Jamison is like a seasoned fisherman who stoically recounts a story of a storm he once experienced. In a routine physical in September 1996, his lab report showed that his liver enzymes were elevated. A series of tests followed—an ultrasound, a CAT scan and finally a liver biopsy performed under anesthesia. Art, then forty-nine, and his devoted wife, Sally, celebrated their twenty-fifth wedding anniversary under a dark cloud waiting for the results. Art was diagnosed with liver cancer. There were three tumors.

The complexity of the liver's functions is second only to that of the brain's.

Almost the entire blood supply from the lower body flows through the liver to get to the heart. The liver is a large organ with a remarkable regenerative ability. As much as 75 percent of a liver can be removed and it will regenerate up to 95 percent within a few weeks. The most common course of action in liver cancer is to surgically remove the cancerous tissue. But Art's tumors were spread too diffusely throughout his liver to attempt surgery.

Art's only hope was a liver transplant. In October 1996, his doctor arranged for him to go through a three-day evaluation program at the UCLA Medical Center in Los Angeles. Art and Sally were relieved when he was accepted and placed on the liver transplant list. But this news came with an additional blow—Art had hepatitis C. The Jamisons tried to take comfort in the fact that Art would soon have a liver transplant. For the next eighteen months, Sally and Art were tethered to their beeper and remained within a two-hour travel distance to UCLA. While waiting for a liver, Art went through a rigorous course of chemotherapy. In June 1997, after nine months of weekly chemotherapy treatments, the Jamisons heard more brutal news. Despite the chemotherapy, Art's tumors had actually *increased* in size.

The next course of action was chemotherapy embolization. A needle or a long, narrow tube called a catheter is inserted into a major artery leading to the tumor. A large dose of a chemotherapy agent is delivered directly to the tumor site. The procedure is designed to minimize the overall impact on the patient's body. As the chemotherapy agent enters the vessels that feed the tumors, it creates a blockage or causes surrounding tissue to wither and die. The blood supply to the tumor will be diminished by the resulting scarring, effectively starving the tumor into regression. Under local anesthesia and sedation, a catheter was threaded up through Art's groin to reach the tumor sites in his liver. But two chemotherapy embolization treatments, one month apart, had no effect on the size of Art's tumors.

During eleven months of chemotherapy, Art had been called three times by the transplant coordinator alerting him to the pending arrival of a viable liver. All three calls turned out to be false alarms.

Art is a tall and lanky man who at six foot two had kept to a steady 175 pounds his entire adult life. He was now suffering from acute ascites—twenty pounds of accumulated fluid in his abdominal cavity. "It was an uncomfortable, hot feeling, having a belly like a tight drum," he said.

The liver, if sliced open, would look like a sponge full of blood vessels. These blood vessels, patterned like fishnets, can contract and relax to allow blood to flow. If the scarring of cirrhosis or a tumor is blocking the main blood vessels, it is like a blocked plumbing system. Blood leaks into the abdominal cavity, where there is room to expand, thereby causing ascites (fluid retention).

In August 1997 it had been one year since Art had gone in for a routine exam and had subsequently undergone chemotherapy. "I had absolutely no energy. I'd get up in the morning, barely make it downstairs to eat breakfast and then slowly climb the stairs and go back to bed to sleep another two hours." Chemotherapy and modern surgical skills had kept Art alive, and he was grateful. On the other hand, staying alive had come at a great cost. When their nutritionist suggested that Art see Dr. Han, the Jamisons did not hesitate.

Art's condition resulted from exposure to the External Cause hepatitis C virus. The medical conditions that resulted from this exposure had clearly affected his internal Energetic systems. Art was suffering from severe Kidney and Spleen deficiency. He also had significant Liver, Qi, Blood and Toxic stagnation. Moreover, Art had a glazed look that indicated that his Shen had been all but worn out.

Within two weeks of taking Chinese herbs, Art began to feel a flow of energy.

"I got a good sixty to seventy percent of my energy back within a month," he said. Three weeks after he began taking herbs, Art was on the beach, throwing a Frisbee. The herbs also resolved his fluid retention, and his weight normalized within two months. Repeated imaging studies demonstrated that his tumors were shrinking.

In March 1998, eighteen months after Art's initial diagnosis, the phone call came from the hospital that a viable liver was available. Art felt conflicted, knowing that the tumors were shrinking from the herbal medicine. He had been called three times before with the possibility of an available liver, but each time there was a problem and he could not have the liver transplant. It was like throwing a drowning person a lifeline and then pulling it away. Art just did not want to go through that again. To accept the liver transplant was a psychological insurance policy.

The liver transplant ward on the sixth floor of UCLA looks like a maternity ward. Both men and women have distended bellies from fluid retention. Art was the exception. "I was in such great shape at that point," he said. "My weight was normal, and I had very little water retention. During the operation the surgeons were able to forgo some of the procedures that they normally do during a transplant."

After Art's surgery, the pathology report of the liver that was removed from his body showed that two of the three tumors had calcified and died.

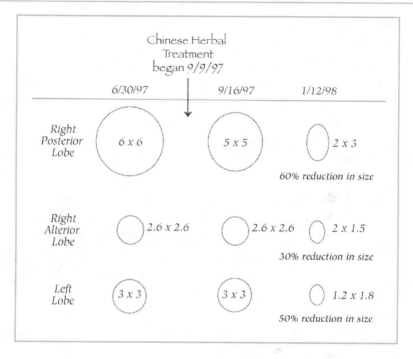

*Figure 22*

*The reduction in size of Art's tumors during the six months he used Chinese herbs (measurements in centimeters)*

As Art's story demonstrates, organ transplants are fraught with complex life-and-death decisions, emotional pressure and physical challenges. The development and advancement of antirejection drugs is the key for the success of transplants. At the same time, it is the best Western medicine can do, and every year thousands of people die waiting for liver transplants—there are simply not enough organs available.

Because of the integration of Chinese and Western medicines, at age fifty-four—five years after being diagnosed with liver cancer, three years after a liver transplant and beginning Chinese herbs—Art feels healthy and is living a normal life. He appears physically normal and strong and radiates strong Shen. "When we go to see Dr. Han, energy and quality of life are so important," Sally said. "Western doctors have only given us drugs to boost our energy. And you know it is only a temporary fix. Chinese herbs made the difference between life and death, and I really do believe that in my heart. Our experience has shown us that Chinese and Western medicine works effectively together. We'll use Chinese herbs for the rest of our lives."

Art will be on immunosuppressants for the rest of his life. Immunosuppressant drugs have certain problems associated with them. No matter how perfect the match, differences will exist between the donor of an organ and the recipient. It is therefore necessary to suppress the recipient's immune response in order to prevent it from recognizing and attacking the donor organ as a foreign invader. Without effective immunosuppression in the recipient, organ rejection is extremely likely. However, immunosuppressive therapy suppresses *all* immune responses, including those to virus, bacteria, fungi and even malignant tumors. Individuals who undergo significant immunosuppression are much more vulnerable to infection by pathogenic organisms that normally reside within our bodies. These organisms normally are kept well in check by our immune system and cause no particular problems. Suppressing the immune system can lead to significant medical problems, often requiring intensive intervention. This intensity of intervention can in itself further challenge the already weakened and highly stressed body.

Chinese herbs do not suppress the immune system but rather support the Energetic systems so that your body can find balance. In fact, there are a group of Chinese herbs that have immune-modulating and -regulating properties. These herbs do not simply enhance or suppress the immune system; they balance it depending upon the direction in which the immune system is out of balance. If the immune system is hyperactive, these herbs will down-regulate it back to a normal range. If it is weakened, these herbs will strengthen and support it back to this same normal range. For example, Cordyceps, an exotic mushroom, has traditionally been considered to be a strong Kidney tonic and has been successfully and widely used in China to treat post-kidney-transplant patients without the need for immunosuppressants.

## The Silver Bullet Versus the Enlightened Shotgun Approach

Western medicine often takes a silver bullet approach by targeting the clearly defined cause of the illness. Using hepatitis as an example, Western medicine will note the symptoms of fever, jaundice, elevated liver enzymes, nausea and vomiting and sometimes take a liver biopsy to make the appropriate diagnosis of hepatitis. When it comes to the treatment, the silver bullet would be interferon to target the virus, which is considered to be the root cause of hepatitis. If this silver bullet (interferon) hits a bull's-eye—in that it is completely effective in treating the underlying hepatitis C virus—then the signs and symptoms may go away. If, however, it misses the bull's-eye just a little, then the patient continues to suffer symptoms.

When you know the exact cause of a disease and have the effective means to target it, then the silver bullet approach can be highly effective. If the cause of a disease is not clearly defined—such as the later stages of hepatitis C, when the nature of the disease has somewhat changed—then the silver bullet approach may be futile. Toward the later stages of hepatitis C there is not just inflammation of liver cells, there is also extensive scarring of the liver, and the patient's immune system is imbalanced. In other words, the target has expanded to such a large degree that a shotgun is necessary to try to cover all the various areas of the disease. Chinese medicine takes an enlightened shotgun approach by targeting many factors that are involved in the various stages and aspects of the disease.

Chinese medicine's approach to treatment does not require the same levels of accuracy as Western medicine. The enlightened shotgun approach will often effectively defuse the disease by interrupting its negative impact on a number of systems. What is diagnosed and treated by Chinese medicine is often not the disease itself, but rather a disease state, which reflects the interactions of the disease and the human body in its entirety. Chinese medicine's treatment is designed to correct, or reharmonize, this imbalanced state. By effectively rebalancing the body, one is able to effectively treat the disease state without necessarily having to focus on eradicating the exact causative factor itself. For example, liver cancer, hepatitis, chronic fatigue, migraine headaches and other conditions can all produce a particular pattern of Energetic disharmony such as Liver Yin deficiency. Thousands of years ago, Chinese medicine developed methods to effectively correct Liver Yin deficiency and rebalance the system. Chinese medicine is able to treat this disorder without needing to exactly identify the underlying causative factor(s).

## Treatment with Minimum Side Effects

By focusing on the specific cause/infection/disease, Western medicine will often be able to eradicate a disorder, but will often produce side effects. Hepatitis C can demonstrate many patterns of disharmony such as Dampness disharmony, Blood stagnation, Toxic stagnation, Spleen, Kidney or Liver Energy deficiency, or Qi, Blood or Yin deficiency, or a combination of any of these. By differentiating these various types of disharmonies and addressing each of them specifically, Chinese medicine is able to tune in the finer points of the disease state and often achieve a better and more comprehensive therapeutic result with minimal or no side effects.

## Ways to Improve Your Immune System If You Are Diagnosed with Hepatitis C

### Focus on your spiritual connection

"During everything I went through I realized that I could die," Art said. "I had to ask myself if my life was in order. Aside from making sure that my family was taken care of, I wanted to make sure that I was at peace and that I had done everything that was necessary without feeling regrets. I read the *Tibetan Book of the Dead* and I realized that there is life after death and that there was nothing to be afraid of. After my surgery I practiced visualization. If you have fear going into a disease like this, you can't conquer it. I had to embrace it and work with it. I did a lot of visualization. I imagined I had a quilt, and every square was a picture of a friend or family member. This gave me the higher power to let the transplant take hold."

"While we were going through this, we would meet other people in trying situations and increasingly we realized that we are all interconnected," Sally said. "It was such a life-altering experience. We now go to comfort people who are dying and feel no hesitation. We can embrace and give comfort to people in such a different way. We are all interconnected and there for each other."

Stress reduction and addressing unresolved emotional issues are crucial. Consider seeing a therapist or finding an instructor who specializes in relaxation and visualization. Regular moderate exercise such as restorative yoga, gentle walking and activities that result in a calm, relaxed state are beneficial and can help you explore your spiritual path.

Make a practice of listening to relaxation tapes, especially before rest times and bedtime. See chapter 16 for more on your spiritual connection.

### Make rest a priority

Proper rest is an absolute necessity for chronic hepatitis C patients in order to assist the restorative process of healing. According to Chinese medicine, overexertion or lack of rest can tax Liver Energy.

Protect yourself from further chemical exposure

Follow the guidelines for environmental illnesses starting on page 166.

Modify your diet

Follow the guidelines for environmental illnesses starting on page 166. Avoid coffee, greasy foods, alcohol, sugar, refined white flour and processed foods. Toxic residues in foods are damaging to your liver, so eating organic foods is especially important. Avoid trans fatty acids (margarine, fried foods, fast foods). Include essential fatty acid supplements in your diet, or eat foods high in essential fatty acids such as fatty fish (tuna, salmon, mackerel, herring, sardines), leafy greens and whole grains.

Quit caffeine, nicotine or other stimulants

Follow the guidelines for raising serotonin levels to quit addictions on pages 151–155.

Practice detoxification under the guidance of a health care practitioner

Detoxification can be hard on the body. Under the supervision of a medical professional, you may follow the guidelines for detoxification for environmental illnesses on pages 291–296. Increase water intake to eight to ten eight-ounce glasses of water per day.

Chinese herbs and Western supplements

The hepatitis A virus is contracted through fecal contamination of food or water. Roughly 200,000 people in the United States are infected each year. Hepatitis A infection usually resolves in time and, according to Western medicine, needs no treatment. Taking Chinese herbs can shorten recovery time and increase your sense of well-being during your recovery.

The hepatitis B virus is transmitted by exposure to infected blood (via transfusions or needle sticks) or through intimate contact with an infected partner. In the United States about 250,000 new cases occur annually, and 0.2 to 0.4 percent of the population is chronically infected. The hepatitis B virus is the leading cause of hepatitis worldwide. A substantial number of cases of hepatitis

B become chronic. The prognosis for this form is generally better than for hepatitis C. In addition, there has been a vaccination in use for hepatitis B for over ten years. Chinese medicine is generally effective in treating hepatitis B by reducing liver cell inflammation and suppressing the viral activities.

You can use Chinese medicinal herbs in recipes to boost your immune system. See chapter 21 for recipes. You can also take Chinese herbal formulas and Western supplements specifically formulated to treat hepatitis A, B and C. Formulas can be purchased online at ancientherbsmodernmedicine.com.

# 14

# Treating Degenerative and Progressive Diseases

*Heart disease, type II diabetes, arthritis and osteoporosis*

Reviewing every degenerative disease would fill volumes, so only a few common conditions are covered in this chapter. No matter what your condition, supporting your immune system is pivotal in treating degenerative disease. An immune-modulating formula is discussed on pages 103–104.

In addition to taking this formula, find a health care professional who can test you for food allergies and dysbiosis. Stool, hair and blood tests can determine if you have (1) high levels of accumulated heavy metals in your system, (2) sensitivities to foods or (3) dysbiosis, which is an imbalance of the healthy and unhealthy bacteria and yeast in the gut, any of which may be weakening your immune system and draining your energy. See page 431 for a laboratory that can refer you to a health care provider in your area who does these types of tests. If you test positive for any of these factors, your health care practitioner can treat you on an individual basis.

In potentially life-threatening situations or when one is seriously ill, however, herbal formulas must be prescribed by a trained and experienced herbalist. To maximize the benefits of your treatment, your herbalist and Western physician should collaborate and communicate throughout the course of your treatment. If you are taking Western drugs, always tell your herbalist what medications you are taking. Likewise, always tell your Western M.D. if you are taking Chinese herbs. Resources on pages 423–431 will help you find a Chinese herbalist to treat you on an individual basis.

You can find patent formulas at your local Chinese herbal clinic or online at ancientherbsmodernmedicine.com. Patent formulas may be used to fill in the gap between the times when you can consult a doctor, or if a doctor is not available in your area.

## Heart Disease

Some people are born with a genetic predisposition to heart disease, but this does not automatically mean that you are doomed. If you are prone to cardiovascular disease because your parents died of a heart attack, but you eat well, do not smoke or use stimulants, if you exercise and deal with your stress, your chances of developing heart disease will be dramatically reduced. Examine the habits you may have learned in your family and take responsibility for the state of your own health. Become an active participant rather than a passive recipient in your health by eliminating the habits that can exacerbate any genetic predisposition you may have to disease.

From a Chinese medicine perspective, life itself can be seen as a giant cycle of Energy fluctuation. Most of us are born with certain constitutional imbalances. The imbalance itself does not mean that we are necessarily going to have problems. These constitutional traits and differences define each person's uniqueness. It is part of who you are as an individual. The imbalances you are born with represent a tendency and play a major role in determining the direction in which your health will evolve as you go through life. The key is to reduce or counterbalance your original imbalances instead of aggravating them, by living a lifestyle that is compatible with your constitutional traits. If you do this, you can maximize your health potential.

### See a health care professional to have homocysteine levels checked

Deficiencies of B vitamins in the diet—folic acid, vitamin $B_6$ and vitamin $B_{12}$—raise the level of homocysteine in the bloodstream. Homocysteine is an amino acid that, when elevated in the blood, has been found to cause arterial damage and plaque. You can reduce your risk by eating foods rich in B vitamins or by taking supplements.

- *Folic acid (folacin):* brewer's yeast, oranges, green leafy vegetables, wheat germ, asparagus, broccoli, nuts
- *Vitamin $B_6$ (pyridoxine):* whole grains, meats, fish, poultry, nuts, brewer's yeast.
- *Vitamin $B_{12}$ (cobalamin):* meat, fish, poultry, eggs, dairy products

Focus on stress management

Follow the guidelines for breathing and movement practices in chapter 16.

Modify your diet

Carbohydrates rapidly turn into sugar in the system and increase the secretion of the hormone insulin. Prolonged high levels of insulin dramatically increase the damage to blood vessels, which results in heart disease. You can regulate your insulin levels by eating regular meals to avoid dramatic blood sugar fluctuations, avoiding sugar and high carbohydrate consumption and eating a balanced diet of real, whole foods. See pages 431–433 for referrals for further reading about balanced diets.

*The Role of Fats in Your Diet:* In 1900, heart disease was rare in the United States. Between 1920 and 1960 the incidence of heart disease rose to become the number one killer in the country. During this time butter consumption fell from eighteen pounds per person per year to four pounds per person per year. Food manufacturers began pushing cheaper processed oils such as margarine and corn oil and other processed foods such as corn flakes. Manufacturers continued influencing the public until Americans' diets consisted primarily of processed foods.

A balanced diet of real, whole foods is the answer to heart disease prevention. Butter and eggs have always been part of a balanced diet. Butter is the most easily absorbed source of vitamin A, which protects you from heart disease. Vitamin A is necessary for thyroid and adrenal gland health—both of which play a role in maintaining the proper functioning of the heart and cardiovascular system. Butter contains lecithin, which assists in the proper assimilation and metabolism of cholesterol and other fat constituents. Butter contains antioxidants such as vitamin A, vitamin E and selenium, which protect against free radicals that damage arteries.

Hydrogenated vegetable oils containing trans fatty acids, such as margarine, shortening and polyunsaturated vegetable oils, which have been transformed from their natural state by heat and chemicals, have been shown to be a major cause of heart disease. For heart health, eat naturally occurring fats and oils and include essential fatty acids (omega-3 and omega-6) in your diet.

*Sources of Omega-3*

| | |
|---|---|
| Chia seeds | Salmon oil |
| Fish oil | Sardine oil |
| Flaxseed oil | Sea algae (spirulina) |
| Hemp oil | Tuna fish |
| Mackerel oil | Walnuts and walnut oil |
| Pumpkin oil | |

*Sources of Omega-6*

| | |
|---|---|
| Butter | Meat |
| Cream | Pumpkin oil |
| Eggs | Safflower oil |
| Fish oil | Sunflower oil |
| Flaxseed oil | Turkey |
| Fowl | Walnuts and walnut oil |
| Grape seed oil | Wheat germ oil |
| Hemp oil | |

**Lose weight**

See chapter 19 for more on weight loss.

**Quit caffeine, nicotine or other stimulants**

Follow the guidelines for raising serotonin levels to quit addictions on pages 148–155.

**Chinese herbs and Western supplements**

You can use Chinese medicinal herbs in recipes for heart health. See chapter 21 for recipes. You can also take Chinese herbal formulas and Western supplements specifically formulated for heart disease.

# Type II Diabetes

Type I diabetes, known as insulin-dependent diabetes mellitus (IDDM), accounts for approximately 10 percent of all diabetes cases, while type II, known as non-insulin-dependent diabetes mellitus (NIDDM), is estimated at over fourteen million cases (90 percent of diabetes cases). Diabetes is generally classified as type I if an individual's pancreas does not secrete insulin. Type II is associated with insulin resistance or abnormal insulin secretion, resulting in obesity. It is believed that more than half of those suffering from type II diabetes have little or no symptoms and often are undiagnosed. Ninety-eight percent of adult-onset diabetes is diet related. You can take steps to avoid diabetes and to reverse insulin resistance (explained on pages 296–299), which leads to type II diabetes. Because the progression from healthy to insulin-resistant to type II diabetes is part of accelerated aging—which is a factor that affects everyone in varying degrees—you will find more on this subject in chapter 19 on antiaging.

## See a health care practitioner to have your adrenal functions checked

High cortisol levels could be driving your sugar up and exacerbating insulin resistance. Cortisol is a stress hormone that is released in response to chronic/long-term stress. One of cortisol's jobs is to mobilize blood sugar as energy for your body to use to deal with the stress. It does this, in part, by breaking down muscle and bone mass into amino acids that are converted into sugar. Insulin will be secreted in reaction to this incoming sugar in your bloodstream, and blood sugar levels will fall. If you are constantly stressed, the dual actions of cortisol and insulin will cause your blood sugar levels to rise and crash throughout the day. Taking 100 milligrams of phosphatidyleserine—available in health food stores—three times a day, with meals, can reduce cortisol levels and thereby decrease frequent blood sugar crashes.

## Focus on stress management

Follow the guidelines for breathing/movement practices in chapter 16. Regular walking lowers stress—and insulin levels.

## Modify your diet

High insulin levels are generally accompanied by high total cholesterol levels. Use monounsaturated fats in your diet. Monounsaturated fats raise HDLs—the good cholesterol. When purchasing oils, always make sure you buy pure cold- or expeller-pressed oils. These oils have not been damaged in the refining process. Oils processed with heat are damaged and in turn will damage your cells, which will contribute to ill health.

*Monounsaturated Fats*

| *Eat at room temperature (do not heat)* | *You may cook with these fats* |
|---|---|
| Almond oil | Extra-virgin olive oil |
| Apricot kernel oil | Safflower oil |
| Avocado oil | Sunflower oil |
| Black currant oil | |
| Grape seed oil | |
| Hazelnut oil | |
| Mustard oil | |
| Oat oil | |
| Rice bran oil | |
| Sesame oil | |

In addition, Energetically Warm and Hot foods are good for type II diabetes if the patient does not have an overly Warm constitution or underlying Yin deficiency. Sulfur, contained in garlic and onions, is thought to lower insulin levels. Cinnamon, cloves and bay leaves have been shown in studies by the U.S. Department of Agriculture's Vitamin and Mineral Laboratory to triple insulin's ability to metabolize sugar and remove it from the bloodstream.

For those with Warm constitutions or Yin deficiency, foods such as asparagus, mung beans, kudzu root, white wood ear mushroom and pumpkin are good.

## Quit caffeine, nicotine and other stimulants

The use of stimulants increases levels of the stress hormone cortisol, which drives up insulin levels. To quit using stimulants, follow the guidelines on pages 148–155.

## Chinese herbs and Western supplements

You can use Chinese medicinal herbs in recipes to balance insulin and blood sugar levels. See chapter 21 for recipes. You can also take Chinese herbal formulas and Western supplements specifically formulated for type II diabetes.

As previously noted, the vast majority of Western pharmaceuticals are uni-directional in their effect—they either raise or lower a biological factor such as blood pressure, blood glucose level or thyroid function level. In contrast, many of the Chinese herbs are bidirectional, meaning that they regulate biological factors. If blood sugar is too low, a specific herb can raise it to within normal levels. If it is too high that same herb can lower it to within normal levels. For example, in the treatment of diabetes, blood sugar regulators raise blood sugar levels of individuals with symptoms of hypoglycemia, and will lower the blood sugar levels of individuals with diabetes.

## Arthritis

Arthritis is one of the oldest and most common disorders that afflict hu-mankind. It is an inflammation of the joint(s) that creates pain, swelling and potential structural damage. From a Chinese medicine perspective, arthritis is a result of invasion of the External Causes Wind, Cold, Damp, Heat and Toxins. It is also closely associated with the disharmony of Kidney, Spleen and Liver En-ergetic systems. At a certain stage of the illness, there can also be Blood and Phlegm stagnation involved. Generally in the earlier stages of the disease the External Causes are more pronounced and dominant. As the disease extends into the later stages, the deficiencies of Kidney, Liver and Spleen start to set in. Certain types of arthritis, such as rheumatoid and osteoarthritis, that are char-acterized by pronounced bone/cartilage destruction are treated with strong emphasis on Kidney Energy. Kidney Energy is responsible for the function and structure of bones. Even though rheumatoid arthritis and osteoarthritis are two distinctively different diseases by Western medical diagnosis, they can be treated with the same strategy as they display the same disharmony—Kidney Energy imbalance.

### Modify your diet

Decrease consumption of tomatoes, potatoes, bell peppers and eggplant, which can cause inflammation. If you do not see any change within one month, you may resume eating these foods.

Ginger reduces inflammatory chemicals called eicosanoids. In clinical stud-ies ginger has been shown to provide better relief of pain, swelling and stiffness than the administration of nonsteroidal anti-inflammatory drugs.

Make regular moderate exercise part of your lifestyle

Exercise can elevate cortisol levels, which causes anti-inflammatory responses. Regular, moderate exercise helps maintain flexibility and movement in your joints and can help you maintain a normal weight to reduce the amount of pressure on your joints. To avoid stressing your joints, do not overexercise.

The ROM-Dance program is endorsed by the Arthritis Foundation, doctors and therapists to help keep joints flexible, promote a general sense of relaxation and reduce pain and limitations. ROM-Dance (range-of-motion exercises combined with the basic principles of Tai Chi) is a unique exercise and relaxation training program for people with pain and other physical limitations. ROM-Dance takes a few minutes a day to perform and is gentle enough for nearly everyone, including individuals in wheelchairs.

Practice regular detoxification

Detoxification can calm your system and reduce inflammation. Detox under the supervision of your health care practitioner. Follow the guidelines for environmental illnesses starting on page 166.

Chinese herbs and Western supplements

If you suffer from digestive discomfort, routinely, before and after each meal, take the digestive formulas on page 102.

You can use Chinese medicinal herbs in recipes to treat the symptoms of arthritis. See chapter 21 for recipes. You can also take Chinese herbal formulas and Western supplements specifically formulated for arthritis.

## Osteoporosis

Osteoporosis is a degenerative disorder resulting from the loss of minerals, particularly calcium, from the structural matrix of the bones. From a Chinese medicine point of view it usually has much to do with the state of Kidney Energy. Kidney Energy not only helps the body to hold on to various minerals, but also helps to absorb and reabsorb these minerals.

See a health care professional to have your hormone balances checked

Progesterone builds bones, and estrogen keeps your bones dense. If you are a woman and your hormones are imbalanced, you are more likely to be losing bone mass. See a hormone expert for hormone balancing. Ask to have your adrenal function checked. High cortisol levels and low DHEA can cause bone loss.

Modify your diet

Get calcium from almonds, kale and parsley. Protein is critical for bone formation. When your blood is acidic, more calcium, which is alkaline, is taken from your bones to neutralize the acidity. Eat protein at every meal and increase your consumption of alkaline foods. Avoid refined foods, caffeine and sugar, which are acid forming, and eat fruits and vegetables, which are alkalinizing.

Make regular moderate exercise part of your lifestyle

Weight-bearing exercise such as walking, yoga and weight training has been shown to increase bone mass.

Get at least half an hour of sun exposure every day

Exposure to sun helps activate vitamin D in the body, which helps to improve calcium absorption in the digestive tract.

Chinese herbs and Western supplements

Minerals need an acid environment in the stomach to be absorbed. Do not take Tums, as it is not an absorbable form of calcium. Tums blocks your stomach's acid production, which is essential for the absorption of the calcium you need to build bone, nails and hair. Instead, routinely, after each meal take 600 to 1,200 milligrams betaine hydrochloride, depending on the size of your meal. If you feel a warm, burning sensation in your stomach, drink an eight-ounce glass of water and discontinue the use of betaine hydrochloride.

You can use Chinese medicinal herbs in recipes to build strong bones. See chapter 21 for recipes. You can also take Chinese herbal formulas and Western supplements specifically formulated for osteoporosis.

# 15

## HIV

*Chinese medicine seeks to treat disease without side effects*

It was the life most of us only glimpse in gossip magazines: the charismatic producer with dark movie-star good looks and magnetic smile, under contract with a major studio, living in a beautiful home in the Hollywood hills with Tinseltown sprawling at his feet. In 1986, thirty-three-year-old Brandon Elliot had it all. He had a glamorous social life. He had maintained the physical edge he had cultivated in college as a competitive swimmer. An accomplished equestrian, he owned and trained Thoroughbred horses. Competing in horse shows was a focal point in his life.

Then he was diagnosed with the human immunodeficiency virus—known simply by its acronym, HIV—which causes acquired immune deficiency syndrome, or AIDS. A virus is a minute parasitic organism that is incapable of growth and reproduction apart from living cells. In simplified terms, HIV invades a type of cell called T cells, which are part of the immune system. Once inside the T cell, the HIV virus infiltrates the cell's ribonucleic acid (RNA), which controls protein production in all cells. The HIV virus is able to convert the RNA into its own DNA—an acid that carries genetic information. In addition, the HIV virus replicates within the cell. As more T cells are invaded and more HIV virus is replicated, the T cell count falls. The immune system is weakened and eventually destroyed.

Stephen Hosea, M.D., is in private practice in Santa Barbara, specializing in infectious diseases.[5] Dr. Hosea said, "I like to think of the helper cells like the

---

5. Stephen W. Hosea, M.D., is the medical director for the department of infection control and the assistant academic chief of medicine at the Santa Barbara Cottage Hospital, professor of medicine at the USC School of Medicine, the director of the AIDS clinic for Santa Barbara Health Care Services and medical advisor for the Visiting Nurse and Hospice Care of Santa Barbara, Inc., board of directors.

conductor of the orchestra. The conductor tells the other cells that are in the orchestra what to do, resulting in a symphonic immune system. When the conductors aren't there, it's just noise and none of the other cells know what to do. They can't work together to create an effective front to fight off infections."

The Centers for Disease Control and Prevention developed a system of categorizing the progression of HIV to AIDS:

1. *Primary infection.* Symptoms of the primary infection start approximately two to four weeks after exposure. The illness is acute and lasts for about one to three weeks. There may be signs of an acute nonspecific viral infection with fever, malaise, rash, joint pain, sore throat, swollen lymph nodes and headache.

2. *Chronic phase.* Patients convert to HIV-positive, which is marked by the absence of the signs and symptoms just described. For the majority of individuals this chronic phase can last anywhere from seven to ten years. There are always exceptions—people who convert from the primary infection to the chronic phase in six months and then rapidly to full-blown AIDS—but typically the chronic phase lasts for years while the virus causes the destruction of more and more T cells and replicates more HIV. This results in a progressive loss of immune function.

3. *Full-blown AIDS phase.* When a syndrome of opportunistic infections occurs—such as thrush (a fungal infection of the mouth or vagina), herpes simplex (a viral infection of the mouth, genitals or anus) or Kaposi's sarcoma (a skin malignancy)—a person is considered to have AIDS.

When Brandon was diagnosed with the HIV virus, he assumed he would be just another statistic in an epidemic of inexplicable, acute suffering and swift death that was sweeping the globe. His physician wanted to put him on AZT, which had just come out. AZT belongs to a class of drugs called protease inhibitors, which are designed to lower the amount of HIV in the body—referred to as the viral load—thus increasing the number of functional disease-fighting T cells. Brandon flatly refused. Instead of going on AZT, Brandon took steps to clean up his lifestyle, eliminating caffeine, alcohol, processed foods, recreational drugs and other toxins. He ate only organic foods, avoided stress and got more rest.

Eight years later, at forty-one years of age, Brandon was at the height of his career. He was nominated for producer of the year by the Producers Guild. A Hallmark television movie he had produced that year received five Emmy nominations and won three. Despite being HIV-positive, Brandon's future seemed paved with gold. Physically he had never felt stronger. He was running, lifting weights and swimming. He was feeling somewhat impervious to the HIV virus. But the turning point would come suddenly and without warning. "I had intentionally lost ten pounds of fat. I was what they call 'ripped,' " he said. "One day at the gym, I looked at myself and thought, 'You know, I really do look incredible.' In fact, I was in such great shape that I thought I'd start training for a triathlon. The very next day I collapsed and couldn't get out of bed. I knew my T cells were dropping, but I never thought that in twenty-four hours the virus would take over my whole being."

In an industry where heterosexual marriage is an essential component to image, and where movie stars and studio executives enter into marriages as arrangements to create an acceptable persona, being gay was one strike; being gay with HIV was anathema. For the next four months Brandon worked at home and lay low in an attempt to hide his illness from his associates at the studio. When a new studio head was hired, Brandon was called in for a face-to-face meeting that he could not avoid. By then he was deathly pale and had begun to lose muscle mass. "I borrowed some makeup from my mother and tried to make myself look healthier," Brandon said. "She drove me there and waited while I went in for the meeting. I thought I did okay and that I had gotten away with it. But after that, everyone knew."

Brandon managed to hang on until his contract ran out at the end of the year. But he could not continue the pretense any longer. His hair had begun to thin. The gum tissue around his teeth had receded, exposing the roots, and he had to have eight molars pulled. He had lost all control over his life. "The effects of the virus kept gathering like moss on a stone," Brandon said. "Once I was headed downhill this illness kept getting bigger and bigger and faster and faster until it rolled over me." He knew that when the disease went into full swing nothing could stop it. Instead of renegotiating his studio contract, Brandon did his best to put on a brave front, explaining that he had been there long enough and that it was time to move on.

Brandon's immune system had begun to fail. He remained in a self-imposed solitary confinement in his Hollywood hills home for several months. His horses languished in their stalls. He had no energy to devote to his dogs. In the spring, his attorney helped him move to Santa Barbara, a resort town 150 miles north of Los Angeles. Brandon settled into a cottage where his horses were corralled right off his bedroom, his dogs were at his side and he had a view of the ocean. His focus shifted to finding good homes for his animals while he steeled himself for imminent death. But he was terrified.

One month after moving to Santa Barbara, Brandon awoke with an intense headache. Slick with perspiration, his heart racing wildly, he crawled on his hands and knees out to his car, then drove himself to the nearest hospital emergency room, where he was diagnosed with meningitis and admitted to the hospital. Dr. Hosea, Brandon's attending physician, started him on antiviral medications and explained that after they cleared up the infection, he wanted to start him on the "cocktail"—the colloquial term for a combination of three or more HIV drugs that work in concert to lower a patient's viral load with the least amount of toxicity.

According to Dr. Hosea, the newer drugs were much less toxic than AZT alone, and the cocktail had proven to be more effective in prolonging life while preserving the best quality of life: "The virus replicates so quickly that it can become resistant to a single drug. It is more difficult for the virus to become resistant to three drugs." The object of the cocktail was to slow down the replication of HIV so that the T cells, which are constantly replicating, could build back up, which correspondingly builds up the immune system. There is much evidence to support the use of these drugs. "I have seen a fair number of patients who had close to zero T cells but who now have normal numbers of T cells because the drugs have successfully suppressed the virus," Dr. Hosea said.

Brandon did not go on the cocktail at that time, but went home from the hospital to recover from meningitis. He returned two weeks later, this time by ambulance, struggling to breathe and running a temperature of 105. He had developed *Pneumocystis carinii* pneumonia, one of the dreaded diseases of HIV. Brandon was given an anti-inflammatory drug and prednisone, a synthetic steroid, to treat the complications of pneumonia.

Though his fever came down, Brandon had severe side effects from the prednisone. "My tongue split open from a reaction to the prednisone. So that I could eat, I had to use this glue stuff [which was denture paste laced with cortisone] that I'd squirt on the split on my tongue that would keep it sealed for an hour so I could get food down." He soon found that he could not discontinue the use of prednisone without suffering from severe muscle ache, chills and fever. "There were times when I had to be held down, I was convulsing so violently. It was like having an exorcism." But nothing else could be done to keep his fever below 105 degrees, and he was forced to keep taking prednisone.

Dr. Hosea is a spiritually minded, empathic man who is committed to helping the terminally ill and dying. Brandon's confidence in Dr. Hosea combined with a feeling of having nothing left to lose gave him the incentive to agree to go on a cocktail of Crixovan, AZT and 3TC in November 1996.

Eight months into his treatment on the cocktail, Brandon had a realization that was to be a turning point. "When you're so traumatized, your mind shuts down. You're just not aware of anything. One day I was having a moment of clarity and looked at myself. There was no doubt that the virus had affected me, but the drugs had completely destroyed any health or vitality I had left. The insides of my cheeks were ripped open as if someone had taken razor blades to the flesh. I had a quarter-sized hole in the back of my throat. My jaw was swollen on one side to the size of half a baseball. I had gone from having a muscular body to cellulite. My waist had gone from a thirty-one to thirty-eight inches, so I looked pregnant. My eyes were sunken and swollen. My hair was falling out in clumps. My skin was itchy and scaly. If I scratched, the bumps would bleed and spread, like leprosy."

The youthful, athletic and dynamic film producer Brandon had once been was a dim memory, replaced with a depressed, ravaged man who had barely the energy to navigate the triangle from his bed to the bathroom and the living room. It was true that his T cell count was improving and that the drugs were saving his life. But it was not enough. "I started contemplating suicide," Brandon said. "I just didn't have the energy or the gusto anymore to live."

## A Combined Treatment Plan of Western Drugs and Chinese Herbs

While Dr. Hosea has seen firsthand the benefits of HIV drugs, he is realistic. "One of the problems with the AIDS drugs is that they get approved soon after they show any efficacy, before we understand the toxicities associated with them." One of the fundamental problems with many Western drugs is the side effects. Although Western pharmaceuticals developed from herbology, as Western medicine became more focused on technology it became less concerned with side effects. Since World War II, more drugs have been made by chemical synthesis—they are chemical imitations of plant medicines. These isolated, pure and extremely concentrated ingredients are highly effective, but they also come with side effects. In spite of efforts by researchers to combat them, side effects can often be an intractable problem. Medication errors and serious side effects account for some seven thousand deaths in the United States each year.

Western pharmacology has constantly searched for an isolated pure substance with the highest degree of potency that will not cause side effects. This ideal has proven to be elusive. What has proven to be true is that the higher degree of purification, the higher degree of side effects. Two thousand years ago,

Chinese medicine had an advanced knowledge of chemistry and made efforts to isolate certain ingredients from natural substances. This stage of Chinese medicine reigned for a couple hundred years and then eventually died down. Doctors came to a consensus that mainstream Chinese medicine was to continue to use natural substances in their whole state. The exploration into isolated active ingredients ended there. Natural substances used in their whole state have fewer side effects. Natural substances in their whole state contain ingredients that are meant to interact synergistically and to counteract potential side effects.

As Chinese herbal medicine gains more attention, researchers are turning toward these drugs to isolate their active ingredients. Isolating active ingredients from herbs runs counter to Chinese medicine's basic philosophy of wholeness. An isolated active ingredient does not have the synergistic and buffering properties that it has when it remains in the whole form of an herb. Isolated active ingredients cause side effects and side effects are not tolerated in Chinese medicine. In fact, if side effects occur, the treatment is considered a failure even when the treatment is effective. By using whole herbs Chinese medicine can avoid and alleviate most side effects. To elaborate: a natural plant can contain dozens of active ingredients that all have chemical or physiological effects on the human body. At the same time, the plant may contain some ingredients that have no effect on the body. Within these ingredients are complex interactions. Take the simple saying "An apple a day keeps the doctor away." The truth in this saying lies in the fact that the many active ingredients within the apple interact within the body. We do not completely understand the synergy that occurs with these active ingredients. But we do know that if we isolate all of the active ingredients from an apple and ingest them individually, we will never get the same health benefits as eating the real apple. It is one of the wonders of nature.

Instead of isolating active ingredients, Chinese medicine takes a holistic approach in using natural substances. In other words, Chinese medicine looks at the overall property of a natural substance. For example, if you have cold symptoms and you eat ginger and you feel better, then ginger must have a worthy property. You do not have to know the exact properties of each active ingredient within the ginger. Herbalists need to know how ginger interacts with other herbs in order to be able to put them together in a formula; because of these interactions, Chinese medicine relies heavily on experience accumulated over thousands of years.

Part of the art of herb combining is controlling and minimizing side effects. The undesired aspects of herbs are canceled or balanced out by another herb. In addition, when herbs are combined there can be certain aspects that are not desirable for the particular treatment purpose. However, when properly combined, these aspects are balanced out by other herbs and the desirable aspects reinforced.

While it is extremely dangerous and inadvisable to self-diagnose and treat with Western medicine, Chinese medicine is more forgiving. Taking the wrong herb or combination of herbs may not solve your problem, but most of the time it will not hurt you.

Brandon's case presents a classic example of how people who would have otherwise quickly perished are being kept alive as a result of the technological advances of Western medicine. Brandon's case also demonstrates how vital the quality of life is to our existence. Chinese medicine gives quality-of-life issues top priority by focusing first and foremost on improving or maintaining a patient's sense of well-being.

In July 1997, Brandon learned about Chinese herbs from an AIDS volunteer and sought out treatment at a clinic where Dr. Han was consulting. Dr. Han recognized that Brandon's illness had been caused by the External Cause HIV virus. The HIV virus is considered Li Qi—a highly contagious External Cause. His External Causes and the medical conditions they resulted in had deeply altered Brandon's Energetic systems. He was severely Kidney Energy deficient. Kidney Energy in Chinese medicine provides the most important part of vitality. Kidney Energy has two sides, Yin and Yang. The Yin side is the Cooling, calming, nourishing side, and Yang is the Warming, active, functional side. Brandon's Kidney Energy was deficient on both sides. Nearly all his Energetic systems were depleted, and on top of that there was a tremendous amount of Toxin stagnation. Part of the stagnation was from the virus, but part of it was clearly from the side effects of the medications he was on.

"Dr. Han gave me herbs to cure my fever," Brandon said. "I thought, oh sure. I'd been to every top doctor on the West Coast and nothing was going to shake this." To his great surprise Brandon began to improve immediately. "I could feel the fever lifting, and I cried with joy. I started feeling stronger every day." During this time, Dr. Han also weaned Brandon off the prednisone. Three weeks after beginning the herbs, Brandon's Shen became strong enough that he accepted an invitation to a party—where he met his current partner. Brandon began living again, and his Vital Energy returned.

Dr. Hosea learned about and was convinced of the benefits of Chinese herbal medicine through the positive experiences of his patients. "My personal approach is to support anything that helps my patients," Dr. Hosea said. "With

AIDS, we can treat the pneumonia and the meningitis, but we can't effectively treat the nausea, the diarrhea or the other side effects of the medicine. I clearly remember when Brandon began the herbal medicines. He tolerated the medicines better, looked better and he was gaining weight." Dr. Hosea is one of the many Western doctors who have learned about the benefits of Chinese medicine from their patients and who are now beginning to consult and work together with Chinese doctors on their patients' treatment plans. "My patients have taught me the benefits of Chinese medicine. It is something we are just not taught about in Western medicine at all. I have been pleasantly surprised to find out that patients have sought out herbal medicines and are getting good results from it when I wasn't able to help them with Western medicine.

"Chinese medicine has been around a lot longer than Western medicine, and they know a lot more about dealing with symptoms than does Western medicine. Western medicine often uses a hand grenade to kill a fly. Eastern medicine does a much better job of paying attention to the subtleties of symptoms and dealing with them to get people back into balance. It is the integration of Chinese medicine and Western medicine, including meditation and prayer, that creates a holistic picture."

Throughout Brandon's illness, a belief in a higher power and purpose stayed with him. Before his HIV progressed to AIDS, he had attended retreats at a Buddhist temple. "I found myself feeling good while I was there, but I knew that my good health was not going to last forever," he said. "On one visit to the temple, I picked up a book in my room. In it was a newspaper clipping from India, dated July 1895—which was the same month I was there, but nearly one hundred years before. It said: *'Dear Sir, We feel bad about your illness, and we know it's considered terminal. But we know that hope is on the horizon, and we know that you will be well. A cure is being developed. Don't hold any fear. Know that we are all thinking about you and that you will be fine.'* Throughout my illness, even when I couldn't get out of bed that message stayed with me."

Brandon and his partner recently bought a ranch in Santa Barbara. Against the window-framed backdrop of the cloudless sky and deep blue Pacific Ocean, Brandon looked very much the athletic, dynamic Hollywood mogul. Instead of producing, Brandon has turned to writing screenplays, which allows him more free time. "When I was really low, I would go to the market and people would step in front of me to reach for something, or push their cart in front of me, or beat me to the checkout line. I was aware that the world was moving so much faster than I was, and I no longer felt like part of the world. But the down-and-outers, the alcoholics, the drug addicts, the old people, the really sick people, were on my frequency. They would be the only ones who would smile or talk to me. Like little voices of the underworld. As soon as I started getting healthy, they disappeared. During everything I went through, it was as if voices were telling me I had more to do with my life. I promised that if I got healthy again, I would do what I could to help people who have fallen through the cracks." Several days a week, Brandon volunteers as a counselor to the homeless. "I see people that are in the shape that I was in. All they need is just a little bit of assistance to get them to that next place where at least they can function to go to the next step."

Six years after Brandon began Chinese herbs, he looks healthy and vibrant—having gone from the brink of death to balance and vitality on a combined treatment plan of Western drugs and Chinese herbs. He also works to raise funds for herbal treatments as part of the recovery process. "Herbs were the major part of my recovery, and I want to share that with others."

## Do not make any changes in your health program without consulting your doctor

If you are seriously ill, you need to see a health care professional to work with you and follow your healing progress. People with HIV/AIDS have varying degrees of sensitivities and must be carefully supervised.

Stool, hair and blood tests can determine if you have (1) high levels of accumulated heavy metals in your system, (2) sensitivities to foods or (3) dysbiosis, which is an imbalance of the healthy and unhealthy bacteria and yeast in the gut, any of which may be weakening your immune system and draining your energy. See page 431 for a laboratory that can refer you to a health care provider in your area who does these types of tests. If you test positive for any of these factors, your health practitioner can treat you on an individual basis.

## Modify your diet

Follow the nutritional guidelines for environmental illnesses on page 168. See chapter 21 for recipes for HIV.

Take extra care to cook foods well to defend against salmonella and *E. coli* bacteria.

Many AIDS patients can benefit from the extra phytonutrients, probiotics and electrolytes from fresh vegetable juices and/or super green food. However, raw vegetable juices can be too stimulating for weakened digestive systems. If you use raw juice or super green food, do so under the supervision of your doctor. See page 294 for instructions on making fresh vegetable juice.

Detoxification can be hard on the body. Follow the detoxification program on pages 291–296 only under the close supervision of a health care practitioner.

The following herbs and foods have been shown to have either antiviral or immune-strengthening properties or to help treat the symptoms of AIDS.

*Antiviral Herbs and Foods*

Aloe vera
Asparagus
Bitter cucumber
Dandelion greens
Fava beans
Garlic
Ginger
Mung beans
Seaweed
Small Chinese red beans
Turmeric

*Immune-Enhancing Herbs and Foods*

Astragalus
Chinese yam
Codonapsis
Lycium fruit
Poria mushroom
White wood ear mushroom

*Herbs and Foods That Have Both Antiviral and Immune-Enhancing Qualities*

Pearl barley
Shiitake mushroom
Water lily

*Herbs and Foods to Treat the Recurring Diarrhea and Digestive Weakness Commonly Seen in AIDS*

Kudzu root
Lily palm
Lotus seed
Pearl barley
Poria mushroom

*Herbs and Foods to Treat the Weight Loss and Dehydration of AIDS*

Asparagus
Mung beans
White wood ear mushroom

*Herbs and Foods That Treat the Loss of Appetite Associated with AIDS*

Bitter cucumber
Hawthorn berry
Lotus palm

Mary Enig, Ph.D., an internationally recognized biochemist in the field of fats and oils and an authority on trans fatty acids, reports that eating coconut is thought to reduce the viral load of HIV. Coconut oil contains lauric acid, which is converted by the body into monolaurin. Monolaurin is thought to solubilize the lipids in the virus envelope, causing its disintegration. According to Dr. Enig's research, some of the pathogens inactivated by monolaurin include HIV, measles virus, herpes simplex virus and influenza virus, as well as several kinds of bacteria. Dr. Enig suggests a diet containing about 24 grams of lauric acid, which can be obtained from 3 $^1/2$ tablespoons of coconut oil, 10 ounces of pure coconut milk or 7 ounces of raw coconut per day. Since allergies to coconut are caused by the proteins, if you are allergic to coconut you can safely eat coconut oil.

## Chinese herbs and Western supplements

Human growth hormone is now being used by some Western doctors to prevent muscle wasting and to rebuild lean body mass in HIV patients. Discuss using human growth hormone injections with your Western doctor. See more about this hormone in chapter 19.

Deer Velvet Antler is an important Kidney Yang tonic that enhances strength and rebuilds lean body mass in HIV patients. Deer Velvet Antler must be used under the supervision of a Chinese doctor. Discuss using Deer Velvet Antler with your Chinese doctor to stimulate the natural production of human growth hormone to rebuild wasted muscle mass. See more about Deer Velvet Antler in chapter 19.

Find a health care practitioner to give you injections of B vitamins, intravenous vitamin C or a "Meyer's cocktail," which is a combination of calcium, magnesium, vitamin C and B complex.

Routinely, take the immune-modulating formula discussed on pages 103–104.

Routinely, thirty to forty-five minutes before breakfast, lunch and dinner take 1,000 milligrams free-form amino acids.

Routinely, before and after each meal, take the digestive formulas found on page 102.

You can use Chinese medicinal herbs in recipes to boost your immune system. See chapter 21 for recipes. You can also take Chinese herbal formulas and Western supplements specifically formulated for HIV. To purchase herbal formulas log on to ancientherbsmodernmedicine.com.

# PART FOUR

## Health Maintenance and Excellence

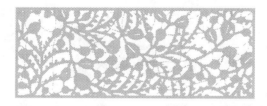

# 16

## Mind-Body-Spirit Medicine

*Disease is a symptom of life out of balance*

On February 28, 1995, Lorne Feldman, a Los Angeles–based oncologist, had just returned from a ski vacation in Utah. His twelve-year-old son had lured him on advanced runs and he had fallen a lot. Back at work, when he noticed his urine seemed dark, he assumed, with all the falling, that he had bruised a kidney.

About to exit the men's room, Feldman ran into a urologist friend and mentioned that his urine looked dark. His friend steered him to the E.R., where a urine sample indicated a lot of blood cells in Feldman's urine. The two doctors went to the X-ray department, where a radiologist did an ultrasound of Feldman's kidneys.

In his mid-forties, Lorne Feldman is impossibly youthful, healthy and relaxed-looking given the story he recounted. "We are good friends," he said of the doctors who were checking him out that day. "They were joking and asking about my ski trip." When the radiologist began the ultrasound of Feldman's left side, the room fell silent. "You could cut the tension with a knife. They said they saw a big tumor in my left kidney."

At three-thirty that afternoon, after seeing patients all day, Dr. Feldman left his office to undergo a CAT scan. The CAT scan showed a tumor twelve centimeters in diameter—the size of an orange—on his left kidney. Prior to seeing the blood in his urine, Feldman had been completely asymptomatic and felt fine. Because cancer tumors are vascular (contain a lot of blood vessels), the bumping and jarring during Feldman's ski trip had caused them to bleed. Kidney cancer is most often deadly because it is discovered too late. Even if the cancerous kidney is surgically removed, cells often have already broken off and metastasized elsewhere in the body. Feldman was well aware that there are currently no chemotherapy drugs to treat kidney cancer. He went home and delivered the painful news to his wife, Sonia.

Forty-eight hours after he first noticed blood in his urine, Feldman underwent a laparotomy and a thoracotomy. An incision was made from his lower back around his ribs to his chest wall, extending down toward his navel. The surgeon inserted a rib spreader into Feldman's chest. The handle of the rib spreader was slowly turned, tearing the ligaments that attach the ribs to the breastplate and spreading his ribs apart. The surgeon worked his way toward Feldman's kidney, tying off the arteries before cutting them along the way to prevent a major loss of blood. The surgeon delicately removed his kidney. The tumor appeared contained there.

After recovering from surgery, Feldman went on a regimen of CAT scan reevaluation and examination every three months. His best hope of survival was to catch any metastasis in the early stages. Two years went by.

In 1997, during one of his three-month evaluations, the CAT scan showed a mass in his chest. Two attempted needle biopsies were inconclusive. As a last resort, Feldman underwent a second thoracotomy, which was the only way doctors could get at the mass. This time he was diagnosed with non-Hodgkin's lymphoma. As odd as it sounds, Feldman was elated. This diagnosis meant that he had gone from the 2 percent survival rate of metastatic kidney cancer to the 95 percent cure rate with stage one lymphoma.

During a grueling six weeks of aggressive chemotherapy, followed by another six weeks of radiation therapy to his chest, Feldman began to consider the fact that he needed to start making some changes in his life. "After the kidney cancer I thought about what could have caused it and I would make myself promises that I would change things—not to drink diet sodas, and things like that," he said. "My promises all lasted about six months. My office administrator, Lorene Cangiano, who has always been interested in holistic medical approaches, started feeding me books. I have always had a scientific, clinical way of thinking, but by that point I was more open to reading them and started to be more open to hearing about other ways of doing things."

Despite this openness, Feldman carried on pretty much the same. One year later, in 1998, a CAT scan revealed a nodule in his left chest. Feldman underwent a *third* thoracotomy. This time the mass taken from his chest was metastatic kidney cancer. In all likelihood, cancerous kidney cells had broken off three years earlier during the surgery in which his kidney had been removed. Cancerous cells had traveled through his bloodstream and attached to his lung (the metastasis), but it had taken years for them to grow to a detectable size. It was the death sentence Feldman had feared.

As he recovered from surgery, Feldman was put off by his surgeon's doom-and-gloom attitude. He sought second and third opinions at Memorial Sloan-Kettering in New York and M. D. Anderson in Houston. "Each time, I was devastated by emotionally bereft oncologists who did not know how to connect with me." Three years after first being diagnosed with kidney cancer, then going through non-Hodgkin's lymphoma and metastatic kidney cancer and undergoing invasive medical procedures, including having his chest cracked open three times, chemotherapy and radiation, Feldman was physically and emotionally spent. Though the new tumor had been surgically removed, he knew that there were probably more tumors developing, and that they would most likely be lethal.

"I am an oncologist," Feldman said. "I knew that I would probably be dead within six months." He resolved to search out his own path to healing and began by learning about a number of nontraditional healing approaches such as nutritional supplements, yoga and meditation. Our focus here is his exploration into Chinese medicine. "A friend of mine asked me if I knew anything about Chinese medicine," Feldman said. "My only experience had been with a few patients who were having acupuncture, who I thought were weird. To me, acupuncture was always one of those California things." Now he was willing to learn. His friend gave him a book called *The Eight Treasures: Energy Enhancement Exercise,* by Maoshing Ni, Lic. Ac., D.O.M., Ph.D. Feldman read the book and then made an appointment to see Dr. Mao, who was a specialist in immunology at the Tao of Wellness Clinic in Los Angeles.

When he went to see Dr. Mao, Feldman did not spend time talking about the trauma of surgery, chemotherapy and radiation, but stuck to the facts about the three diagnoses and focused primarily on what he was searching for. "He was starting to understand and be curious about the relationships between lifestyle, diet and especially the mind/body connection," Dr. Mao said. "Prior to his illness he was geared in the Western medical thinking that disease has little to do with outside processes or any connection between mind and body. He assumed the cancer occurred as a result of some genetic predisposition. As a physician, Dr. Feldman was trained to eradicate cancer with surgery, chemotherapy and radiation. When the cancer was gone, it would be the end of the treatment. When he came to see me, he was looking hard at his life and realizing that if he didn't make changes, it might be the end.

"Dr. Feldman had built a busy oncology center with four oncologists on staff. The effort involved took a toll on his Kidney Energy. Then his surgeries, chemotherapy, radiation and chronic worry had further depleted his Kidney Energy. His Lung Energetic system was also weakened, which manifested in asthma and allergies. His Spleen Energetic system was also deficient." Dr. Mao focused on boosting Dr. Feldman's Kidney Energy as well as balancing his other Energetic systems through a program of acupuncture, herbs, lifestyle and dietary changes.

"In the past, for me to have confidence in a drug it had to be subjected to randomized, double-blind clinical trials where several trials all show the same result," Feldman said. "When pharmaceutical representatives come to my office and try to get me to prescribe their products, I'm always cynical. So for me to take a Chinese herb and not even know what it is or what it is supposed to do was a really big leap. But after I saw Dr. Mao, I began taking the herbs willingly and open-mindedly."

Herbal and acupuncture treatments resulted in an improvement in Feldman's chronic asthma, allergies and back pain. These positive experiences were encouraging. Still, he felt as if he was making his way across a vast uncharted wilderness. "I was at a loss for what to do. I was in a phase where I had to make some plans—given that my Western medical prognosis only gave me six months to live. But I only felt comfortable making decisions that fell within the ninety-day window between CAT scans."

Shortly after his first visit to Dr. Mao, Feldman had an epiphany while walking on the beach. "I started praying, 'God, please help me with all of this. It has gotten to be too much, and I don't know what to do, and I feel paralyzed.' I said that I would really appreciate it if He could show me some kind of a sign. 'If we are communicating, then show me a whale.' I was walking along, and at first I thought that I was seeing the waves crashing against the rocks, but then I noticed that the rocks were moving." Thirty yards out in the kelp beds were two whales, spouting and playing. Feldman picked up a piece of driftwood and wrote in the sand *Thank you, God*.

"Universal spirituality crosses all boundaries of religion and faith," Dr. Mao said. "It doesn't matter if you are Buddhist, Jewish, Christian, Muslim, Hindu or Taoist. Part of a balanced life is establishing a connection with God—to connect with the divine within and understand that you are a divine being. We are spiritual beings on a human path, not human beings on a spiritual path. When I treat an atheist I say, 'You don't have to believe in God. But do you believe that there is a rhythm in the universe that says summer always follows spring, and that after a harsh winter, spring will come?' They say yes. This is universal truth. So there is a higher power that they can connect with. They may not believe in a monolithic male sitting on a throne, but everybody relates to the power of the universe. In Chinese medicine, having a spiritual connection is important because it is part of the balance, part of the whole, but also this connection allows you to transcend suffering."

Feldman pursued his spiritual outlet by turning to prayer and worship in his Jewish faith. He also went on a spiritual sojourn to India and continued daily yoga and meditation and prayer. "These practices lead to a peaceful, serene beginning to each morning," Feldman said. "This was in stark contrast to my life before cancer, when I tore out of bed and compiled a to-do list several pages long. It also helped me consider the circle of life and the inevitability of death. This understanding and acceptance helped to replace fear with comfort."

The mind/body connection in Chinese medicine includes nurturing a spiritual outlet. Dr. Mao said, "At the onset of the Cultural Revolution in China in 1966, Chairman Mao Tse-tung forbade religious practice. The Cultural Revolution ended in 1976 with Mao Tse-tung's death, and by the 1980s the communist government loosened its taboo on religious practice. During this time, many schools of Qigong sprang up in China, including the Falungong. (Qigong can be described as a preventative healing system comprised of breathing, movement and visualizations that are designed to master the Vital Energy or Qi that permeates all of nature and humanity.) The practice of Qigong became increasingly popular in China as a spiritual outlet and, for many people, became a substitute for religion. The founder of the Falungong school was a Qigong Master who was said to have extraordinary supernatural power. He and other Qigong teachers proceeded to conduct Qigong forums that drew half a million people. What communist government would allow half a million people to congregate? But Qigong was allowed because it was practiced under the pretense of health. In other words, as long as the Falungong congregated to practice Qigong and did not become politically active, the communist government could live with it."[6] The inception and growth of the Falungong is a testimony to the fact that people have a drive to find a spiritual outlet.

Dr. Mao also worked with Dr. Feldman to help him learn to express his emotions, which would give him some relief from the pressure cooker of fear

6. In 1999, after it became apparent that the Falungong was politically active, China's government banned the Falungong as an "evil cult" and passed laws making such groups illegal. China's government fears Falungong's organizational abilities, as it has been estimated to have up to a hundred million followers in the country.

and apprehension that had gripped him for three years. "There is Energy behind each emotion. Because he had controlled his emotions during this trying time, his Liver Energetic system was somewhat hardened and stagnant. He needed to learn to express his emotions. At the same time, it is important to maintain some control and calmness. In Western culture it is more acceptable to be expressive and even melodramatic to make a point or to get what you want. Since our cells are suggestible, we need to remain peaceful and calm. Five thousand years ago Chinese physicians understood the importance of keeping emotions calm and peaceful. *The Yellow Emperor's Classic Book of Internal Medicine* says that when you remain peaceful within, then your Wei Qi—which is your defense Energy, in this case your immune system—will remain strong and healthy, therefore preventing illness from developing." In addition to his daily meditation and prayer, Feldman allowed himself more relaxation and pleasure time, even taking up the saxophone and starting dance lessons.

Feldman's personal experiences began to influence the way he practiced medicine. "I knew that there had to be better ways to care for patients. I had learned that when you are told that there is nothing more that can be done, it just means that there isn't anything more that Western medicine can do for you. We physicians look at a person with a sickness and say that they have a disease, and we treat that body dysfunction. Chinese medicine treats the person with an illness—not just a symptom, but all of the different parts of the body and aspects of that person's life that have influence. When I was sick I did not want to *be* kidney cancer. Kidney cancer was my disease, not me. My illness was the sum total of all of the influences and occurrences of the forty-six years that I had lived to that point that had led to kidney cancer and lymphoma. Treating the kidney cancer by surgically removing it didn't change whatever genetically or environmentally, emotionally, spiritually had led to the occurrence of the kidney cancer. It took me three tough kicks in the rear to take a look at that."

Feldman successfully beat metastatic kidney cancer for more than six years by integrating alternative complementary methods of healing with traditional medicine. His own journey redefined his approach to treating cancer. He and his office administrator developed BIOS—B'shert Integrative Oncology Services. *B'shert,* a Hebrew word, means "the path," "God's way" or "destiny." BIOS integrates Western medicine with complementary medicines. BIOS has on staff doctors of Chinese medicine who work with patients with acupuncture, guided imagery, polarity and herbs. BIOS also has on staff a nutritionist; a therapist who works with patients using techniques such as biofeedback, counseling, massage and healing touch; and group support such as journaling, a reading club and life issues discussions. The Odyssey program, an ongoing experiential program, offers workshops throughout the year in many modalities including arts and crafts, scrapbooking and cooking. Feldman gives patients a preliminary plan that involves the standard traditional approach with chemotherapy, radiation and surgery. He presents their information at a group meeting that includes the entire faculty of BIOS. "All of us talk together," he said. "BIOS breaks down all of the formalities of the way that oncology care had been delivered. I never dreamed medicine could be this rewarding.

"Fifteen years ago, if you would have come to me as a patient and said that God would work through my hands, I would roll my eyes. It was something that did not resonate well with me. All I wanted was to get the patient to accept that they had an incurable disease and they needed to take chemotherapy and just forget about all that other stuff. I now look at this experience as God directing me to make changes so that I can maybe show other people and other physicians a different way that medicine can be practiced, particularly oncology."

Your spiritual connection is highly personal. Cultivating a spiritual life is part of the balance that is fundamental to Chinese medicine, in which mind, body and spirit are one.

In the fall of 2001, Dr. Feldman underwent a fourth thoracotomy to remove a kidney metastasis from his lung. He is currently in remission.

## Tapping Into Your Power to Heal

The human body is made up of energy. In physics, energy is the ability to do work. It can be found in two forms: potential (at rest) and kinetic (in motion). From a Chinese medicine point of view, Energy is the Life Force (Qi). Your human body is more than a shell that houses organs, tissues and bones. Your body is a circulating Energy system that links every part within you to every part of the environment, thus creating a whole. The goal of healing is to promote and support this Energy system's innate tendency to strive for balance. *Healing is to restore balance.*

Combined practices of breathing and meditation such as Qigong, Tai Chi and yoga are ways to connect and tap into the healing power of your inner Qi. These practices build and store more Qi than the actual physical exercises use up. The first step in realizing the potential of this Energy is to recognize and harness the power of your own breath.

## The Power of Breath

In this stressful world, it is common to actually hold your breath when tense. Qigong, meditation, yoga and Tai Chi are all practices that teach controlled breathing. However, outside of these practices, regular deep breathing can be cultivated so that it becomes an unconscious habit. Rather than holding your breath, you can find yourself shifting into deep breathing in response to stress.

From a Western scientific point of view, every time you breathe, oxygen floods your lungs, filters into your bloodstream and is pumped into your arteries and capillaries to reach every part of your body. Cells utilize this oxygen and create the waste product carbon dioxide ($CO_2$). In cellular metabolic processes, the oxygen in your blood is exchanged for $CO_2$, which is carried in your bloodstream back through your veins to your heart and lungs, where it is expelled each time you exhale.

When you are tense and breathe shallowly or hold your breath, your blood is not being properly purified or oxygenated. $CO_2$ is kept in circulation in your system, creating an acid environment. This acid environment encourages your autonomic nervous system to remain in a sympathetic state. (Please see pages 141–143 for an explanation of the sympathetic and parasympathetic states.) Remaining in an acidic state of sympathetic dominance contributes to the progression of chronic illnesses and eventually degenerative disease.

Getting into the habit of deep breathing is a way to help your body move from the uptight sympathetic mode to the calming parasympathetic mode. By breathing deeply you signal your brain that you are not in danger. Simply experimenting with deep breathing the next time you face a stressful situation will convince you of the benefits of deep breathing.

Infants and children breathe into their bellies. As we mature into adults, the tendency is to breathe shallowly into our upper chests. Practice abdominal breathing by breathing deeply and slowly, allowing your abdomen to inflate on the inhale and deflate on the exhale.

## Taking Breath to Another Level

Historically, it has been firmly fixed in the collective mind of the Western medical establishment that the mind and body are two separate entities. The mind is thought to intentionally control such functions as the musculoskeletal system, allowing us to flex our muscles and move our arms at will. Other processes of the body, such as our heartbeat, blood pressure, the secretion of hormones, the regulation of antibodies by our immune system and so on are viewed as completely out of our control. These processes are controlled by various mechanisms such as the autonomic nervous system, the neuroendocrine system and the immune system. It is believed that we cannot cross the conceptual and physiological chasm between these two aspects of the body. For example, it has been conventionally believed that our conscious mind cannot influence our immune system.

In the past three decades the Western medical establishment has come to understand that, when the body and mind are in harmony through practices that combine breathing and meditation, the mind *can* control physiological processes. The secret tool for self-healing and Energy balancing that lies within each of us is our breath. Maybe we underestimate our breath because it is so obvious.

Linking your breath with meditation or with gentle synchronized movements, such as Qigong, Tai Chi and yoga, has been shown to have an effect that can be seen on the electroencephalogram (EEG), a common measurement device found in every hospital. There are four types of brain waves: beta (fast)—highly focused, for problem solving and learning; alpha (medium)—tranquil, creative and most relaxed; theta (slow)—unfocused, daydreaming/early dream state; and delta (slowest)—deep sleep. Practices that combine breathing, meditation and gentle movement bring one into alpha state. As your practice deepens, you enter a combination alpha and theta state wherein your body heals most effectively.

The practices of meditation, Qigong, Tai Chi and yoga have also been shown to lower blood pressure and pulse rate and to improve endocrine and immune system function, among other benefits.

## Meditation

Meditation has been practiced all over the world for thousands of years. In China, meditation was defined by Taoism as a way to cultivate mental discipline in which the devotee attempted to channel every thought to Tao, the oneness of the universe, which includes all gods, deities, divine beings, spirits and souls. Taoist master Hua-Ching Ni has devoted his life to continuing his family lineage of spiritual masters dating back seventy-four generations to the Han dynasty (206 B.C.–220 A.D.). He is an acknowledged master of all aspects of Taoist arts and philosophy, including Chinese medicine. In his book *Entering the Tao,* he describes the effect of Taoist meditation thus: "Serenity unfolds itself as a calm inner happiness, and it is enduring and completely independent of external conditions."

In the 1960s meditation was introduced to the Western mainstream when hippies started making spiritual pilgrimages to India. Transcendental meditation (TM) captured the attention of the press. At that time researcher and clinical cardiologist Herbert Benson, M.D., became interested and began studying the then highly unorthodox theory that stress had something to do with hypertension. In 1969, at Harvard Medical School, Dr. Benson and his mentor A. Clifford Barger, M.D., published a study in the *American Journal of Physiology* in which they were able to train monkeys to control their blood pressure with light cues. After the study was published, several TM devotees asked Benson to study them, claiming that they could decrease their blood pressure through meditation.

During stress, your body—in a sympathetic dominant state—releases stress hormones to ignite heart rate, breathing, blood pressure, increase metabolic rate and blood flow to your muscles as immediate preparation for fight or flight. Benson's studies concluded meditation could mediate the effects of stress by shifting your body into a relaxed parasympathetic state—the exact opposite of the fight-or-flight response. Heart and breathing rate decrease, blood pressure drops (if high to begin with), and body temperature and metabolism rates also fall.

"The mind must be peaceful for quality of life," Dr. Mao said. "You must get to a point when you can focus on the present moment. Anxiety comes from either being in the past or being in the future and not being in the present moment. If you are present you can focus and can deal with life's issues. It is the uncontrollable that makes us anxious. Taking twenty minutes a day for meditation will empty your mind. When you become very still it is like water in a pond—you can see very clearly. Otherwise there are too many rocks being thrown in there and the water is muddied and you can't see anything. Stillness brings clarity, which brings better decisions in life, which means fewer regrets and fewer worries. We make mistakes when we are not clear."

As a meditator sits and his or her mind quiets, alpha brain waves are increased. People commonly experience a feeling of well-being. Meditation can be a valuable part of any therapy for illness. It is also a way to connect with the aspect of yourself that is steady and unchanging. This aspect is referred to as mindfulness of your Shen in Qigong, the Self or Atman in the yogic scriptures of India, the Buddha-mind in Buddhist philosophy, the presence of the Holy Spirit in the Christian belief, the presence of God in Judaism, among others.

Spending time in meditation on a regular basis eventually leads to feeling a divine connection throughout the day, not just when meditating. Practicing meditation begins to have profound effects on the way you interact with other people and the way you feel about yourself. Old traumas are forgiven; old neurotic patterns of behavior can be more easily dropped; you will feel more love and joy in life.

Beginning a meditation practice is like beginning any discipline, from playing a musical instrument to training for a marathon. It is called *practice* for a reason. The payoff for perseverance can be enormous. There are many styles and techniques of meditation. The following is a basic practice:

- *Sit in a steady posture, in a quiet, darkened room.* Find a position that is comfortable for you. It is important that your spine be relatively straight and that you are somewhat grounded—either by sitting on cushions on the floor or, if seated in a chair, by having your feet firmly planted on the floor. Find a position that is comfortable enough that you will not be distracted by tension or pain in your joints or muscles.
- *Turn your attention within.* Some traditions advise keeping the eyes partly open, some closing the eyes completely. Experiment and decide what is best for you.
- *Focus your mind on the incoming and outgoing of your breath.* Allow your belly to inflate. Follow the flow of your breath from its innermost place in your chest or abdomen to the full extent of your exhalation.
- *Or you can focus on a mantra—one or more sacred words.* Lists of mantras can be found in many meditation texts. There are no hard-and-fast rules for choosing a mantra. You are free to choose any word or words that resonate with you.
- *Some traditions advise visualizing a specific deity or memorizing a prayer or passage of scripture.* There are many variations on the meditation practice, and it is important to find the one that suits your own individual personality, needs and beliefs.
- *Allow the normal busy activity of your mind to slow.* If your mind remains active, do not worry. Continue to return your attention to your breath or to your mantra. It is not possible to stop the activity of the mind by force of will. But as you continue to turn your attention away from thoughts that arise, and guide your attention back to your breath or to your mantra, your mind will eventually quiet.
- *When your mind comes to a complete rest, a state of pure awareness or pure*

*absorption arises.* This is often described as a sense of blissful emptiness or of union with the divine.

When first starting a meditation practice, sit for short periods—say fifteen minutes—until you feel physically comfortable sitting for longer. As you practice you will go into a meditative state more easily. Meditate at the same time each day if possible—early morning and twilight are considered best. Meditating for a short period during a busy day is better than not meditating at all because you missed your chosen time.

# Qigong

Qigong is a system of deep breathing, with or without slow movements combined with mental focus to control one's Vital Energy (Qi), which brings the body, mind and spirit into alignment and balance. Qigong is said to have been originated by mountain hermits in ancient China and can be traced to inscriptions on tortoise shells dating back to 2,500 B.C. and to silk drawings found in tombs four thousand years old.

Chinese philosophy considers living beings and the environment part of the same whole. The Qi force continually fluctuates in an attempt to harmonize the Yin and Yang Energies of this whole. Air connects the body and the environment. The air you draw into your body will be converted into Qi. The air that becomes the body's internal Qi is the same Qi of the environment. In fact, in the Chinese language "air" and "Vital Energy" are the same word: *Qi.* Air and Vital Energy are merely a different concept of Qi. One is inside and the other outside the body. Breathing joins the environmental Qi with the internal Qi.

Qi is constantly circulating in Meridians throughout the body. This circulation of Qi weaves every component and function of the body into a harmonized whole. Practicing Qigong taps into this Energy flow, engages and invigorates Qi, to dissolve stagnation and break through blockages. In Qigong, movement and stillness are cultivated to create an awareness that guides you through the process of achieving calmness and harmony of your Qi. A calm mind and spirit lead to higher levels of skill and self-knowledge.

Practicing Qigong will loosen your joints, increase flexibility and suppleness and strengthen your sinews and tendons. Qigong has been shown to improve the function of the internal organs, delay aging and prolong life.

Kenneth Cohen is an internationally renowned author, lecturer, health educator, China scholar and master of Qigong healing. Cohen began Qigong training in 1968 and apprenticed with Taoist priests from China's sacred mountains. Cohen divides Qigong into three main categories:

- *Healing Qigong* teaches how to cleanse, gather and circulate healing Energy. Qigong for healing promotes general vitality and well-being and teaches techniques to treat specific problems. In addition to practicing healing Qigong for your own benefit, healing Qigong can be practiced as therapeutic touch. You can learn to project healing Qi through your hands into another person to restore his or her balance.
- *Spiritual Qigong* emphasizes meditation to cultivate self-awareness, awareness of your place in nature and your surroundings.
- *Sports Qigong* uses dynamic exercises to improve strength, endurance, balance and flexibility.

If you engage your breath, every activity can be a way for you to strive for balance and harmony. Overwork depletes Qi and Blood. A sedentary lifestyle stagnates the movement of Qi and Blood. Physical activity helps to promote the flow of Qi and Blood and helps your body develop and/or keep its vitality.

Qigong can be as simple as taking a few purposeful breaths every day, or it can be extremely complex and involving. The beauty of Qigong is that you can conform your practice to suit your needs and desires. While the subject of Qigong fills entire books, the focus here is to simply make the philosophy of Qigong a part of your daily life as a way to help you maintain good health or to heal.

## Making the philosophy of Qigong part of your everyday life

"One of the greatest benefits of learning Qi healing is that you awaken your own hidden potentials and learn more about who you are," Kenneth Cohen said. "As you tap into the well of universal Qi, you increase your sense of belonging—of being at home in the world. Qi, like breath, is the foundation of life. We use it every day but are seldom aware of it. It is the most ordinary thing in the universe, yet it is the source of the most extraordinary insight and energy."

Just as you can cultivate the simple habit of deep breathing, you can learn to breathe, focus your thoughts and emotions, relax and get in touch with your internal Qi by practicing Qigong in an unstructured manner. In other words, it is not necessary to become a master at Qigong to experience its healing and preventative health effects. You can begin by taking your deep breathing practice one step further by visualizing Qi flowing through your body as you breathe. Become aware of yourself and your behaviors. For example, when you walk, become consciously aware of the steps that you are taking. Link deep breathing to your walk. Perform each step—or any other action—deliberately. This deliberateness will bring you to a deeper connection with the present moment and with your inner Energy (Qi). This awareness will help restore balance.

Qigong breathing

Qigong practice teaches deep abdominal breathing, which expands your lung capacity, promotes circulation of oxygen in the blood, massages your internal abdominal organs and aids in digestion and assimilation of nutrients.

* As you reach the top of each inhalation and/or the bottom of each exhalation, hold your breath for several seconds, and then continue breathing. This will help you to focus your mind on your breathing. While practicing Qigong, respiration rate naturally decreases and the duration of each breath increases.
* Maintain smooth, deep, silent respirations, and, at the same time, "listen" to your respirations. Continue your focus until you do not hear, see or connect with any extraneous thought that comes into your mind.
* As you practice awareness of the tendency to hold your breath when you are fearful, worried or otherwise stressed, you can take this awareness to another level. When you are in a stressful situation, breathe deeply and evenly in through your nose, allowing the breath to distend your stomach rather than breathing into your chest, then imagine healing Qi flowing through your body. This is Qigong breathing. You may exhale out of your nose or mouth.

You can practice Qigong breathing while sitting or lying down. It has been shown that Qigong practice lowers the body's consumption of oxygen by about 30 percent and the metabolic rate drops by 20 percent—accompanied by a drop in the respiration rate. This state of lowered metabolism aids in reducing your body's consumption of Energy, allowing the gradual accumulation of Energy, which promotes your body's strength to heal.

A simple Qigong breathing practice for sitting, standing or lying down

Francesco Garri Garripoli, author and lecturer, left a full scholarship in premed at the University of Colorado to study Eastern healing in the mid-seventies. He has practiced and taught Qigong and other Eastern healing techniques for over twenty years. "Qigong can be done sitting, standing or lying down," said Garripoli. "The beauty of this system is that it is as flexible as you wish to make it." If you are pressed for time, are trapped at work, or if you are simply a bit tired but are not ready to fall asleep, try the following Qigong technique.

◆ Visualize that you are holding a small ball between your hands. Bring your complete focus and attention to this ball.
◆ Feel its roundness and breathe into the ball, giving it shape and substance. The more you are able to do this, the more you are engaging your mind into a game of releasing itself from other duties, and in doing so releasing much stress.
◆ Slowly expand the size of this ball as you inhale. As you inhale through your nostrils, focus your breathing on your diaphragm, pushing your belly outwards, minimizing the use of any other muscles, to make this an efficient, minimal-effort process.
◆ When you have reached the full extent of your inhale—and along with it, the full expansion of your imaginary ball—slowly begin to exhale through your mouth to fully empty your lungs.
◆ As you exhale, gently shrink the ball back down to its starting size and position it in front of your belly.

Combining Qigong breath and meditation

When you feel you have mastered the focus on your breath, begin to practice centering your mind. As in many other forms of meditation, you can select a word to repeat and focus on as you continue to focus your mind. Continued practice will allow you to reach a state in which you are conscious yet not conscious, aware yet not aware.

Qigong meditation lessens the intrusion of the emotional ups and downs, allowing your body to reach a state of high physiological and biochemical efficiency through greater relaxation and concentration. In this state of mind,

Qigong enables the cerebral cortex to prepare to meet any urgent need and re-duces the consumption of Energy, thus providing optimal conditions for healing.

Simple exercises derived from ancient Qigong forms

Once you feel comfortable with the combined Qigong breathing and medi-tation, you may wish to add gentle, synchronized movements. A few funda-mentals are important.

### Preparation for Qigong Postures

* *Relax your mind and let go of worried thoughts.* Practice keeping your body and mind relaxed and peaceful. The practice of Qigong, unlike many other forms of exercise, is intended to be without expectations or demands.
* *Get comfortable.* Wear comfortable, loose clothing and remove anything that is restrictive. Remove jewelry and eyeglasses.
* *Practice in a peaceful place.* Find a warm and comfortable spot away from traffic or other noises, preferably with natural light.
* *Align your posture.* Stand with your back straight and your body erect but not stiff, arms hanging down naturally. Your whole body will be relaxed, though not limp, so that your mind and body are comfortable and aligned.
* *Unite your breath and your mind:* There are three Dan Tian regions, or En-ergy centers, upon which to focus the mind or consciousness in Qigong. The Lower Dan Tian is located below the navel about two cun (cun is de-scribed on page 56) above the pubic bone, which is the central gathering point of Qi; the Middle Dan Tian is located behind the navel, which is an-other important gathering point of Qi; and the Upper Dan Tian is located between your eyebrows and is thought to aid in gathering Shen Qi and re-inforcing your connection with the universe. Unite your mind and breath by concentrating your mind on the Lower Dan Tian. By focusing on your Lower Dan Tian, you will reach a state in which your breathing is led by your mind, deep and controlled.
* *Develop your skills gradually.* Practice according to your physical ability and strength, allowing your practice to develop and progress naturally. Do not force your practice or be anxious for quick results.
* *Choose the practice that is right for you.* There are many variations of Qigong. Respect your individual state of health or state of illness when choosing a form of Qigong.

* *Practice regularly.* Qigong skill must be developed. The longer you perse-
  vere, the more profound your results.
* *Give up habits that prevent you from achieving results.* Smoking, the use of
  stimulants, and excessive work and play exhaust the body and are not con-
  ducive to a balanced life.

The following exercise, provided by Garripoli, is a simple movement that
can be easily mastered. You can get up from your chair at work and engage in a
quick stress-relieving practice. It takes very little time and the benefits last
throughout your day.

*The Swimming Dragon*: The Swimming Dragon is in the family of Qigong
moves that can be thought of as a whole-body workout in a single move. Rather
than isolating any single body/Energy region, the Swimming Dragon is designed to help promote Qi flow throughout the whole body, effectively minimizing stagnation that leads to stress and disease. Begin by standing with knees
unlocked and slightly bent.

As you engage in the following movements, inhale when a hand moves toward the Lower Dan Tian and exhale when that hand moves away. As you move
through the exercise, imagine a dragon swimming through a field of Qi. This
field is thick and viscous, infinite in size and density, and Qi is ever-present and
in limitless supply.

* Begin by reaching outward with your right hand, sweeping to the right,
  then forward in an arc. Keep your palm facing slightly upward during this
  phase, focusing on gathering Yang Qi, the masculine, active, light, formless
  Energy, from the heavens.
* Pull your palm in toward your belly region, toward the Lower Dan Tian,
  keeping your palm facing slightly downward. This downward-facing aspect is to enhance the gathering of Yin Qi, the feminine, nurturing, dark,
  solid energy, from the Earth. Your hand should pass by your abdomen
  without touching it, continuing on its trajectory directly behind you.
* Your hand reaches straight behind you, palm facing upward to heaven.
  Lock your gaze onto your palm as it moves to its outstretched position.
  This will help ensure that you are getting a good stretch in your neck and
  spine, one of the important features of this move. This twisting action of
  your neck and spine is critical to good health as it helps promote good flow
  of the cerebrospinal fluid and Qi, of course, which is carried in all bodily

Fluids. Imagine that this spinal twist is akin to wringing out a wet rag—moving stagnant energy and liquids from their pockets.

◆ The fourth and last phase brings your palm and outstretched arm from directly behind you and sweeps in around to the right, meeting up with where you started.

◆ To swim in the infinite field of Qi, it is best to use both arms. Once you have mastered this movement with your right hand, add the movement of your left hand. The left arm begins reaching out when the right palm is nearest to your belly in phase two. Your arm movements will mirror each other, just offset in time to create the beautiful balance of this move.

"Watching this form reminds us of the Yin and Yang forces in the universe," Garripoli said. "When one hand is closest to the body, the other is at its farthest. When one palm is facing upward, the other is facing downward, complementary forces working together to create balance. Each move in this form is a metaphor, a window into the truth of life. Our body is simply a mirror of how Energy flows in the universe."

Healing others with Qigong

Once you have developed your own Qigong practice, you are ready to learn to project healing Qi through your hands, which was called Bu Qi, "spreading the Qi," by ancient Chinese healers. Energy healing, or the laying on of hands, dates back to the Yellow Emperor in China and hieroglyphic recordings from Egypt's Third Dynasty. Hippocrates referred to the force from the healer's hands. "Energy healing is part of the common heritage of humanity," Kenneth Cohen said. "It is still practiced by American Indians, African tribes and Australian aborigines." Cohen recommends that one practice self-healing Qigong before attempting to heal others.

Qigong healing is effective and simple to learn. Since the 1950s it has traditionally been used by hospitals and clinics throughout China to ease pain and other symptoms and accelerate healing. In addition to performing Qigong healing on another person, Qigong can be practiced by the ill individual. Qigong healers both in China and in the West work with people who are too sick to get out of bed or their wheelchairs, assisting the very ill in performing simple Qigong movements to restore Energy balance. Although easy to learn, healing Qi is beyond the scope of this chapter. Please go to ancientherbsmodern medicine.com for instructional courses by Kenneth Cohen on video that demonstrate how to practice self-healing Qigong to build your own abundant reservoir of Qi—the essential foundation of any successful Qigong healer—as well as every step of administering healing Qi energy to others.

## Tai Chi

Dr. Mao and his brother Dr. Dao (see chapter 17 for more on Dr. Dao) are part of a close-knit family who trace their lineage in the Chinese medical healing arts back thirty-eight generations and their family tradition of spiritual masters back seventy-four generations to the Han dynasty (206 B.C.–220 A.D.). Their father, Hua-Ching Ni, was chosen as a youth to spend years living with and learning from Taoist masters in the high mountains of mainland China. He devoted his life to continuing the family's spiritual tradition and is internationally recognized as a master of all aspects of Taoist science and metaphysics. Master Ni passed this tradition on to his sons, Drs. Mao and Dao, who were trained in all aspects of Chinese healing arts, including Tai Chi.

"The most memorable images of China in the media often include the Great Wall, the Forbidden City and people doing Tai Chi in parks," Dr. Mao said. "Tai Chi is as integral to many Chinese people's way of life as rice is to their daily diet. Increasingly, the tradition of Tai Chi has spread outside of mainland China and today people can be seen practicing Tai Chi in parks everywhere around the world.

"Why are so many people mesmerized by Tai Chi's graceful, dancelike movements? What is Tai Chi? Tai Chi was originally conceived by ancient Taoist hermits in China and was first mentioned in the ancient philosophical text *I Ching* as the source and union of Yin and Yang. Ancient masters studied and observed the natural laws, which they called Tao, and created a series of fluid, circular movements to express the polar and yet complementary Energies of Yin and Yang, and to experience these Energetic patterns and cycles. In modern times, Tai Chi is practiced as a fitness exercise for its healthful benefits, but up until the end of the nineteenth century it was also practiced for its potent self-defense, martial-art application.

"As an expression of natural laws, Tai Chi teaches the principles of harmony, balance and regeneration in one's life. So, in a way, practicing Tai Chi is not merely a fitness exercise, but a spiritual quest as well.

"As a popular fitness exercise, Tai Chi is practiced by an estimated hundred million people worldwide. Its health benefits have been studied and confirmed widely in China, which include promoting the healthy function of one's immune system, metabolism, hormonal system and nervous system. Consistent practice can help normalize blood pressure and blood sugar, increase energy and stamina and reduce stress. It also has been shown to be beneficial for the cardiovascular system without the strain on the joints.

"The practice of Tai Chi allows one to profoundly experience the planetary movements of the infinite universe within your personal miniuniverse. As a tool for spiritual cultivation, Tai Chi is a meditation that elevates one's spirit above the mundane and unites one with the divine. As a tool for healing, Tai Chi is a therapeutic modality within Chinese medicine that restores balance of functions. As a tool for life, Tai Chi is a living philosophy that helps people achieve happiness, harmony and inner peace.

"Like Qigong, practicing Tai Chi replenishes your inner Qi by harmonizing Yin and Yang, improving the quality of your inner Qi and ensuring that your inner Qi flows freely and is not blocked. Also like Qigong, Tai Chi is practiced with flowing, rhythmic, deliberate movements in carefully prescribed postures combined with breathing and mental focus.

"Qigong is quicker and easier to learn and is more specific in its effects," Dr. Mao said. "For example, someone might choose to practice the Swimming Dragon Qigong to strengthen the Middle Warmer, which includes the digestive system, and increase metabolism, whereas Tai Chi is a more complex choreographed set of movements that is considered a generalized practice for the benefit of the whole body. I suggest that beginners start with any simple Qigong form and graduate into Tai Chi as their interest and understanding grows.

"There are several styles of Tai Chi. Among the Yang, Chen and Wu styles, the most popular is the Yang Style. In our family tradition, at Yo San University of Traditional Chinese Medicine in Los Angeles, we teach the Style of Harmony, or Trinity Style, which synthesizes the Yang, Chen and Wu styles."

If you are interested in learning Tai Chi, many recreation or parks departments or community centers offer Tai Chi classes. You can find more information on Qigong and Tai Chi at ancientherbsmodernmedicine.com.

# 17

## Women's Health

*Infertility, PMS, perimenopause and menopause*

In 1980 twelve-year-old Meredith Rosen was diagnosed with a strangulated ovary. A grapefruit-sized dermoid cyst on her left ovary was twisting her fallopian tube, resulting in a cutoff of the blood supply to the ovary and acute inflammation of the affected tissue. Meredith underwent emergency surgery with a complete ovariectomy—removal of her left ovary—as well as partial removal of her right ovary, where more cysts were found.

In 1989, at twenty-one years old, Meredith was back in the hospital for another emergency surgery to remove another dermoid cyst that had developed on what was left of her right ovary. Aside from the fear of surgery, Meredith was terrified that she would lose the small piece of ovary she had left and never be able to have her own biological children. Her fears were justified. After the second surgery, Meredith was left with a mere remnant of ovarian tissue. Within a few weeks she began suffering from hot flashes. Her follicle-stimulating hormone (FSH) levels indicated she was in perimenopause.

When ovarian function begins to decline, preceding menopause, the pituitary gland secretes follicle stimulating hormone (FSH) in an attempt to stimulate the ovary to ovulate. If the ovary does not respond, the FSH levels will continue to rise. In a postmenopausal patient with unresponsive ovaries, levels of FSH will typically be above 60 to 80, while a fertile woman with regular menstrual cycles who ovulates monthly will have an FSH level of less than 20. Therefore, lower levels of FSH indicate ovulation, while very high levels of FSH suggest the ovaries are not responding. High levels of FSH can be seen in menopause or in premature ovarian failure.

For the next seven years, Meredith was under medical care for hormone maintenance of her estrogen levels. In 1996, at age twenty-eight, she married

David, her high-school sweetheart. "Two years later, when I was thirty, David and I began discussing raising a family," Meredith said. "I had never given up on having my own children. If I had a piece of ovarian tissue and I wasn't menopausal, then I was determined to find a way. I had faith that God would send me in the right direction. I believed that God would provide so that I could be a mother." Meredith became singularly focused on ovulating. She also became "very aware of pregnant women, menstrual cycles, babies and anything else that had to do with having a baby."

She went to an infertility clinic and shared her story with the specialist. "I was told that I had a zero percent chance of becoming pregnant. I would not listen to the doctor and insisted on starting fertility treatment." Meredith began by using an estrogen patch to see if any ovarian follicles would develop as a result of increased estrogen. During the early follicular phase of a cycle, FSH stimulates the growth of ovarian follicles and increases luteinizing hormone (LH) receptors. Receptors are sites on all living cells that respond to a specific agent such as hormones, neurotransmitters or proteins. In other words, receptors are like the lock and the specific agent is the only key that will unlock the receptor. FSH and LH work synergistically to increase follicle size. As it grows, the follicle secretes estrogen. One follicle outgrows the others and becomes the dominant follicle destined for ovulation. About ten to twelve hours before ovulation LH and FSH secretions peak, causing the follicle to reach maximum size. The follicle releases the ovum (egg) into the fallopian tube. The follicle then decreases estrogen secretion.

Following ovulation, cells within the ruptured ovarian follicle undergo a process called luteinization, forming a small mass called a corpus luteum. The corpus luteum secretes progesterone, which is responsible for ripening the endometrial lining, preparing it for implantation of a fertilized egg. If conception does not occur, progesterone and estradiol (estrogen) levels decline, leading to the sloughing off of the thick and highly vascular endometrial lining of the uterus resulting in menstrual flow.

"I think the doctors at the fertility clinic were trying to show me—without making me spend all my money and waste my time and theirs—that if the patches did not cause a follicle to develop, then obviously there were no eggs on my ovary," Meredith said. When the estrogen patch failed and Meredith did not get any encouragement from the doctors at that clinic, she began shopping for a new fertility doctor, but every doctor she saw attempted to discourage her.

Meredith finally managed to talk one doctor into prescribing Pergonal shots—synthetic high-dose estrogen—in the hopes of stimulating follicular development. It was expensive, time-consuming and painful. Two cycles on Pergonal produced no results. The doctor at the clinic advised Meredith to see a psychiatrist to deal with her denial and to see a gynecologist to receive hormone replacement maintenance to manage her menopausal symptoms. Although Meredith agreed to see a gynecologist, she did not give up. "If my FSH levels indicated that I was in perimenopause, not menopause [when the ovaries are completely depleted of follicles that can develop and release eggs], it meant that I had one egg in what was left of my ovary. One egg meant one baby, and nothing would stop me from finding that egg."

The gynecologist Meredith went to see was sympathetic. "She told me that she thought it would be a rough road for me to get pregnant but it was certainly worth the effort. I thought, 'Finally—a doctor who isn't throwing my hopes in the garbage.' It felt wonderful." The doctor recommended Meredith try natural remedies to help with her perimenopausal symptoms. "I thought she was kind of nuts," Meredith said. "She told me about Chinese herbal teas and acupuncture and referred me to a doctor of Chinese medicine. I thought, 'This is the first time a doctor has really listened to me,' but at the same time I thought, 'I'm not coming back here and I'm not going to any Chinese doctor.' But when I went home and told my husband, he said, 'If you don't try, you may turn around someday and say, "What if Chinese medicine could have worked?"' I knew I would be eating myself alive for the rest of my life wondering."

On February 23, 1999, Meredith went to see Daoshing Ni, Lic. Ac., D.O.M., Ph.D. a thirty-eighth-generation Chinese doctor and cofounder of the Tao of Wellness clinic in Los Angeles. Dr. Dao specializes in gynecology and reproductive medicine, including infertility, pregnancy, postpartum issues, dysmenorrhea, endometriosis, pelvic pain, perimenopausal symptoms, postmenopausal symptoms, aging issues and other issues of women's health as well as male infertility.

Dr. Dao sees approximately three thousand infertility patients a year and estimates his overall success rate is as high as 60 percent when a patient follows the complete treatment protocol. He treats infertility patients with herbs, acupuncture, acupressure and massage. Chinese medicine has been shown to be helpful in the treatment of endometriosis, uterine fibroids, tubal blockage, premature menopause, male infertility, sperm antibody conditions, irregular ovulation, pituitary imbalances, hypothyroidism, recurrent spontaneous abortion, luteal phase defects and unexplained infertility. "Chinese medicine can work miracles with women who have become overly anxious about conceiving," Dr. Dao said. "Unfortunately, most women seek out Chinese medicine as a last resort, after years and many thousands of dollars spent in Western infertility clinics. When Meredith came to see me, she had not had a period in ten years and had been on hormone replacement therapy for almost that long. She had a history of ovarian tissue removal and had very little ovarian tissue left. She exhibited symptoms of menopause—hot flashes and night sweats."

"After reading my medical file, Dr. Dao took my pulse," Meredith said. "Then he asked me to show him my tongue. I remember his words exactly: 'May I see your tongue, please?' I was completely perplexed. I thought, 'Where's the lab? Doesn't he need some vials of blood to look at?' "

"In Chinese medical terms, Meredith's pulse was thready, her tongue tip was red with a thin white coating," Dr. Dao said. "She had Kidney Qi and Kidney Essence deficiency syndrome. Our goal was to replenish her Kidney Qi and Kidney Essence by utilizing acupuncture points that can nourish the Kidney system. From a Western point of view, the goal was to stimulate and facilitate her ovarian function."

Meredith was skeptical but liked Dr. Dao's team mentality. "Meredith and I did not know whether or not she would ever get pregnant," Dr. Dao said. "We set a very conservative goal—to resolve her menopausal symptoms and to get her off hormone replacement therapy." Dr. Dao's plan of action was to put Meredith's body back in balance. This meant stimulating ovarian function to increase her own estrogen production, eliminate hot flashes and night sweats, and facilitate ovulation so that Meredith would begin menstruating again.

Meredith has a highly allergic, reactive and sensitive constitution. She had been hospitalized in the past for allergic reactions. She was worried about taking herbs. She and Dr. Dao mutually agreed not to introduce herbs at the beginning of her treatment and to first see how she responded to acupuncture treatments. Meredith went off the estrogen patch and began acupuncture treatments.

In the beginning, Meredith did not feel confident with acupuncture as a treatment for infertility. But she agreed to the treatments and went twice a week. "Acupuncture moves and draws in Qi," Dr. Dao said. "In this case, Meredith's hypersensitivity became a plus for her. The points that I used are very gentle but powerful. She felt the needle greatly, so the efficacy of acupuncture treatments became heightened. One often doesn't feel pain or discomfort from the acupuncture needles. Meredith responded very favorably to acupuncture treatments, and within the first few treatments her hot flashes decreased dramatically."

After three months of treatment, on May 30, 1999, Meredith told Dr. Dao she was having discomfort where her ovary used to be. He needled her to minimize the discomfort but she still felt something in that area. "I had a funny feeling," Meredith said. "I thought, what if my ovary remnant was actually being stimulated? I decided to get an ovulation test. As I was driving to the pharmacy I was laughing and crying at the same time. I thought, what am I doing? I'm going to buy an ovulation test? Who am I kidding?" Meredith's ovulation test showed a blue line indicating ovulation. Disbelieving, she tried another test and got the same result.

She had an appointment with Dr. Dao the next morning and showed him the test results. He suggested she go to her gynecologist to have a blood test to check her estrogen levels. "I could not control the tears when I got the results," Meredith said. "I had ovulated. Not only were my estrogen levels good, they were great. They were completely normal. My blood levels indicated no sign of perimenopause at all!"

Acupuncture treatments had successfully stimulated Meredith's ovarian function, and she was ovulating. Given the scar tissue in her fallopian tube and other complications, Dr. Dao recommended she work with a Western infertility specialist. Meredith went home and began waiting for her period to start so that she could count the days until midcycle, when she would ovulate again and could begin working with an infertility specialist. When her period did not start, on a whim she purchased a pregnancy test. "Once again, I laughed and cried as I took the test. My heart started beating really fast. 'Oh my God!' I yelled. There were two pink lines!" Meredith and David rushed to the lab in the morning. "The lab technicians all knew me and were also eager to find out if I was really pregnant. They drew my blood and told me they would call me by noon. That was it. It was the day I had been waiting for. I would find out if I was going to have a baby. I would find out if I was going to be a mommy." The lab called at noon and connected Meredith with the doctor's office. The nurse said, "You have us all baffled here. Congratulations, Meredith, you are pregnant!" It was three months after Meredith began acupuncture treatments.

Meredith had a perfect pregnancy with no morning sickness. On January 25, 2000, Hannah Danielle, seven pounds, eight ounces, was born by cesarian section. It appeared that Meredith had been correct in her quest for the one egg that would produce one baby. After the follicle had matured and produced that egg, the remaining shred of ovarian tissue left from Meredith's two surgeries had been absorbed by her body—when Meredith's abdomen was opened, the surgeon could not find a trace of ovarian tissue.

"The Chinese medical approach to infertility is similar to Western medicine's in that we try to stimulate and increase the probability of conception before a woman's eggs get too old," Dr. Dao said. "Age plays a role. Eggs act as if they have an expiration date on them. We try to improve the quality of the follicles. Success has a lot to do with the woman's family history of fertility and how well she has taken care of her body. In some instances, conception requires stimulation to the reproductive system. So you push it a little bit, but sometimes you have to be realistic and careful not to push a woman's body toward perimenopause. We don't want to exhaust the body when there are few or no more eggs to squeeze out."

Dr. Dao often works closely with Western infertility doctors when women choose to use Western infertility drugs. "I advocate the integrative approach," he said, "combining both Chinese and Western medicines to enhance the likelihood of conception. But if a woman comes in who I don't think needs artificial reproductive technologies [ART] to conceive, I will advise her to delay for a few months and to try Chinese medicine alone. If a woman doesn't want to wait, I will refer her to a reproductive endocrinologist and we will work together with her. There are other women who come to my office and I actually think they need ART right away. In that case I will tell them that Chinese medicine might help, but it would take too long.

"I ask that women have a fertility workup to see if there are problems that can be repaired by Chinese medicine. I use Chinese medicine for three months or longer to prepare the woman's body before she takes infertility drugs. A woman needs to be judicial when she uses infertility drugs. She needs to have a plan before she enters into treatment to decide what kind of drug protocol she will do and how many cycles. During her treatment with Western drugs, I watch her responses, monitor her for side effects and adjust my treatment accordingly. Some of the adverse reactions to infertility drugs are low energy, moodiness, depression, bloating, puffiness, breast pains, cramps and headaches."

From Dr. Dao's point of view, Meredith's positive attitude played a role in her success. "Obviously, when you are positive, you can frequently elicit positive outcomes from your body," Dr. Dao said. "We should never underestimate the power and importance of our mind and our spirit, and what they can do for our body. Mental attitude plays a huge role in the success of fertility treatments."

## Premenstrual Syndrome (PMS)

In a woman's fertile years, estrogen is produced by her follicles, peaking at ovulation. Estrogen helps to build up the endometrial lining of the uterus.

Progesterone is produced by the ovaries after ovulation. Progesterone is responsible for ripening the endometrial lining, preparing it for implantation of a fertilized egg. If no pregnancy occurs, estrogen and progesterone levels drop, causing the lining to be sloughed off (menses). A woman can begin to experience PMS during the last two weeks of her cycle. When a woman does not ovulate every month, she does not have the level of progesterone her body needs. Without adequate progesterone, there is too much estrogen left unchecked, which results in symptoms of PMS such as bloating, breast tenderness, crying jags, decreased tolerance to pain, difficulty coping with life, food and stimulant cravings, headaches, irritability and rage. Symptoms of PMS usually stop abruptly with the onset of menstrual flow.

From a Chinese medicine point of view, females have a different Energetic pattern than males. Women possess a special type of Kidney Jing, called Tian Kui (pronounced *tea-en kway*). Due to the cyclical pattern of menstruation, once a female reaches puberty, her Kidney Energy and Blood fluctuate, creating a unique tendency toward certain imbalances. For example, menstruation, although part of the normal physiology of females, also produces a cyclical loss of Yin and Blood. Consequently, females have a tendency to develop Liver Blood and Kidney Yin deficiencies—which result in PMS symptoms. There is a saying in Chinese medicine, "Women tend to lack in Yin and therefore are unable to counterbalance Yang, causing relative excess in Yang." This phrase plays a strategic role in determining treatment for women, which tends to almost always emphasize protecting, supporting and nourishing Yin and harmonizing Liver.

When treating women, Chinese doctors are usually cautious in using herbs that can be overly drying and Warming, to prevent drying out the already deficient Yin Essence. Since Blood is part of Yin, the cyclical loss of Blood obviously tends toward a relative Yin deficiency. Since Yin is Cooling, the relative Yang excess further dries the Yin, causing a certain pattern of internal Heat within a woman's constitution. This is true during a woman's menstruating years.

From a Chinese medicine point of view, PMS symptoms are also tied to Liver Qi stagnation—blood flow is slowed to the pelvic cavity. Reproductive organs depend on blood supply. Herbs, acupuncture, nutritional changes and massage are all used to treat PMS-related Liver Qi stagnation. If Liver Qi stagnation is left untreated, more serious disorders, such as endometriosis and uterine fibroids can develop.

Chinese medicine herbal therapy addresses the individual's unique constitution, medical history and current condition. The treatment may not be the same, even with the same diagnosis of endometriosis. Dr. Dao treats endometriosis with herbs and acupuncture to release the stagnation and circulate Qi.

## Perimenopause and Menopause

During perimenopause and menopause, Tian Kui—the special Kidney Jing—diminishes. Women will therefore develop some acute Kidney Yin deficiency. The loss of the Cooling effects of Yin creates a relative excess of Yang, which leads to hot flashes, emotional fluctuations and insomnia. Normally when one sleeps, Yang is submerged into Yin, Yin thereby having a somewhat more dominant role. Upon awakening and throughout the day, Yang emerges out of Yin and takes a somewhat more dominant role. This is part of the normal perpetual dance between Yin and Yang. In perimenopause or menopause, because of an acute deficiency of Yin, Yin is unable to adequately engage Yang and hold the Yang submerged. As a result, Yang has a tendency to flare up and float toward the top, leading to menopausal symptoms, including insomnia.

Due to the intimate relationship between Kidney Energy and the bones, the Kidney Energy imbalance during perimenopause and menopause significantly increases the risk of osteoporosis in postmenopausal women. The relative lack of Yin Energy and its Cooling and moistening properties also explains why postmenopausal women have a tendency toward dry skin and vaginal dryness.

From a Western point of view, women begin to experience symptoms when ovarian function (estrogen, progesterone and testosterone) declines and sex hormones fluctuate during perimenopause. The cardiovascular system, bones, skin and certain cognitive functions begin to deteriorate. Perimenopause begins when your ovaries are no longer secreting adequate amounts of progesterone because you are no longer ovulating every month. Regular or irregular menstrual cycles may have heavier flow.

*Some Perimenopausal Symptoms Due to Declining Ovarian Function*

Hot flashes and night sweats
Sleep disturbances
Fatigue
Spontaneous crying jags
Irritability
Headaches
Foggy-headedness
Rage

When a woman has not had a period for one year she is considered in menopause. The mean age for menopause is 51.2 years. A woman's ovaries are now only producing very low levels of estrogen. As her ovaries are no longer releasing eggs, there is no progesterone. Testosterone production also declines.

*Some Menopausal Symptoms Due to Decreased Ovarian Function*

| | | |
|---|---|---|
| Acne | Hot flashes | Memory loss |
| Breast tenderness | Inability to have | Night sweats |
| Brittle/ridged nails | orgasm | Night obsessions |
| Constipation | Incontinence | Numbness and |
| Decreased sex drive | Increased facial hair | tingling |
| Degenerative diseases | Increased/decreased | Pain with intercourse |
| Dry skin | breast size | Reduced sex |
| Fibrocystic breasts | Insomnia | drive |
| Fleeting joint pain | Intolerance to | Vaginal dryness |
| Fluid retention | cold/heat | Weakness and fatigue |
| Hair loss | Loss of body hair | Weight gain/loss |

Also, bone loss may accelerate. See pages 212–213 for information on osteoporosis.

## Using Chinese herbs to alleviate perimenopausal and menopausal symptoms

"In treating perimenopause, the goal is to boost and maintain ovarian function," Dr. Dao said. "However, ovarian and other reproductive functions decline naturally in menopause. In menopause the objective is to try to balance the body and slow down the aging process. We use acupuncture and herbs and other traditional Chinese medicine modalities such as Qigong, meditation, massage and acupressure to relieve menopausal symptoms."

From a Chinese medicine point of view, menopausal symptoms are the body's panic reaction to the sudden decrease of Tian Kui. A woman can use Chinese herbs and acupuncture to stimulate the ovaries in a controlled fashion so that sex hormones decline gently over a period of time. This allows the body's withdrawal symptoms from sex hormones to diminish gradually over a period of time without as much discomfort. In the meantime, additional herbs are used to support and protect your heart and bones. Many symptoms can be resolved without bringing up and maintaining the high level of sex hormones.

"Some women are concerned that they will have to take herbs for life," Dr. Dao said. "But most women feel better within a couple of weeks of using herbs and acupuncture. Some women take two or three months to feel balanced and vital. Using hormone replacement is a personal choice that we do not try to discourage women from if that is what they need or if that is their personal choice. Of course, the earlier a woman addresses her symptoms, the more successful the outcome of the treatment. If a woman requires a complete hysterectomy, it's difficult to be without hormone replacement therapy. Whenever possible, I encourage women to request that at least a portion of one ovary be left in when having a hysterectomy."

Hormone replacement

Some women will choose to take Chinese herbs when they experience the symptoms of perimenopause and menopause. Others will use Chinese herbs along with hormone replacement therapy (HRT) and a third group will use only HRT.

Increasingly, over the past fifty years, the stress of eating processed and refined foods, ingesting stimulants and drugs and being exposed to environmental toxins and other poisons has affected women's ovarian function, often leading to sex hormone imbalances (estrogen, progesterone and testosterone). From a Western perspective, the goal is to maintain ovarian function to preserve hormone balance by focusing on nutrition and lifestyle. Once you have done everything you can to balance your hormones and you still feel symptomatic, it may be time to consider hormone replacement therapy.

Some women do not feel symptomatic during menopause. A lack of symptoms, however, does not mean that a woman will not develop a degenerative disease such as cardiovascular disease or osteoporosis due to a lack of hormones.

Herbs and acupuncture can stimulate your ovaries to produce more hormones as well as support your system so that they work better to alleviate symptoms. Taking herbs is not replacement therapy. No matter how well you do at balancing your nutrition and lifestyle, and no matter how many herbs you take to stimulate your ovaries, there is going to come a point where your ovaries are not going to produce any more hormones.

Premarin, PremPro, PremPhase and Prempac-C are estrogen drugs made from the urine of pregnant mares. These drugs are not bioidentical to naturally occurring estrogen in the human body and therefore cannot be called hormone replacement therapy. They are FDA approved only to alleviate hot flashes and to prevent osteoporosis—not as hormone replacement. Synthetic progesterone, called Provera, is made only in part with natural progesterone. Since a natural substance cannot be patented, manufacturers have changed the molecular configuration so that it is unlike anything found in nature. Methyltestosterone is a synthetic drug that has created a bad reputation for testosterone replacement because it can cause hair growth in unwanted places, high cholesterol and aggressiveness.

Estrogen, progesterone and testosterone must be replaced with a hormone that fits into that receptor to mimic what the ovaries once supplied. Bioidentical hormones are hormones that fit into your body's hormone receptors. By using bioidentical hormones in appropriate doses, most symptoms can be relieved without side effects. Problems and side effects do not occur if you use physiological doses of bioidentical estrogen, progesterone and testosterone—in other words, when you replace what the woman is lacking and no more. The goal is to find balance in all hormone levels.

## Ways to preserve or restore ovarian function

*Avoid Processed and Refined Foods:* These foods contain toxic chemicals, pesticides, hormones and damaged fats that lead to cellular damage, decreased ovarian function and premature aging. Likewise, women can maintain healthier ovarian function longer by not using stimulants such as caffeine, nicotine, alcohol and Ma Huang. Recent research has demonstrated that smoking may also lead to premature decline of ovarian function.

Please see chapter 21 for recipes for women's health.

*Avoid Exposure to Toxins:* Exposure to toxins results in earlier ovarian function decline. See more about toxins on pages 166–172.

*Reduce the Amount of Prescription and Over-the-Counter Drugs You Are Taking:* Discuss the necessity of your prescription drugs with your doctor to determine if you are taking any drugs that you can safely eliminate. Instead of automatically reaching for over-the-counter drugs, consider taking herbs and having acupuncture as alternatives.

*Choose Herbs and Acupuncture to Alleviate Symptoms—or Take Hormone Replacement Therapy:* If you are experiencing symptoms of ovarian function decline, a health care professional can work with you and follow your healing progress. If you suffer from PMS, herbs and acupuncture can balance ovarian function, or you can begin herb and acupuncture treatments or begin using an over-the-counter progesterone cream with the supervision of your health care practitioner. When symptoms of menopause increase, you can choose acupuncture and herbs to alleviate your symptoms, or you can see a hormone replacement expert for bioidentical progesterone, estrogen and testosterone replacement therapy.

*Chinese Herbs and Western Supplements:* When you do not provide your body with adequate vitamins and minerals, your body—including your ovaries—will age more rapidly. You can take Chinese herbal formulas and Western supplements specifically formulated for women's health.

For women, the Chinese herb Deer Velvet Antler has been shown to be effective in treating gynecological problems due to hormonal imbalances, particularly low estrogen, excessive menstrual bleeding or amenorrhea (lack of menstrual period), as well as excessive vaginal discharge due to depressed ovarian function. See page 290 for more on Deer Velvet Antler. Deer Velvet Antler should be taken under the supervision of an herbalist.

Routinely, take the immune-modulating formula described on pages 103–104.

## Female Infertility

Female infertility is defined as the inability to conceive with a normal sex life without using contraceptives for two years. Statistically, in relationships where the male has a normal sperm count and no other abnormalities, 60 percent of women become pregnant within six months without using contraceptives, 80 percent within nine months, up to 90 percent within a year.

Female infertility can be generally divided into two categories: structural and functional. Structural problems include (1) blocked fallopian tube(s) resulting from severe scarring from past pelvic inflammatory disease (PID), endometriosis, extensive surgery, obstruction from tumor or congenital abnormality, (2) completely blocked cervix, (3) destruction of the linings of the fallopian tube(s) or uterus and (4) congenitally deformed or nonexistent uterus or ovaries.

Functional problems include (1) obesity, (2) certain hormonal imbalances, (3) inflammation of the pelvis, uterus or vagina, (4) certain immune disorders such as antibodies against sperm protein and antibodies to certain hormone receptor sites and (5) fallopian tubes kinked or blocked by mucus.

Infertility in Chinese medicine can generally be divided into two classes: deficiency primarily involving Kidney Energy, which is roughly equivalent to hormonal imbalances, and stagnation primarily involving Liver Energy, which is often equivalent to a functional blockage in the Western sense, such as decreased libido and hormone imbalance resulting in decreased ovarian function. Some structural problems obviously cannot be resolved by Chinese medicine.

The main therapeutic goals in treating infertility are to balance and support Kidney Energy and Jing, resolve stagnation, especially Liver Energy stagnation, and build Blood.

## Avoid overwork

Overwork depletes Kidney Yin, which is the basis for menstruation and the health of your ovaries and uterus. Excess physical work or exercise in adolescence injures Kidney and Spleen Energies, which are required for the development and continuation of the menstrual cycle. This can create a fundamental weakness or imbalance in these Energies (which carry hormone cycles) by undermining the ovarian function before it is mature. Adequate rest nourishes Yin.

## Avoid long-term use of contraceptives

Such use can interfere with your normal hormonal balance and ovarian function.

## Practice safe sex

Unsafe sexual practices can result in sexually transmitted diseases (STDs), which weaken Kidney Energy. Abortions also weaken Kidney Energy.

## Avoid extreme cold

Avoid exposure of your body to extreme Cold and Dampness. The uterus is sensitive to Cold, which affects the flow of Energy. This is especially true during the menses. Exposure to Cold and Dampness usually occurs during exercise or through sports activities.

Modify your diet

Avoid excess intake of Cold, iced foods and drinks to prevent Cold invasion of the uterus. Excess sugar, processed foods, fried foods and dairy can lead to Damp stagnation, which can affect ovarian function and even result in ovarian cysts and blockage of fallopian tubes.

Chinese herbs and Western supplements

You can use Chinese medicinal herbs in recipes to improve your overall health. See chapter 21 for recipes. You can also take Chinese herbal formulas designed to address mild cases of functional problems. For more information, log on to ancientherbsmodernmedicine.com.

## Uterine Fibroids

Fibroids are knots of muscle tissue typically found in smooth muscle such as the muscle of the uterus. While they are never cancerous, fibroids are sometimes called fibroid tumors because of their shape. Fibroids cause problems simply due to their size and their physical compression of other pelvic organs. If they penetrate into the endometrial cavity of the uterus, they can cause irregular and heavy bleeding; this is a common reason for women seeking treatment for their fibroids. They can sometimes cause infertility. Studies have shown that up to one-third of all women have at least some small fibroids in their uterus at the time of death. Most are completely asymptomatic. When fibroids grow and begin to cause either pain or irregular bleeding, they may require treatment. Fibroids can be removed while leaving the uterus intact in a myomectomy, but this is usually only a temporary treatment, as the likelihood that the fibroids will grow back is quite high. Therefore, myomectomy is generally reserved only for those women who are trying to conceive and give birth. The only definitive treatment for fibroids is a hysterectomy. Occasionally, medications such as Lupron (synthetic progesterone) can be used to shrink fibroids. This again is typically only a temporary measure and is used in preparation for surgery to make the procedure easier and safer; on occasion, the medication can shrink the fibroids prior to conception.

From a Chinese medicine point of view, fibroids are a type of stagnation that can involve Qi, Blood and Dampness.

See a hormone expert

If you are experiencing symptoms of PMS and you have fibroids, you may benefit from bioidentical progesterone replacement therapy.

Focus on your emotional health

See a therapist to resolve emotional strain, especially repressed anger, frustration, hatred and resentment. Negative emotions stagnate Qi; left unresolved, they can result in stagnation of the Blood.

Avoid estrogen-stimulating herbs

Fibroids are stimulated by estrogen. Herbs such as Dang Gui, Lu Rong, Ren Shen and Black Cohosh can stimulate estrogen production and should be avoided.

Manage habits that lead to high insulin secretion

High insulin secretion—which is a growth factor—will contribute to the development of uterine fibroids. Factors that raise insulin levels include eating a low-fat, high-carbohydrate diet, stress, dieting, caffeine, alcohol, aspartame (an artificial sweetener), tobacco, steroids, stimulants and other recreational drugs, lack of exercise, excessive or unnecessary thyroid replacement therapy and all over-the-counter and prescription drugs. Once you have fibroids these factors will stimulate their growth. From a Chinese medicine point of view, these factors create Heat, Damp and stagnation.

Modify your diet

Excess consumption of raw, cold foods or drink results in stagnation of Qi. Irregular eating habits such as skipping meals and poor diet upset Spleen and Liver Energy, which also leads to Qi stagnation. Avoid fried foods, dairy, sugar and processed foods, which create Damp and Phlegm accumulation. Do not eat chicken skin, which contains xenoestrogens—molecules that exert an estrogenic influence on your body. Avoid commercial chicken broth, which is processed with chicken skin. Be aware that restaurants often use chicken broth, and order accordingly.

Get adequate rest

Overwork, overexercise and lack of rest leads to Qi deficiency. All abdominal masses involve Qi deficiency.

Chinese herbs and Western supplements

You can use Chinese medicinal herbs in recipes to strengthen your Qi. See chapter 21 for recipes. You can take Chinese herbs and Western supplements to strengthen Qi.

Surgery

Hysterectomy is surgery in which the uterus is removed. In a total abdominal hysterectomy, the entire uterus including the cervix is removed. A subtotal hysterectomy is sometimes performed, in which the cervix is left behind but the rest of the uterus is removed. The subtotal hysterectomy is a much easier surgery, and is performed when a shorter surgery is optimal. It is also performed in a laparascopic procedure when removing the cervix would simply be too difficult. A major drawback in the subtotal hysterectomy is that leaving behind the cervix leaves the woman at risk for cervical cancer. One of the benefits of a hysterectomy is the removal of tissue that commonly develops cancerous cells. Leaving behind a nonuseful organ fragment that can develop cancer is not thought optimal by many experts in the field.

There are three methods currently used for performing a hysterectomy. The first and most common is a transabdominal hysterectomy. This surgery involves taking the uterus out through an abdominal incision. The gynecologist will try to use a bikini incision if possible, but many factors play a role in making the decision of where and how to perform the operation. The second and often preferred method is a vaginal hysterectomy. This method involves taking the uterus out through the vagina. This method is technically more difficult and requires an experienced surgeon but is generally preferred when possible, as the recovery time and discomfort are significantly less than with the abdominal procedure. It also does not have the drawbacks of leaving visible scars. The vaginal hysterectomy is a dying art in this country, and there are too few physicians experienced in this procedure due to its technical and dexterity requirements. The last method for hysterectomy is called laparoscopic surgery, a newer technique that involves performing surgery with the use of tube-shaped cameras and instruments that are inserted through small incisions in the abdominal wall of the anesthetized patient. This surgery commonly takes much longer than the previously mentioned methods but offers the benefits of much smaller incisions and in some cases faster recovery. While techniques are rapidly changing, it is clear that the future of surgery in all specialties will be the minimally invasive surgical laparoscopic techniques. Currently, however, the laparoscopic approach should be reserved for cases where it is deemed appropriate. Using this type of procedure in the wrong type of surgical candidate can lead to a much more difficult and potentially dangerous surgery.

Whether or not the ovaries are taken out during a hysterectomy is a complicated decision. The conservative approach is to remove the ovaries at the time of hysterectomy if the risk of cancer is thought to outweigh the benefits of leaving them. Today women are more informed, engage in more research before surgery and are more involved in decision making than in the past. More women are opting to have their ovaries or part of one ovary as well as their cervix left in place when having a hysterectomy. Since every woman's case is different, this decision is best made with the advice of your doctor.

## Thyroid Decline

In addition to healthy ovarian function, healthy thyroid function is crucial for health and well-being. Hypothyroidism, or low thyroid function, affects as many as 40 percent of the population, though many people go undiagnosed—and it can affect you at any age. The thyroid is a small, butterfly-shaped endocrine gland located just below your Adam's apple. Every cell, tissue and organ of your body is affected by the actions of your thyroid gland. The thyroid controls your metabolism, regulates your body's thermostat, helps maintain your circulatory system and blood volume, heightens the sensitivity of your nerves and is necessary for building and maintaining lean body mass (muscle and bones).

Some symptoms of hypothyroidisim and menopause are similar, so the two can often become confused. A patient may have one and be labeled as having the other. There can also be multiple interactions between hormonal disorders, further complicating the situation. Patients with menopausal symptoms will sometimes benefit from screening for thyroid disorders.

Secreted by the thyroid gland, T4 is converted into T3 in the liver, heart and kidneys. Thyroid-stimulating hormone (TSH) stimulates the thyroid gland when it is not making enough thyroid hormone. When a thyroid blood test shows an elevated TSH, hypothyroidism is indicated even if T3 and T4 levels are normal.

*Symptoms of Low Thyroid Function*

Bruising easily

Coarse hair or hair loss

Constipation

Dry, coarse, leathery or pale skin

Emotional instability with
crying jags

Feeling cold all the time,
particularly hands and feet

Fluid retention

Impaired memory

Increased susceptibility to colds
and other viruses

Infertility

Lethargy

Loss of appetite

Mental sluggishness

Migraine headaches

Mood swings

Weakness

In a hypothyroid individual, body temperature falls below normal. You can easily check your thyroid function at home by using a basal (mercury) thermometer. Shake the thermometer down before you go to bed and leave it at your bedside, within reach. Immediately upon awakening in the morning take your temperature. Reach for the thermometer and put it under your tongue. Do not get up to use the bathroom, and avoid movement. Remain still for ten minutes. If your temperature reads below 97.8 degrees, you may well be suffering from hypothyroidism.

From a Chinese medicine point of view, those suffering from hypothyroidism manifest classic Yang deficiency.

See a hormone expert

If you are experiencing symptoms of hypothyroidism, you may benefit from thyroid hormone replacement therapy.

Focus on your emotional health

Focus on resolving emotional strain, especially anxiety and fear. Anxiety and fear injure the Yang. Think of the expression "frozen with fear." When Yang Energy is deficient, the body turns Cold.

Modify your diet

Avoid overconsumption of Cold, iced or raw foods. Eat a diet that is generally Warm. See pages 310–326 for the Energetic temperature of foods. Eat a whole-food diet, which does not create Dampness. Regulate your weight within ideal limits. Obesity is usually a reflection of Damp stagnation and Spleen deficiency.

Chinese herbs

Chinese medicine does not use a substance to replace the functions of thyroid hormones, but rather works to stimulate thyroid function. Mild to moderate hypothyroid function can be restored by using Chinese medicine to regulate Kidney Yang deficiency. You can purchase Chinese herbal formulas to stimulate thyroid function at a Chinese herbal clinic or online at ancientherbsmodern medicine.com. You can also use Chinese medicinal herbs in recipes to stimulate thyroid function. See chapter 21 for recipes.

# Menstrual Cramping

Uterine pain and cramping during the menstrual period is called dysmenorrhea. Dysmenorrhea is extremely common and can vary in women from hardly noticeable to severe and disabling. Extreme pain is not normal and is usually associated with an underlying medical condition. There are a variety of gynecologic conditions that can lead to disabling pain before and during menses. Pain present since a woman's first period or pain that develops early in the teen years is considered primary dysmenorrhea and is usually caused by excess prostaglandin production. This type of menstrual pain is characterized by onset prior to menstrual bleeding and can be treated with nonsteroidal anti-inflammatory drugs such as ibuprofen (Motrin, Advil) or naproxen (Aleve).

Pain that begins with bleeding or after bleeding has begun is usually considered secondary dysmenorrhea and is usually associated with an underlying anatomical problem such as endometriosis or adenomyosis (benign invasive growth of the endometrium into the muscular layer of the uterus). Treatment of this condition is more complex and diverse and ranges from hormonal therapies to hysterectomy.

In Chinese medicine, menstrual cramps can be of five different origins, depending on the nature of the imbalance. It can be caused by excess or deficiency, and is commonly associated with the stagnation of the Liver and Kidney Energy systems.

### Focus on your emotional health

Repressed anger, frustration and hatred constrain Liver Qi. Negative, unresolved emotions stagnate Qi, which can lead to menstrual cramping.

### Modify your diet

Alcohol, sugar, caffeine, dairy and oily foods create stagnation. Avoid physically and Energetically Cold foods and drink.

### Avoid overuse of drugs

Unnecessary over-the-counter and prescription drugs or recreational drug use upsets your body's balance and can create stagnation.

### Avoid overexertion

Overwork or overexercise can create Qi and Blood deficiency so Liver and Kidney Energies are undernourished and do not have the force to move the menstrual blood, which stagnates and creates pain.

### Chinese herbs and Western supplements

You can use Chinese medicinal herbs in recipes to ease menstrual cramping. See chapter 21 for recipes. You can also take Chinese herbal formulas to relieve menstrual cramping. Herbal formulas can be purchased online at ancientherbs modernmedicine.com.

## Bladder Infection

Urinary tract infections are extremely common in women due to the relatively short length of the urethra (the tube draining the bladder). The short urethra in women allows bacteria to more easily swim upstream and infect the bladder. Many additional factors increase the risk of infection, including sexual activity, pregnancy, and dehydration or decreased bladder drainage. Treatment includes aggressive hydration to flush out the bacteria, antibiotics and acidifying the urine with acidic foods such as cranberry juice.

In Chinese medicine, acute bladder infection, or urinary tract infection (UTI), is usually considered to result from Heat and Dampness, which disrupts normal bladder functions, creating discomfort and irritation. Chronic or recurrent bladder infection often results from Kidney or Spleen deficiencies or Liver Energy imbalance.

### Modify your diet

Avoid sugar, dairy, fried foods and processed foods, which create internal Dampness and Heat and make the bladder vulnerable to infection. Excessive Cold such as iced foods and drink, especially ice cream, can create Dampness, precipitating Damp/Heat.

### Avoid unnecessary drug use

Unnecessary over-the-counter and prescription drugs (especially antibiotics) or recreational drug use interferes with your body's balance and can result in Heat and Dampness, making the bladder vulnerable to infection.

### Focus on your emotional health

Constrained emotions, particularly jealousy and suspicion or paranoia, can transfer to the bladder via Heart and Small Intestine Energy.

### Keep cool

Exposure to Damp and Heat can arise from your living situation. To avoid Dampness, take care to stay cool and dry if you live in a tropical environment.

### Be responsible in your sexual activity

So-called "honeymooner's syndrome" results from sustained sexual intercourse, or intercourse that is unsanitary (anal and genital during the same encounter).

Chinese herbs and Western supplements

You can use Chinese medicinal herbs in recipes to ease the symptoms of a bladder infection. See chapter 21 for recipes. You can also take Chinese herbal formulas to treat bladder infections. For more information log on to ancient herbsmodernmedicine.com.

## Vaginal Candida

Vaginal yeast infections are caused by *Candida albicans,* an organism that is normally present in relatively small numbers in the vagina. A yeast infection occurs when yeast multiplies rapidly. This can be due to a change in the vaginal environment, injury, sexual transmission or HIV. Common environmental disruptions that favor yeast include increased pH, increased heat and moisture, allergic reactions, elevated sugar levels, hormone fluctuations and reductions in the populations of bacteria that are normally present to counterbalance the yeast. Symptoms include intense itching, a burning sensation in the vagina and vulva, a yellowish-white cheesy discharge and a yeasty odor.

Primarily classified in Chinese medicine as Dampness, vaginal candida also involves the External Causes Wind and Heat.

Ways to address vaginal candida

*Modify Your Diet:* Reduce the consumption of fried foods, dairy, sugar and refined white flour products, which create Dampness that can manifest as candida. Skipping meals or eating too much (even if it is a well-balanced diet) can create Dampness. After menstruation or childbirth, women are susceptible to Damp invasion, which often combines with Heat in the vagina. It is crucial to eat a well-balanced diet of whole foods at these times.

*Avoid Unnecessary Drug Use:* Contraceptive pills and steroids can encourage yeast infections. Excessive use of antibiotics and antibacterial soaps can result in Dampness that can manifest as candida. Antibiotic soaps kill unwanted bacteria but can also kill good bacteria, upsetting the balance in your vaginal tract and allowing yeast to take over.

*Wear Cotton:* Wear unbleached, undyed cotton underwear and breathable clothing. Synthetic fabrics, tight or soiled underclothing trap heat and moisture. Do not sleep in underwear.

*Practice Safe Sex:* Candida can be sexually transmitted. Women with compromised immune systems due to HIV or Lyme disease are prone to yeast infections. Maintain scrupulous hygiene and practice safe sex.

*Avoid Perfumes and Dyes:* Chemicals, such as those in inks, dyes and perfumes, can upset vaginal balance and/or trigger allergic reactions that lead to yeast infections. Commercial douches damage mucous membranes. Perfumed toilet paper, bubble baths, bath salts, scented tampons or sanitary pads, feminine deodorant sprays, detergents and fabric softeners contain allergenic dyes and perfumes. Use environmentally safe, fragrance-free products that can be purchased at your health food store.

Condoms are packaged with a lubricant that contains nonoxynol-9, a spermicide that may kill HIV. Several recent studies have shown that nonoxynol-9 is linked to yeast infections.

Injury to vaginal membranes from lack of lubrication during sexual intercourse can lead to a yeast infection.

*Focus on Emotional Healing:* Worry, anger, frustration and resentment all can imbalance Liver Qi, which can further compromise Spleen Energy's ability to digest properly, resulting in the accumulation of Dampness in the intestine and causing Damp vaginal conditions.

*Chinese Herbs, Western Medications and Supplements:* Effective over-the-counter FDA-approved medications to treat vaginal candida can be purchased at any pharmacy. You can use Chinese medicinal herbs in recipes to treat vaginal candida. See chapter 21 for recipes. You can also take Chinese herbal formulas to address vaginal candida. Formulas can be found online at ancient herbsmodernmedicine.com.

# 18

## Sports Medicine

*Excel in sports like world-class Chinese athletes—without the use of drugs or steroids*

Ma Jun Aren was born on October 28, 1944, in a humble village in China. At age fourteen he dropped out of school and worked to help his struggling family survive. After a short stint in the army he returned to the countryside, where, like generations before him, he scraped a living out of the soil. In 1970 the Chinese government began seeking out qualified lay people to fill the shortage of teachers. Ma had little education, but because of his army experience he was recruited into a training program to become a physical education teacher. He was assigned to work at a middle school in an impoverished rural region, where he immediately established an all-girls athletic team.

When his athletes turned up at their first track-and-field event with no uniforms or shoes, they were the laughingstock of the opening ceremony. The girls had the last laugh when they won most of the medals and collectively placed number one. Ma and his team were dubbed the Barefoot Troops.

After this initial success, Ma was regularly transferred from school to school. Wherever he went he made champions. His reputation for being a miracle worker in athletic competition grew. Unconventional, often abrasive and hardworking, Ma was controversial. His critics argued that though he had had some success at lower-level competitions, he could not succeed in more advanced national or international competitions. Ma proved them wrong. Throughout the eighties Ma's farm-girl athletes broke records in track and field throughout China. Ma was eventually promoted to the position of professional coach.

By 1991 his athletes were winning in national championships, breaking national records and winning international competitions. By the end of 1991 his girls had won over a dozen domestic national medals. In 1992 they consistently won national championships, minor international championships and Asian championships. The highlight came in the Barcelona Olympic Games. In track and field two of his girls placed third and fifth in the 1,500-meter run. Both girls broke the Asian records. By this time Ma's girls had positioned themselves to be competitive in the major international competitions.

Coach Ma Jun Aren had become a national hero in China and something of a curiosity among sports enthusiasts worldwide. How could someone who hailed from a long line of peasant farmers take center stage in global sporting events? By 1993 Ma's athletes had won too many domestic and international competitions to list—five out of eleven of his girls broke the world record thirteen times in three fields. In August 1993 at the World Track and Field Tournament in Germany, Ma's athletes took the gold medal in the 10,000-meter race and the 1,500-meter race in addition to all three medals in the 3,000-meter race. On September 8, 1993, in Bejing, Wang Jung Xia, Ma's best athlete, broke the world record in the 10,000 meters by 41.99 seconds—a record that had been unchallenged for seven years. A few weeks later, Wang Jung Xia and Qu Wun Xia both broke the world record in the 1,500 meters—a record unchallenged for thirteen years. Another world record, for the 3,000-meter race, was broken by five of his girls at the same time. The same record was broken by the same girls *again* in the finals of that game. In October 1993, Ma's athletes appeared in Spain in the fifth World Marathon Games and took all the medals for first, second, third and fourth places. Wang Jung Xia, known as the Oriental Deer Goddess, was selected as the United Press International Female Athlete of the Year. She was invited to accept the award in New York accompanied by Coach Ma. The male athlete of that year was Michael Jordan. In 1994 Wang Jung Xia joined the ranks of Carl Lewis, Marion Jones and Lance Armstrong in receiving the Jesse Owens Award.

## What Makes Ma's Girls Run

Because of Coach Ma's unlikely success, there was speculation that he used stimulants to increase the athletic abilities of his Barefoot Troops. The athletes were repeatedly checked and rechecked for traces of stimulants. The tests came out clean. The most often used performance-enhancing drugs (steroids and testosterone) increase muscle mass tremendously and thereby increase body weight, which is undesirable in mid- and long-distance running. In fact, Ma intentionally recruited girls who were light, with smaller, leaner musculature.

Ma had grown up in a poor peasant family that could not afford medication and used Chinese herbs to treat illness and to maintain health. In Chinese culture the herbs overlap with food. Foods may have both nutritional value and strong medicinal qualities. The secret to Ma's success was his focus on the relationship between training and recovery as well as on nutrition and supplements. He developed a unique method to help his athletes recover from high-intensity training which included nutritional programs—especially herbs. Coach Ma said, "Chinese medicine is really a great treasure. I literally grew up in a pile of herbs, and they are in my blood."

Many years earlier, when Ma was first promoted to head track-and-field coach in Liao Ning province, he often took his athletes for high-altitude training. Blood in the urine usually signals the limit of high-altitude training. Ma pushed his athletes beyond that limit and wanted to figure out a way to solve this problem. He consulted an herbalist who told him about Cordyceps—one of the most peculiar herbs in Chinese herbology. Its Chinese name is Dong Chong Xia Cao, meaning "winter worms and summer grass." Cordyceps is typically found only on the China/Tibet border. It is two life forms—a fungus grown on the head of a caterpillar. It is considered one of the ultimate Kidney tonics. It is also used to treat lung problems such as chronic asthma. For that reason it can be used to enhance the body's ability to breathe deeply. Coach Ma began using Cordyceps for his girls, and the blood in their urine quickly cleared up. To his surprise, Cordyceps also seemed to help enhance the girls' endurance, particularly helping them to recover quickly from the high-altitude training. From that point on, Ma consulted a panel of sports medicine experts and herbalists who further developed his recovery system.

## The Five Major Energetic Systems and Sports

Sports medicine as a specialized field of study in Chinese medicine has been explored in depth in the past three decades. Each of the Five Major Energetic Systems is involved in promoting athleticism. On the most basic level, Chinese medicine can increase energy and endurance and can reduce fatigue and recovery time following intensive training. The next level of effectiveness involves specific and well-targeted support, depending on exactly what the athletic activity requires. For example, certain athletic performance requires powerful muscle strength to be utilized over a very short period of time, such as in power lifting, wrestling and sprinting. Other activities require endurance and the availability of sustained energy, such as long-distance running and swimming.

In the first group, one strives for increased muscle bulk and explosive strength. In the latter group, the goal is to develop small, tight, lean muscles while at the same time keeping the athlete's total body weight as low as possible.

## Heart Energy

Heart Energy is a dynamic source that delivers the blood supply to the various muscles and critical organs. Therefore, cardiovascular capacity is a critical component. Although Western medicine and Chinese medicine both consider the heart in a very similar way—that its main function is to act as a pump, circulating life-giving blood throughout the body—Western medicine's view is that the heart is an electomechanical device, whereas Chinese medicine views the heart's pumping action as being the result of life's Energy source stimulating the action as well as carrying the circulation. In Chinese medicine, when working with patients who suffer from poor circulation, the master herbalist will prescribe not only an herb that dilates the blood vessels, thereby improving circulation, but also herbs that increase the vital Energy of the Heart and other Energetic systems, thereby producing a much greater improvement in overall circulation.

Furthermore, in Chinese medicine the Heart is the "monarch." Heart Energy empowers and coordinates the optimal expression of the whole being. It also endows the love and joy required to excel at any endeavor. The closest association from a Western point of view is the use of the word *heart* to describe someone with great skill and courage.

## Lung Energy

According to Chinese medicine, the Lung Energetic system takes in air and converts the air in our environment into Qi (within our body). By supporting Lung Energy, we provide the body with an ample supply of Energy source. This is consistent with Western medicine's view of promoting lung capacity in the athlete in order to enhance performance.

## Liver Energy

Liver Energy regulates Energy flow and circulation. The theory in Chinese medicine is that Liver Energy stores the blood when in a state of rest and relaxation, and releases the blood and redistributes it to the skeletal muscles when in a state of activity. Liver Energy is also responsible for maintaining the structure and function of the body's ligaments and tendons, which is a critical part of an athlete's ability to maintain muscle strength and flexibility without sustaining joint or soft-tissue injuries. In Chinese medicine Liver Energy has much to do with endurance. Liver Energy is involved in the coordination and gait of movement. Graceful, powerful movement requires balanced Liver Energy. Liver Energy regulates the steady and adequate supply of Blood and Qi to the tissues during strenuous activity, thus providing endurance. Liver Energy also endows us with the insight to be subtle and harmonious in our relationship to our internal Energies. This is crucial for refining physical performance to high levels. Stress and emotional imbalance, which impact Liver Energy, are acknowledged to inhibit peak performance.

Chinese medicine attributes acuity of vision to Liver Energy. This is consistent with the Western understanding that eyesight endows us with approximately ninety percent of our spatial information and coordinated balance for skillful movement.

## Spleen Energy

According to Chinese medicine, Spleen Energy converts nutrients into the nourishment required by the body. It is responsible for developing and maintaining muscle mass. Strengthening Spleen Energy will improve all functional and structural components of the digestive system, which is consistent with optimal nutrition being the foundation of physical training.

## Kidney Energy

Kidney Energy is the ultimate source of energy and vitality. It is also responsible for the structure and functions of the bones and joints. Ligaments, muscles and joints are the three primary components of the body's athletic makeup. This is consistent with the Western anatomical understanding that the adrenal glands (located just above the kidneys) mobilize our resources for strenuous activity. By balancing and strengthening our sympathetic response, the body can develop greater capacities for physical performance.

## Interaction of the systems

Kidney, Spleen and Liver Energies are all involved in the processes that make blood. Oxygen delivery capacity of blood is critical for any athletic performance.

Western medicine and Chinese medicine share the perspective that there are three major areas of focus of sports medicine: (1) the body's capacity to transport and utilize oxygen via hemoglobin (a component of blood), (2) the training and shaping of muscles and (3) cardiovascular and pulmonary (lung) conditioning.

In Chinese medicine, the strength of Blood Energy is particularly important for endurance competition in female athletes, because Chinese medicine considers women to be more vulnerable to Blood deficiencies. This too is consistent with Western medicine, whereby normal hemoglobin values for women are considered to be lower than for men—along with the fact that most women experience routine periodic loss of blood through menstruation. Some of the more commonly used herbs that Tonify or strengthen Blood are: Dang Gui, He Shou Wu, Dan Shen, Shu Di, and A Jiao. Some of the more commonly used foods are mulberry fruit, Notoginseng, longan fruit, dates and chicken broth (made without chicken skin). These herbs and foods help strengthen Blood. Other herbs, such as Chuan Xiong, Ji Xue Teng and Tao Ren, and foods, such as turmeric, wood ear mushrooms and safflower, promote circulation.

The strength and shape of muscles is maintained by the Liver, Spleen and Kidney Energetic systems. The Chinese medical concept of muscle includes muscles, ligaments, bones and joints, not just the muscles themselves. Therefore, by supporting and strengthening critical underlying Energetic systems Chinese medicine is able to enhance athletic ability and performance without the need for use of dangerous steroids or other performance-enhancing drugs.

## Ways to Enhance Athletic Endurance, Stamina, Reduce Recovery Time and Ease Muscle Soreness

Avoid overtaxing your system

Many people feel that their exercise program is lacking—even when they are exercising adequately. Our culture has developed an unfortunate mind-set about the *quantity* of exercise needed to be healthy. In fact, regular moderate exercise is optimal.

As you begin to exercise, your adrenal glands produce adrenaline, which raises your heart rate and directs the blood flow to your working muscles. Adrenaline also releases blood sugar into your bloodstream for your muscles to burn for energy. As you continue to exercise moderately, your pancreas releases the fat-utilizing hormone glucagon. Glucagon releases fat from your fat cells to be turned into sugar and burned as fuel. The entire time you are exercising, your adrenal glands continually release the stress hormone DHEA, which also stimulates your body to burn fat for fuel. Because of the release of these hormones during regular moderate exercise, your body will burn fat.

However, if you increase the intensity of your exercise without training gradually—such as weekend warriors do—your body will switch into alarm mode. The stress hormone cortisol will be released from your adrenal glands to deal with this emergency fight-or-flight signal. High cortisol leads to muscle wasting, lowered metabolism and weight gain. The better trained you are, the further you can go without getting into cortisol production. That is why gradual athletic training is important.

Protein is an important component of your diet. When you do not eat sufficient protein, your glucagon production will decline. Then when you exercise, your brain will be forced to call on cortisol to release blood sugar from your muscles for energy. No fat will be burned.

## Vary your athletic activities

To maintain balance (physical symmetry), always stretch and strengthen in opposition. For example, if you swing a golf club, swing it backward to work the opposite side of your body. If you play tennis, it is important to work your opposite arm. If you weight train, incorporate stretching to lengthen the muscles that have been contracted by your training. If you are a runner, incorporate yoga to stretch your hamstrings. Endurance, strength and flexibility are factors that are important to consider when training in any sport or athletic activity.

## Incorporate mind/body breathing exercises into your program

No matter what your sport, you will benefit from incorporating a mind/body breathing practice into your program, such as Qigong, yoga or Tai Chi. These practices bring Life Force (Qi) and healing into your life. They cultivate strength, vitality and longevity. See chapter 16 for more on these practices.

## Use Chinese herbs in cooking to enhance your performance

You can use Chinese medicinal herbs in recipes to promote athletic endurance. See chapter 21 for recipes.

*Supports Muscle*

> Astragalus (Huang Qi)
> Dan Shen
> Deer Velvet Antler (Lu Rong)
> Ginseng
> Poria mushroom (Fu Ling)

*Supports Ligaments*

> Bai Shao
> Chai Hu
> Huang Qi
> Nu Zhen Zi

*Strengthens Bones and Joints*

> Du Zhong
> Niu Xi
> Sang Ji Sheng
> Xu Duan

*Improves Cardiac Functioning*

> American ginseng
> Dan Shen
> Gan Cao
> Gui Zhi

*Promotes Pulmonary Functioning*

> Astragalus (Huang Qi)
> Bei Sha Shen
> Cordyceps
> Mai Meng Dong
> Yu Zhu

Obviously, the success of Ma's Barefoot Troops was partially determined by herbs. Ma also pays a great deal of attention to nutrition, especially foods that have medicinal qualities.

*Enhances Athletic Performance*

Astragalus
Bee pollen
Codonopsis
Cordyceps
Ginseng
Lycium

*Supports Muscle*

Chinese yam
Codonopsis
Licorice
Poria mushroom
Royal jelly

*Supports Ligaments*

Beef and pork tendons

*Supports Bones and Joints*

Black sesame
Lycium fruit
Turtle soup
Walnuts

*Improves Cardiac Functioning*

Chinese date
Cordyceps
Licorice
Longan fruit

*Promotes Pulmonary Functioning*

Almonds
Asian pears

Asparagus
Lily bulbs
Walnuts


## Chinese herbs and Western supplements

Vitamin B is depleted through exercise. If you are a serious athlete, ask your doctor to have your homocysteine levels checked. High levels of homocysteine are a risk factor for heart disease. See page 206 for more on homocysteine.

The stress of athletic achievement can increase the production of the stress hormone cortisol. Taking 100 milligrams of phosphatidylserine before a workout can help keep cortisol levels from rising too high.

Prolonged high cortisol levels will result in a decrease of the stress hormone DHEA. High cortisol and low DHEA leads to muscle wasting, lowered metabolism and weight gain. DHEA can improve your overall health and athletic performance, but it must be prescribed and monitored by a doctor.

Ask your doctor to have your sex hormone levels checked. Overexercising can result in decreased testosterone, estrogen and progesterone. Hormone replacement can improve your strength and endurance, help you lose body fat and improve insomnia and mood.

Super green food every day in a protein shake will provide your body with phytonutrients and probiotics to nourish your cells as well as the electrolytes necessary to replace those lost during exercise. Electrolytes are minerals required by your cells to regulate the electric charge across cell membranes. Electrolytes are lost through sweating. See page 104 for more on super green food.

As you age, your body repairs less effectively and much more slowly. Regular moderate exercise slows the aging process and prolongs your life. When you exercise moderately the release of human growth hormone (hGH) from the pituitary is stimulated. hGH helps activate all the metabolic and repair systems in your body. hGH is the longevity hormone. It accelerates repair of all tissues, stimulates immunity, increases muscle building and fat burning and therefore gives more energy. (See page 289 for more about hGH.)

Ma's recovery system had several basic components. He used herbs such as ginseng, which is considered to be a Qi tonic and therefore strengthens Qi Energy. He also paid a great deal of attention to Blood tonics. These are the herbs that help strengthen the blood by keeping the hemoglobin and red blood cell counts up, which supports the body's ability to utilize and process oxygen at a cellular level.

Routinely, three times a day, thirty minutes before meals take two or three capsules of free-form amino acid complex.

You can take Chinese herbal formulas and Western supplements specifically formulated to enhance athletic performance. Formulas may be purchased on-line at ancientherbsmodernmedicine.com.

# 19

## Antiaging

*Improving your health and extending your life by*
*combining ancient herbal formulas and modern medicine*

Wars, invasions and the ravages of nature have turned many of ancient China's wood and rice-paper structures to dust. The Forbidden City—named because no commoner or foreigner was allowed to enter without special permission from court officials—was constructed of stone and has survived since 1421. Surrounded by a wall thirty-five feet high and extending two and a half miles on each side, the Forbidden City contains hundreds of buildings, many of which served as the Imperial palaces of the emperors of China until 1911.

Within the Forbidden City are dozens of museum rooms housing ancient records. In 1976, an archaeological student entered one of the rooms and stepped into the dark shadows. Although it was not acceptable behavior to touch the artifacts, her curiosity took over. She opened one of the dust-covered leather sacks that had sat undisturbed for over a century. The sack turned out to be one of many that contained meticulously prepared and preserved medical archives of thirteen generations of emperors and their families. This happenstance find was considered to be by far the most complete and detailed set of Chinese medical history records to date.

The newly rediscovered manuscripts afforded the Chinese medical community an unprecedented opportunity to examine the works of some of the greatest Chinese physicians in the past three to four hundred years. The modern Chinese medical community was able to learn and understand their ancient techniques and formulations. They were also able to re-create many of the formulations and test them under modern medical protocols.

In examining the manuscripts, it quickly became evident that health maintenance and preventive medicine were favored topics among the royal families. Among the plethora of formulations developed over the ages was a group of formulas designed to promote youthfulness.

In August 2000, forty-five-year-old Alana Mays, a nationally known yoga instructor, was preparing to shoot another yoga video for her series. "I was born and raised in Miami, Florida, and had years of sun damage," Alana said. "I work in the field of fitness, doing videos and public appearances, and I felt I looked haggard. My career was blossoming and I wanted to take advantage of it. So I had scheduled cosmetic surgery."

The surgery did not take place as planned. Alana was in demand and had to reschedule five times. Under the stress of the hectic pace and juggling of her schedule she developed shingles on her face. Her plastic surgeon prescribed Valtrex. "After six weeks on Valtrex the shingles had cleared," Alana said. "But before surgery they give you antibiotics for infection. Then, of course, there is the anesthesia during surgery. Afterwards I took Vicodin for pain." For three days after surgery, the nurses in the aftercare facility kept Alana on soft, cold foods such as applesauce. "What I was really craving was something hot to eat. After three days of that my body blew up with water. I couldn't get my clothes on. I had a rash from my neck to my kneecaps. My body hurt worse than my face, which looked like I had been in a train wreck. I went to the plastic surgeon, and he wanted to give me medication to take away the inflammation. I said, 'No, that's what got me here.' I went home and drank lots of water, vegetable broth and herbal remedies. Over the next six months I couldn't do my yoga practice, I put on weight, and my face was still very painful." Eight months after surgery, Alana was asked to relocate to Los Angeles by the company that produces her yoga videos. Hesitant, Alana shared her story with her producer, who suggested she go ahead with the relocation and see Dr. Mao as soon as she arrived.

"When Alana first visited my office, she was suffering from complete exhaustion," Dr. Mao said. "The cosmetic surgery she had had eight months prior had affected her vitality to the point where she was nonfunctional. Her hormones were imbalanced, causing an irregular menstrual cycle and a sharp drop in libido. She was suffering from pain in her neck, chest and face. Ironically, the procedure that was supposed to restore youth had caused her decline.

"When formulating a treatment plan, I took into account her condition previous to the surgery—she had been constantly working and traveling. Her Kidney system—her vitality—had become depleted. Her inner fire—what we call Kidney Yang—was deficient. In Chinese medicine, the Kidneys are considered to be the storehouse of life Essence. Chinese medicine enjoys a long tradition of antiaging research from which developed methods to slow down and even reverse the aging process. Acupuncture, for example, can be used to improve circulation, immune functions and muscle tone—such as in the face—and enhance and balance overall body function. Specifically, there are many herbs that are used and possess known antiaging properties. This group of herbs was documented in *Shen Nong's Herbal Materia Medica.* Shen Nong was thought to have lived five thousand years ago, and his *Medica*—written by scholars using his name—purportedly dates back to the time of Christ. These antiaging herbs belong in a category called superior herbs, also known as tonic herbs. Examples include Ginseng root, Cistanche root, Schisandra fruit, Chinese wild yam, Lycium berry, Angelica root, Fo Ti root, Lotus seed and Longan fruit. Special formulations consisting of carefully prepared combinations of various tonic herbs were created by ancient Taoist physicians specifically for increasing energy, longevity and enhancing quality of life."

Alana was treated with acupuncture and given Chinese herbal antiaging formulas. "In the beginning preparing the herbal decoction seemed like a chore," she said. "It's not the most pleasant-tasting drink in the world. But I feel very nourished when I drink it. So it's become a pleasure to smell the herbs cooking.

"Before I started Chinese medicine I was getting out of bed after ten hours of sleep, feeling exhausted. I had to take a two-hour nap every day. I have more energy now and don't need to nap. I am mentally alert. I've begun exercising again. Chinese herbs supported my body's balance so that I could rebuild muscle mass. I'm getting ready to do a video production, and I need to be the best I can. It's been very easy to get myself into shape to do that. I don't think yoga, exercise or diet would have brought me back. Once you are depleted you have to go deeper to bring yourself back to optimum."

## Antiaging from a Western Perspective

The sale of prescription drugs in this country rose 40 percent from 1998 to 2000. Drugs, surgery and other sophisticated scientific modalities have great value and much to offer medical care. At the same time, the goal of good health is to prevent the necessity of taking drugs, having surgeries and so on. In the past, Western medicine had little or no interest in fostering wellness. Western medicine has traditionally been crisis- or illness-focused. Patients generally are not treated until a diagnosable illness develops or a trauma occurs. A person had to be stricken with an affliction before a doctor could intervene. This premise infiltrated the public's mind-set, and a dangerous attitude resulted: Eat, smoke, drink and generally live it up. When a person got sick, he or she went to the doctor to get "fixed." Fortunately, this attitude is being revised as the concept of preventative medicine has begun to creep in and take hold within the common mind-set and within the Western medical establishment.

Today, scientists now agree that prevention is as important as treating illness and that wellness begins on the cellular level, within the interconnected, interdependent systems of your body. Prevention, from a Chinese point of view, is based on the philosophy of balance. Antiaging medicine, a newly emerging field in Western medicine, parallels the philosophy of Chinese medicine more than any other specialty.

In addition to the progressive Western doctors who are working in the areas of antiaging, clinics devoted solely to the specialty of antiaging have sprung up across the nation. Physicians who incorporate antiaging medicine into their work often practice both sickness and wellness medicine. Specialized antiaging clinics do not treat disease. Instead they target hormonal imbalances and educate patients on nutrition and exercise as a way of maintaining the body in the most optimally functioning state—thus thwarting the aging process to the degree possible with current scientific knowledge.

Cenegenics, a premiere antiaging clinic located in Las Vegas, was founded by Alan Mintz, M.D., and John E. Adams in the early 1990s. Mintz and Adams organized a team of professional health care specialists ranging from neurologists and pharmacists to internists, nutritional experts and exercise physiologists. "Over eighty percent of medical costs in this country are incurred during the last few years of life," said Dr. Mintz. "That doesn't make sense. Why wait until something goes terribly wrong to try to make repairs? In makes more sense to invest in preventing illness early on, so that your middle and older years can be vigorous and productive."

David Leonardi, M.D., medical director of Cenegenics, takes his own medical advice. "At twenty-nine, I was single and used to vacation at Club Med. My buddy Roger and I could get up at six-thirty in the morning, eat an eighteen-hundred-calorie breakfast and be on the tennis court at eight. After three vigorous sets of singles, we'd shower and devour an eighteen-hundred-calorie lunch—starches and desserts prevailing. The afternoon was spent learning to windsurf, which is a sport with a steep learning curve. By four-thirty we'd drag ourselves to the shower. But by dinnertime we were miraculously rejuvenated. Dinner was twenty-five hundred calories—a thousand of which came from alcohol—followed by dancing and debauchery till two in the morning at the nightclub. After four and a half hours of sleep, we'd repeat the performance the next day.

"Fifteen years later, at age forty-four, tennis was doubles from ten to eleven-thirty followed by a light lunch. After a few hours of relaxing, we might get in one hour of windsurfing. A nap was necessary to make it to dinner. We'd have a glass of brandy at the table in lieu of four hours of dancing and hit the sack by ten."

At age fifty, Leonardi feels closer to how he felt as a twenty-nine-year-old than to how he felt as a forty-four-year-old. He credits his recovery to judicious application of hormone replacement therapy, optimal nutrition and regular sensible exercise. "Aging progresses swiftly between ages twenty-nine and forty-four, yet by age fifty I'd learned state-of-the-art 'age management.' Aging is a preventable disease. We simply don't have all the answers necessary to prevent it. At our current state of the art, we are able to slow the aging process and to a significant extent reverse many of the symptoms. Supplementing hormones as levels decline is one of the most effective methods for reversing the symptoms of aging and for improving the quality of life. Hormone modulation is not a simple endeavor, as it affects our physiology in a multitude of ways. It should be undertaken only under the care of a physician knowledgeable in the nature of these hormones and their interactions, and one who will monitor not only their levels but their effect on all aspects of well-being. Hormone modulation should accompany lifestyle improvements in nutrition, exercise, stress reduction and the avoidance of environmental toxins. This comprehensive program can maintain a remarkably slower rate of aging, enhancing quality of life and, we believe, an extended lifespan. We feel confident that we can make a ten-year difference, and if they're quality years, that's a lot of tennis."

New patients at Cenegenics are put through the thorough diagnostic Medical Biological Age Comprehensive Evaluation, or MedBACE. A day of diagnostic evaluation provides baseline information on the patient's general state of health, metabolism, level of fitness, hormonal status and biological age—including memory and cognitive tests, reaction time, muscle motor tests, lung function and capacity and sensory tests of vision and hearing. Patients' bone density, body fat and muscle mass are also evaluated. Included in a full day of evaluation are one-on-one consultations with a staff physician, nutritional counselor, exercise trainer and care coordinator.

The Cenegenics team individualizes a program for each patient comprised of nutrition, exercise, nutritional supplements, prescription medications and hormone replacement therapy. Follow-up evaluations and consultations are scheduled regularly so that prescriptions can be adjusted. Hormones, medications and supplements are shipped monthly to your home. Antiaging clinics such as Cenegenics do not take over your medical care. These clinics offer wellness programs and communicate with your regular doctor and specialists.

## Develop Your Own Program by Following the Principles Taught in Antiaging Clinics

Consult with a doctor who specializes in antiaging medicine to have your hormone levels checked

Studies on hormonal therapy for the aging are ongoing. "So far, evidence suggests that appropriate advanced hormonal, metabolic and exercise physiology interventions can slow down, maybe even turn back, the biological clock," Dr. Mintz said. The following hormones collectively contribute to energy, strength, stamina, large muscle mass, lower body fat, greater libido, and the more optimistic outlook of youth.

- *DHEA.* A male sex hormone that is critical for men and women's well-being. It is important for your immune system, for your mood and to maintain muscle mass, which decreases body fat.
- *Testosterone.* The primary male hormone, which is also crucial for women's health and well-being. Testosterone is important for lean body mass and to decrease body fat. It is a critical component for your brain (mood), heart, and sex hormones, and for the formation of bone. A lack of testosterone is associated with decreased sex drive. In men, from age thirty to fifty, testosterone levels decline on the average of 30 percent.
- *Melatonin.* A hormone that is synthesized and secreted by your pineal gland. It regulates circadian rhythm, aids in sleep and is an antioxidant. By age thirty-five, melatonin levels in both sexes decline to the level of an eighty-year-old. Keeping melatonin levels at a more youthful level will provide benefits in sleep, energy levels as well as providing antioxidants.
- *Thyroid hormones T3 and T4.* Every cell, tissue and organ of your body is affected by the actions of your thyroid gland. The thyroid controls your metabolism, regulates your body's thermostat, helps maintain your circulatory system and blood volume, heightens the sensitivity of your nerves

and is necessary for building and maintaining lean body mass (muscle and bones).

- *Estrogen and progesterone.* Sex hormones produced in the ovaries. When ovarian function declines during perimenopause, sex hormones fluctuate. The cardiovascular system, bones, skin and certain cognitive functions begin to deteriorate. Bioidentical estrogen and progesterone replacement therapy is associated with prevention of osteoporosis and heart disease, maintaining strength and a youthful appearance, among other benefits.

- *Insulinlike growth factor (IGF-1).* Human growth hormone (hGH) is produced by your pituitary gland. In response to the presence of hGH, insulinlike growth factor (IGF-1) is released. Your level of IGF-1 will determine your need for hGH. HGH and IGF-1 decline progressively with age. By raising the levels of these two hormones by hormone replacement of hGH, you can see such improvements as:

  Increased skin thickness and elasticity
  Diminished wrinkling from sun damage
  More lean body mass and less body fat
  Improved cholesterol panel
  Less recovery time between workouts
  Better mood and a sense of well-being
  Better sleep and improved energy levels

These effects can take up to six months and diminish once you discontinue use. Side effects such as joint pain and stiffness from hGH replacement can almost always be avoided by using conservative doses. HGH may only be absorbed via injection. It must be obtained by prescription and must be used under the supervision of a licensed physician. Currently under patent, hGH is very expensive, running between $300 and $600 per month.

No studies to date have proven that using hGH replacement has caused disease. Studies have pointed to possible links between higher levels of IGF-1 and the risk for prostate cancer and breast cancer. Other studies have demonstrated that higher levels of IGF-1 are not a risk factor for these cancers. At this time there is not enough data to draw reliable conclusions. As with other types of hormone replacement, many doctors and individuals feel the benefits are worth the potential risks. The decision to use hGH or any other hormone replacement is up to the individual. When researching hormone replacement, it is always best to consult with a physician trained in antiaging medicine.

Deer Velvet Antler, Chinese medicine's answer to hGH

If you want the benefits of increased human growth hormone without using the injectable hormone, you can talk to your doctor of Chinese medicine about the benefits of using Deer Velvet Antler. Deer Velvet Antler has been known for centuries as "the Emperor's tonic." It is one of the most important medicines in Chinese herbology. Deer Velvet Antler is the very tip of the new male deer antler growth, which has not yet become the hardened calcified bone of the antler. Deer Velvet Antler is harvested in China and New Zealand in deer farms that have been developed for the sole purpose of acquiring this substance as a supplement. The animal is not hurt or killed, and it takes about one year for the antler to grow back.

Deer Velvet Antler is considered an important Kidney Yang tonic. It enhances strength and accelerates metabolism. Energetically, it is Warm and can even be considered Hot, so it is not suitable for everyone. For example, people with a Yin-deficient constitution need to be careful using it, and people with an excess Yang condition will most likely experience some side effects such as headache, nosebleed, insomnia, irritability, heart palpitations and elevated blood pressure.

Considered an adaptogen (antistress substance), Deer Velvet Antler strengthens the immune system to combat the effects of physiological and psychological stress. Deer Velvet Antler is rich in minerals, amino acids, anti-inflammatory agents, glucosamine and chondroitin sulfate.

Deer Velvet Antler Tonifies Jing (Essence). Recent research has demonstrated that Deer Velvet Antler contains IGF-1, which increases muscle mass. For this reason Deer Velvet Antler has become popular with bodybuilders and other athletes to increase muscle tone and lean muscle mass.

Deer Velvet Antler is considered one of the most effective remedies for male impotence. It is used for so many conditions that it would be impossible to list them all. Deer Velvet Antler must be used under the supervision of a Chinese doctor.

Depending on the grade or quality and the form (powder, extract or tincture), an antiaging dose of Deer Velvet Antler would cost between $30 and $160 per month.

See a health care professional to have homocysteine levels checked

High levels of homocysteine are a risk factor for heart disease. See page 206.

Take care of yourself on a cellular level

Medical science today is just beginning to understand the importance of caring for our bodies on a cellular level. The key to good health and vitality is to provide regular nourishment for your cells and to regularly take toxins out of your cells by detoxification.

Many Western doctors and scientists are beginning to view the human body as a whole, interconnected picture. Like Chinese medicine, they are also recognizing that this wholeness is connected by a pattern of energy that must be kept flowing. Gary Tunsky, Ph.D., a naturopathic doctor, nutritional biochemist and independent research scientist in private practice at Precision Health Systems in Dallas, Texas, explains how the process of disease, when viewed on a cellular level, corresponds with the Chinese view. "The human body contains more than seventy-five trillion cells," Tunsky said. "You have seventy-five trillion libraries of information containing genetic information. These seventy-five trillion cells communicate like a wireless fiber-optic network. Picture all six billion people on earth simultaneously picking up a wireless phone and making a phone call. That's six billion conversations at the same time. Then picture everyone hitting conference call. That's what happens in your body's communication system twenty-four hours a day.

"Each healthy cell has an electrical current of one-thousandth of a microvolt. When seventy-five trillion cells are all lighting up at a thousandth of a microvolt, you have a healthy body. When cells are diseased, the voltage decreases to half that or less. Every living food we eat has an electrical current. Every apple, orange or vegetable has a certain microvolt or life force. This electricity is necessary for vibrant health at the cellular level.

"If you ingest processed foods with zero microcurrent, your cells will not receive the electric current that is necessary for cellular communication. Eating processed foods results in a toxic coating around the cell membrane, similar to a car battery covered in oil. If you tried to hook up cables to this oil-covered battery, the electrical charge would not be able to pass through the cables because of the oil coating. When the cells are diseased or contaminated from processed foods, their voltage decreases. With this decrease in voltage, energy levels decrease, causing a lower metabolic rate in the cells and susceptibility to disease."

This view of the human body as a pattern of dynamic energy parallels Chinese medicine's view of Qi. Like Qi flowing through Meridians to deliver nutrients and remove toxins and metabolic waste, it is necessary for the electric current of the cells of the human body to flow freely—and when the flow is obstructed, stagnation occurs. "The human body has a filtration system that keeps the river flowing," Tunsky said. "Cells are constantly burning fuel and producing metabolic waste, like an automobile giving off carbon monoxide. In addition, you're breathing, eating and drinking toxic substances, and your cells become further contaminated. When your seventy-five trillion cells are bathing in toxic sewage—called toxemia—cells begin to die from suffocation. Then the next generation of cells is weaker than the one before and if you don't clean up the toxic waste, the next generation will be weaker than that one, and so on. This is progressive stagnation. Picture a stagnant swamp or pond where there is no movement. Algae and fungi begin to form. This stagnation is going to attract scavengers. Then germs, bacteria, parasites and cancer cells begin to breed.

"Western medicine treats health problems by attempting to attack these problems with a kill-mode mind-set. That's like blaming algae and fungus for killing off fish in a stagnant swamp. But if you clean up the swamp and get it flowing again like a vibrant river, the algae and fungus go away." Like Chinese medicine, getting the systems moving (as in moving your Qi) will remove stagnation, restore balance to your body and correct disease. "The seventy-five trillion cells flow like a river. When the filtration systems are working, there will be no buildup of toxic residue within your cells to cause stagnation. The goal in treating illness is to break up stagnation and get systems moving freely again. In treating illness, you don't treat the system or the organ, you treat the cell, because healthy cells make healthy tissues, healthy tissues make healthy organs, healthy organs make healthy systems and healthy systems make up a healthy body."

Recent modern scientific research has revealed that herbs work on a cellular level to nourish cells and to remove toxins. Looking at healing from under the microscope of Western science, we understand that putting nutrients into the cells and taking toxins out will allow the cellular system to become dynamic and vital again, which will counteract the degenerative diseases of aging.

In addition to avoiding processed foods, toxins and sugar, detoxification is essential in preventing illness and promoting youthfulness. One of the most effective ways to do this is to drink fresh vegetable juice.

Whole foods and vegetables must be digested before your body can absorb the nutrients. Because most people's digestive systems begin to weaken by the time they reach forty, no matter how nutritious their diet, many of the nutrients they eat are not fully absorbed. When you drink fresh vegetable juice, the juicer does part of the digesting for you by taking out the fiber and leaving only live liquid nutrients containing enzymes that signal your pancreatic juices that digestion has already taken place. These juices go directly through your portal vein into your liver, where toxins are filtered out and nutrients put directly into your bloodstream and then carried to your seventy-five trillion plus cells. "Imagine your arteries as a river, your veins as streams, and your capillaries as trickling brooks," Tunsky said. "A flowing river with abundant growth with healthy trees and vibrant flowers at its banks."

Dr. Tunsky recommends what he calls the "Einstein drink," which is a mixture of nine different vegetables—of your choice—which provides thirty-five thousand phytonutrients. "Through a technology called chromography, researchers have found twelve thousand phytonutrients in one spinach leaf. Science has only studied and identified a hundred and fifty-one of these micronutrients. You can't get this full spectrum of vitamins, minerals, enzymes and nutrients in a supplement." It takes one to one and a half pounds of fresh vegetables to make eight ounces of juice. If you drink fresh juice twice a day, you are getting the phytonutrients of two to three pounds of fresh vegetables.

The human body strives for a delicate pH balance. Maintenance of the delicate acid-base balance in the body is critical. As previously noted, the acid-base system is measured by what is known as the pH system. On a scale of 1 to 14, a measurement of 7 is neutral. The human body strives to maintain a mildly alkaline state of approximately 7.4, give or take 0.05. This alkaline environment allows all the repair processes such as making new cells, membranes, tissues, enzymes, hormones and neurotransmitters to take place. Normal metabolic processes, stress, toxins, acidic foods and beverages and ingesting stimulants all make your body more acidic. Excess acid in your system causes degeneration of normal cellular function, or stagnation from a Chinese medicine point of view. In addition to providing your body with nutrients, drinking fresh juice helps change the pH of your body from an acid state to a slightly alkaline state and cleanses your body's cells, tissues and organs.

Because many toxins are fat-soluble, the heavier you are, the more toxins you carry in your fat cells. A juice detox releases these toxins from cells back into your bloodstream before they are eliminated. You may feel the effects of this blood toxicity the first four or five days with mild flu-like symptoms. After a few days, you will begin to experience an improvement in energy. From then on, you can see improvements in sleep, memory, concentration, vitality, fewer cravings for sugar, weight loss and improved skin and hair.

In addition to drinking juice for detoxification, if you are ill, you can benefit from drinking four to eight ounces of fresh organic vegetable juice twice a day until your illness resolves. If you are healthy, you can benefit from drinking four to eight ounces of juice several times a week.

*Seven- to Fourteen-Day Detoxification Program:* To make fresh juice you will need a juicer. Select up to nine different vegetables of your choice. As you try different combinations, you will find those that you prefer. A mixture of nine different vegetables of your choice provides thirty-five thousand phytonutrients. Avoid fruits in your juiced drinks, as fruit juice is pure sugar. One exception is to use up to one-fourth of a green apple for flavor. You may also use up to two carrots and one-half to one beet, as these foods raise the sugar content of the juice. Avoid citrus fruits in your juiced drinks. Juice every part of the vegetable, including skins, rinds, seeds and leafy tops. Vegetables are considered to be Energetically Cool or Cold because the cellulose (fiber) in vegetables takes Stomach Fire and Qi to digest, which uses up Yang Energy. If the vegetable in juice form is at room temperature, it can be absorbed with less demand on your digestive Energy. However, excessive amounts of fluids could eventually create Dampness and bring about an imbalance at some point in the future. The purpose of drinking vegetable juice is to feel better. If you experience gastrointestinal distress or any other adverse symptom, add Energetically Warm ingredients to balance the Cold Energy and reduce the amount you are drinking or discontinue and begin again, with moderation, at another time. In addition, always drink your juice within ten minutes after juicing. Some of the phytonutrients will oxidize and be lost after that point. If you must store it, do so in a thermos—not in the refrigerator.

*Examples of Juice Combinations*

| | | |
|---|---|---|
| Arugula | 1/4 green apple | Fresh parsley |
| Asparagus | Crookneck squash | Fresh turmeric |
| 1/2 to 1 beet | Cucumber | Kale |
| Broccoli | Daikon radish | Mustard greens |
| Brussels sprouts | Dandelion greens | Red bell pepper |
| Burdock root | Fresh basil | Red cabbage |
| Cauliflower | Fresh ginger | Spinach |
| Cilantro | (use sparingly) | Swiss chard |
| Collard greens | Fresh kudzu root | Zucchini |
| | Fresh oregano | |

Among these ingredients, several are or are closely related to Chinese herbs and have particularly strong medicinal properties.

| *Vegetable* | *Closely Related Chinese Herb* |
| --- | --- |
| Asparagus | Tian Men Dong |
| Burdock root | Niu Bang Zi |
| Daikon radish | Lai Fu Zi |
| Dandelion greens | Pu Gong Ying |
| Fresh basil | Zi Su Ye |
| Fresh ginger | Sheng Jiang |
| Fresh kudzu root | Ge Gen |
| Fresh parsley | Yuan Sui |
| Fresh turmeric | Jiang Huang |
| Swiss chard | Da Huang |

Ginger root, parsley, basil, oregano, kale, daikon radish, mustard green and red bell pepper are Warming and active in their Energetic temperature, and are important for those with a Cold constitution or sensitive digestive system. These vegetables have extremely strong tastes. Experiment by using a pinch and add more as desired.

The following ingredients in powder form can also be added to the juice to counterbalance the Cold or Yin nature of other ingredients:

Cardamom *(Bai Dou Kou)*
Cinnamon *(Rou Gui)*
Clove *(Ding Xiang)*
Dried orange peel *(Chen Pi)*
Fennel *(Xiao Hui Xiang)*
Fresh garlic *(or odorless garlic powder)*
Galangal *(Gao Liang Jiang)*
Nutmeg *(Rou Dou Kou)*
Turmeric *(Jiang Huang)*

For people with particularly sensitive stomachs who do not do well with Warm ingredients, adding a piece of raw potato to the juice can help.

For breakfast, lunch, dinner and snacks, choose from organic eggs, cottage cheese, plain whole yogurt, raw nuts, fresh fish, poultry, cooked and raw vegetables, legumes and grains, coconut oil, butter, flaxseed oil and other essential fatty acids and extra-virgin expeller-pressed olive oil—which is available in your health food store. Avoid red meat and dairy products, as they are hard to digest and can harbor toxins in the fats.

> Breakfast: *4 ounces juice with 1 tablespoon flaxseed oil. Choose foods from list. Take 600 milligrams of milk thistle and 1,000 milligrams N-acetylcysteine.*
> Midmorning snack: *Choose foods from list.*
> Lunch: *Heavy Veggie Detox Broth 1 or 2. See pages 345–346 for recipe. Choose foods from list.*
> Midafternoon snack: *4 ounces juice with 1 tablespoon flaxseed oil.*
> Dinner: *Heavy Veggie Detox Broth 1 or 2. Choose foods from list.*
> Bedtime snack: *Choose foods from list.*
> Throughout the day: *Drink eight to ten eight-ounce glasses of water*

If you do not want to juice or do not like the taste, or if your digestive system is particularly sensitive, bioavailable vegetable pills can provide you with the active plant food enzymes and other vital nutrients found in fresh, raw fruits and vegetables. Product recommendations can be found online at ancient herbsmodernmedicine.com.

Another option is super green food. See page 104 for more on super green food.

## Eat a low-sugar diet to maintain a normal weight and to prevent degenerative disease

Chinese medicine focuses on balance. A high-sugar diet causes imbalances and stagnation in the body.

Aging is a degenerative process. We start out healthy and everything we eat and how we live our lives determines the rate at which we will age. If you eat a balanced diet of real, whole foods, your body will degenerate more slowly than if you eat a diet of chemically processed foods. Type II diabetes is an example of degeneration within the body that is almost solely due to an imbalanced diet of too many carbohydrates (sugar).

*From Healthy to Insulin Resistance to Type II Diabetes:* One of the most important factors in extending your lifespan is to keep your insulin levels low and even. When you eat, your body converts some of the food into amino acids for building blocks for lean body mass and some into sugar as energy to fuel your body. When you eat carbohydrates, they are immediately broken down by your gastrointestinal system into sugar and absorbed into your bloodstream. For that sugar to be burned as fuel, it must get into your cells. Cells have receptors that act as portals that can only be opened by the hormone insulin. Insulin is secreted from the pancreas and stows away the sugar molecules into cells for use as energy. Removing sugar from your bloodstream causes your blood sugar levels to fall.

If you eat too much sugar as a child, teen and young adult, your cells will become filled to near capacity with sugar. At that point, your cells will reduce the number of insulin receptors, so that insulin cannot upload as much sugar into the cells. This is known as insulin resistance. As you continue to eat sugar, your pancreas will secrete even more insulin in an attempt to overcome this resistance in order to lower your blood sugar. Too much insulin in the bloodstream is known as hyperinsulinemia. Your cells react to this excess by further reducing insulin receptors, leading to further insulin resistance. Extra sugar in the bloodstream will continuously be diverted into fat production and deposited in your fat cells. When your fat cells are filled, the sugar has nowhere to go and remains in the bloodstream, damaging vital organs. This state is referred to as type II diabetes.

In summary, prolonged consumption of high levels of carbohydrates leads to prolonged high insulin levels, which leads to insulin resistance, which leads to even higher insulin levels, which leads to increased insulin resistance, which leads to type II diabetes.

While type II diabetes is advanced insulin resistance, everyone will arrive at a certain level of insulin resistance as they age. No matter what your stage, you can reduce the amount of fat stored in your cells by reversing insulin resistance (emptying cells of sugar). This is accomplished by systematically reducing the amount of sugar you eat so that your body can have the opportunity to burn the stored sugar, and then begin to burn stored fat as energy.

In addition to added weight, sugar degrades the body in many ways. Sugar, which is Energetically Damp, provides no nutritional value, yet it depletes your body of minerals necessary to interact with vital metabolic enzymes. It is a known immunosuppressant. All illnesses have their roots in an imbalanced immune system. Sugar has been proven to destroy the germ-killing ability of white blood cells for up to five hours after it is eaten. Eating sugar reduces the production of antibodies, which destroy or deactivate foreign invaders in your system. Sugar interferes with the transport of vitamin C, which is a key nutrient for your immune system. Sugar neutralizes the actions of essential fatty acids.

Without essential fatty acids, your cells become more vulnerable to invasion by allergens and microorganisms.

In addition to stagnation caused by processed foods and toxins, excessive sugar consumption also causes stagnation in the body on a cellular level. "Eating excess sugar results in prolonged high glucose levels in your bloodstream, resulting in higher rates of glycation," Dr. Leonardi said. "Glycation is the process by which sugar attaches protein molecules. When protein molecules are glycated, they stick together in your cells. This results in decreased cellular efficiency and begins the process of degenerative disease."

*The Glycemic Index:* The glycemic index is a numerical system of measuring how fast a carbohydrate food triggers a rise in blood sugar level. The glycemic index was arrived at by feeding 50 grams of glucose to test subjects. The subjects' blood sugar levels were tested, and the average level was assigned a value of 100. Subjects were then fed individual foods and their blood sugar levels that resulted from eating those foods were compared to the standard 100. A subsequent index used white bread to achieve a baseline measurement of 100, which demonstrates that because refined white flour products are highly refined, they turn rapidly into sugar in your system.

Carbohydrates are absorbed into your blood as glucose, or sugar. When you eat a balanced meal, or a low-glycemic-index meal, your blood sugar rises gradually over two hours, which causes insulin levels to rise gradually over the same amount of time. Sugar and fatty acids (from fat cells) are burned as fuel. You will feel more energetic, will not suffer from blood-sugar-related mood swings or energy-level fluctuations and will not have the urge to snack. Likewise, eating low-glycemic-index foods for dinner will mean that you go to bed with low blood sugar and insulin levels, allowing for fat burning while you sleep.

You can keep your body in tune by eating low- to medium-glycemic-index foods and by always eating protein, fat or high-fiber foods with carbohydrates. For a Web site containing a complete glycemic index, go to www.mendosa.com.

### A Basic Guide to the Glycemic Index of Foods

*Low-Glycemic-Index Foods*

> Proteins *(meat, fish, fowl, eggs, cheese)*
> Fats and oils *(olive oil and other liquid oils, butter, cream, sour cream, cheese, cottage cheese)*

Nonstarchy vegetables *(green leafy vegetables and other low-carbohydrate vegetables)*

## Medium-Glycemic-Index Foods

Beans and legumes
Fruits
Nuts
Starchy vegetables *(corn and tubers)*
Whole grains *(barley, buckwheat, bulgur, millet, quinoa, rye, wheat, wheat bran, wheat germ, brown rice, wild rice)*

## High-Glycemic-Index Foods

Refined white flour products
Sugar
Processed and imitation foods

There are four basic food groups: proteins, fats, nonstarchy vegetables and carbohydrates. In addition to eating low-glycemic-index foods, eating proteins, fats and nonstarchy vegetables lowers the glycemic index of your meal by slowing down the digestive process. This prevents sugar from rocketing into your bloodstream.

We used to believe that dieting was the way to reduce body fat. We now understand that balanced nutrition will allow your body to gradually reach its optimal body weight and ideal body composition. If you want to lose body fat, focus on becoming healthy and balanced. Fat loss occurs cell by cell as your cells become healthy and your body becomes nourished. Some ways to heal on a cellular level to achieve your ideal body composition:

◆ Eat real, whole foods that are in their natural state.
◆ Eat low-glycemic-index foods.
◆ Reduce carbohydrate consumption (see *The Schwarzbein Principle* by Diana Schwarzbein, M.D., and Nancy Deville for further reading on metabolism and weight loss).
◆ Avoid sugar and refined white flour products.
◆ Eat frequent smaller meals. Stop dieting.

- Drink eight to ten eight-ounce glasses of water per day.
- Give up or reduce stimulant intake (caffeine, nicotine, alcohol, herbal stimulants).

## Avoid bad fats and eat good fats

Hydrogenated vegetable oils containing trans fatty acids, such as margarine, shortening and polyunsaturated vegetable oils processed out of their natural source through heat and chemical processes, have been linked to the dramatic rise in degenerative diseases of aging such as osteoarthritis, some cancers, cholesterol abnormalities, coronary artery disease, high blood pressure, osteoporosis, stroke and type II diabetes.

Eat naturally occurring fats and oils and include essential fatty acids (omega-3 and omega-6) in your diet. Omega-3 and omega-6 blends can be purchased at your health food store in liquid or capsules to supplement your diet. See page 208 for a list of oils containing omega-3 and omega-6 and page 210 for a list of monounsaturated oils. Monounsaturated oils raise HDLs—the good cholesterol.

Eating coconut oil can help you stay healthy and lose weight. One teaspoon of coconut oil three times a day (it can be used in cooking) contains many health-giving properties, among which is the promotion of thermogenesis, which means to boost your metabolism to burn calories. Coconut oil is a non-hydrogenated, naturally saturated oil with no trans fatty acids. It will not raise blood cholesterol.

## Maintain a positive outlook

Developing a spiritual connection, having healthy relationships, letting go of grudges, engaging in forgiveness and maintaining a general positive attitude have been proven to extend longevity. Tyrannical confidence, which is a negative influence on others, has not been shown to extend longevity. A positive attitude is reflected in confidence that uplifts others as well as yourself.

## Chinese herbs and Western supplements

Manufacturers are adding herbs such as ginkgo biloba, kava, St. John's wort and Ma Huang and nutritional supplements such as glucosamine to processed foods as a way of making their products appear healthful. Consuming more processed food products will not give you the benefits that you would enjoy from a diet of real foods and from taking added nutritional supplements. The Chinese were probably one of the first peoples to recognize the association between the lack of certain nutrients and specific illnesses. As early as 307 A.D., there were descriptions of treating beri beri (a vitamin B deficiency illness) in ancient texts written by scholars of Chinese medicine. By 465 A.D. Chinese medicine had made observations that the individuals who were susceptible to beri beri were the aristocrats, whose food was more refined than that of the commoner. In 652 A.D. a famous physician, Sun Si Miao, studied several deficiency diseases, such as beri beri, osteoporosis (calcium deficiency), night blindness (vitamin A deficiency), goiter (iodine deficiency) and others, and developed appropriate treatments for them. These treatments consisted of specific foods and herbs that were high in the appropriate nutrient. Beri beri was treated with the husks of various grains and legumes, osteoporosis with Tortoise Shell, night blindness with Goat Liver and goiter with seaweed.

There is no pill in the world that can cure your body. You can only give your body the materials it needs so that it can heal itself. The old adage "You are what you eat" has never been as true as it is today with the proliferation of junk foods devoid of nutrients that are either intentionally or inadvertently adulterated with toxic substances. Naturally, your body is best served when it receives nutrients from the foods you eat. Unfortunately, this is not possible today, with depleted soil and with the undue demands our bodies are under—creating an even greater need for nutrients such as vitamins, antioxidants, minerals and enzymes. Regardless of your health concerns, you will benefit by taking a daily multiple vitamin-mineral supplement. Vitamins and minerals are critical in supporting your basic biochemistry and in neutralizing and excreting toxins from your body. It is important to take vitamins and minerals in certain combinations so that they can work synergistically with the metabolic and enzymatic systems in your body. A multiple vitamin-mineral supplement that contains small amounts of each vitamin and mineral with food three times a day is optimal. Vitamin/mineral supplements are absorbed best when taken with food, when digestive juices are secreted. Spreading out your vitamin-mineral intake allows the absorptive surfaces of your digestive system to take in more of each nutrient. Less is wasted, and your body receives a more consistent flow of nutrients. A well-formulated multiple supplement is designed to help fill in the missing nutrients that your body needs, in addition to providing antioxidants to neutralize free radicals.[7]

Routinely, on an empty stomach 20 minutes before breakfast and lunch, take 1,000 milligrams of free-form amino acids.

Routinely, take the immune modulating formula described on pages 103–104.

Routinely, take the digestive formulas found on page 102.

In 1980, a team of Chinese medical experts specializing in aging-related illnesses from Longhua Hospital of Shanghai University of Traditional Chinese Medicine analyzed thousands of ancient herbal formulas that had been developed over a fourteen-hundred-year period between the Sui and Qin dynasties (circa 500 A.D. to 1900 A.D.). These researchers identified 124 classic formulas that claimed to have antiaging properties or to promote longevity. A dozen formulas were eventually selected and then integrated into a single formula. This new formula was put through extensive clinical and laboratory testing involving over two thousand patients.

The studies concluded that the formula had remarkable therapeutic effects on a wide range of symptoms associated with aging, such as weakness and fatigue, degenerative changes in the spine and joints, dizziness or lightheadedness, frequent urination or weakened urinary control and insomnia. The formula significantly improves cellular immune functions, increases muscle strength, delays the occurrence of osteoporosis, and counteracts hypertension. Laboratory studies also confirmed that the formula markedly extended the lifespan of laboratory mice and silkworms, and slowed down the degeneration of sex organs, thymus and liver cells due to aging.

Restoring Essence I was designed to be a comprehensive tonic that addresses all of the major aspects of vital energy—Yin, Yang, Qi and Blood. The formulation focused on the core of Kidney energy known as the Essence—the fluctuations of which dictate vitality and aging according to Chinese medical theory. Restoring Essence I is a revitalizing formula emphasizing treating weakness and fatigue. It fortifies multiple biological functions, including the immune, endocrine and nervous systems. It has also been used successfully in the United States to treat certain types of chronic fatigue syndrome.

---

7. Free radicals are molecules with at least one unpaired electron. Since electrons must be paired, free radicals bounce around your body trying to pair with other electrons by stealing electrons from other molecules. This creates oxidation, which leads to premature aging, degenerative diseases and abnormal weight gain. We live in a world rife with free radicals from exhaust, cigarette smoke, insecticides and other toxins. An antioxidant is a substance, such as vitamin E or C or beta-carotene, that prevents or slows oxidation.

Restoring Essence II was formulated to retard the aging process and promote youthfulness. It is considered one of the most significant findings in the exciting and active field of aging research in the past two decades. The formula can regulate blood pressure and blood sugar levels, lower cholesterol and triglycerides, strengthen the back and joints, enhance sexual function and desire, moisten skin, improve eyesight, reduce frequent urination and promote regular bowel movements. These and other Chinese herbal formulas as well as supplements formulated with a combination of Western nutraceuticals and Chinese herbs can be purchased online at ancientherbsmodernmedicine.com.

You can also use Chinese medicinal herbs in recipes for antiaging. See chapter 21 for recipes.

# PART
# FIVE

## Recipes

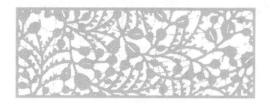

# 20

## Your Individual Constitution

*Foods that suit your constitution*

From the Chinese medicine point of view, we all have different nutritional needs based on our individual constitutions. Just as an individual's constitution can be divided into Yin and Yang (Hot and Cold), Energy from food can also be classified as Yin and Yang (Hot and Cold). Yin foods are Cooling, Calming and nourishing. Yang foods are Warming, stimulating and Energetic. In addition, there are foods that can balance or support each individual Energetic system.

In Western nutrition there are healthy and unhealthy foods. Chinese medicine goes further. You must have the right balance in many different nutritional groups, as well as the Energetic pattern that agrees with your system. Eating foods that agree with your constitution will go far in preventing the imbalances that lead to disease.

At the most basic level, constitutions can be divided into two types, Yin and Yang.

## Yin Type

The Yin type results from either a Yang deficient or Yin excess imbalance. You have a cool constitution if you:

* Use thick or several layers of covers at night while sleeping
* Always keep hands and feet inside covers
* Wear warm clothes (bundle up)
* Love warm weather—cannot tolerate cold
* Have hands and feet that get cold easily
* Do not usually feel thirsty

* Like warm drinks and hate icy drinks
* Retain fluid
* Tire easily

## Yang Type

The Yang type results from either a Yin deficient or Yang excess imbalance. You have a hot constitution if you:

* Use thin or few covers at night while sleeping
* Tend to throw covers off
* Stick hands and feet out of covers
* Dress lightly
* Prefer cooler weather—hate hot weather
* Hands and feet are always warm
* Tend to be thirsty and like icy drinks
* Have a high metabolism
* Have erratic energy levels

In general, if you tend to run Warm, Cooling foods will be most agreeable to your constitution. If you run Cool, Warming foods will be most agreeable to your constitution. If you are more or less Neutral, a balance of Warming and Cooling foods is best for you. Neutral constitution people can fluctuate from Warm to Cold, depending upon the season.

It is possible, however, to overdo a good thing. Again, you want to attain balance in the types of foods you consume. If a Warm constitution individual consumes too many Cooling foods, his or her body will gradually turn Cold, resulting in lethargy, fluid retention, weight gain, and a persistent feeling of bloating. If a Cool constitution individual were to overconsume Warming foods, he or she might experience a feeling of being overheated, especially at night, increasing thirst and dry mouth, irritability and sometimes disturbed sleep.

## The Seven Flavors

Like herbs, foods have Energetic properties that are referred to as Sour, Bitter, Sweet, Spicy, Salty, Bland and Stringent. The term used to describe each flavor does not necessarily correspond with what would be considered its usual taste, but rather the flavors are defined by how your body responds to them Energetically.

- *Sour.* The basic property of this flavor is contracting—a pulling/holding back of Energy. For example, foods with Sour properties are used to treat certain types of diarrhea because of this contracting property. It can also be used to treat problems of spontaneous sweating.
- *Bitter.* The basic properties of this flavor are clearing and drying. Clearing is the opposite of Tonifying. In other words, bitter foods can be used to treat excess conditions such as Heat and Toxin, both of which can be cleared. Drying is the opposite of moistening, and therefore foods with this flavor can be used to treat Damp stagnation.
- *Sweet.* The basic properties of this flavor are Tonifying, Harmonizing and relaxing. Tonifying is to support or strengthen. Harmonizing is to bring into balance. And relaxing is to counteract spasms and tightness.
- *Spicy/Pungent.* The basic properties of this flavor are dispersing and moving. Dispersing is to break up and distribute a concentrated stagnation; for example, to release a cold and push out the pathogens. Moving is to activate and mobilize Energy flow and circulation. It is useful in the treatment of Qi or Blood stagnation.
- *Salty.* The basic properties of this flavor are softening and purging. Softening is to counteract hardness, such as a nodule or mass. Purging is to vigorously promote elimination, primarily of the bowels. Therefore foods that possess this flavor can be used to treat certain types of constipation.
- *Bland.* The basic property of this flavor is draining—essentially promoting urination.
- *Stringent.* The basic properties of this flavor are similar to Sour, but more intense and stronger.

In the chart below you will see that many foods are considered tonics in Chinese medicine. Tonic foods possess strengthening properties. Rather than stimulating or transferring already existing Energy, tonic foods actually generate new Energy. Therefore, tonic foods can be used to treat any sort of weakness or deficiency condition that requires production of Qi. Tonic foods strengthen the body, including the immune system, hematological system (blood), endocrine system and nervous system. Tonic foods help correct deficiencies and replenish what is lacking in the body.

# Vegetables

| Vegetable | Temperature/ Flavor | Action | Good for |
|---|---|---|---|
| Alfalfa sprout | Cool | dries Dampness | arthritis, obesity |
| Asparagus | Cool/slightly Sweet | benefits Kidney Energy and Lung Yin | hypertension, dry cough, cancer |
| Bamboo shoot | Cool | generates fluids | dry cough |
| Beet | Neutral | calms spirit | menopause, nervousness |
| Bell pepper | slightly Warm/ Pungent | soothes Stomach Energy | upset stomach |
| Bok choy | Cool | heals wounds | ulcers, constipation |
| Broccoli | Cool/slightly Pungent | brightens eyes, anticancer | irritated eye, nearsightedness, cancer |
| Burdock root | Cool/Pungent/ Bitter | clears Internal Heat and Toxins | sore throat, infections, gas |
| Cabbage | Neutral/slightly Sweet | benefits Stomach Energy | ulcers, parasites |
| Carrot | Cool/Sweet | dissolves stagnation | tumors, heartburn |
| Cauliflower | Cool/slightly Pungent | disperses nodules | tumors, cancer |
| Celery | Cool | benefits Lung Energy/ Pancreas | appetite control, diabetes |
| Chard | Neutral/slightly Bitter | benefits Liver Energy | eye inflammations, headache |
| Chinese cabbage | Cool | lubricates colon | constipation |

# Vegetables (cont'd)

| Vegetable | Temperature/ Flavor | Action | Good for |
|---|---|---|---|
| Chinese chive | Warm/ Pungent | counteracts blood coagulation | injuries, poor circulation |
| Chinese cucumber | Cold | benefits Fluids | thirst, painful urination |
| Chinese yam | Neutral/ slightly Sweet | strengthens Spleen and Kidney Energies | weak digestion, diarrhea, menopause |
| Cucumber | Cool/slightly Sweet/Bland | cleanses Blood | bladder infection, acne, Internal Heat |
| Daikon radish | Cool/slightly Pungent | reduces mucous discharge, promotes Qi movement | laryngitis, cough, indigestion, gas, bloating |
| Dandelion greens | Cool/Bitter | clears Internal Heat, detoxifies, promotes lactation | irritability, infections, breast-feeding |
| Eggplant | Cool/Sweet | benefits Large Intestine Energy | painful diarrhea |
| Endive | Cool/slightly Bitter | benefits Stomach Energy | stomach discomfort or pain |
| Garlic | Hot/Pungent | promotes Energy circulation, enhances immune system | common cold or flu, poor circulation, whooping cough, viral infection |
| Kale | Warm/slightly Bitter | benefits Stomach Energy | peptic ulcers |

| Vegetable | Temperature/ Flavor | Action | Good for |
|---|---|---|---|
| Leek | Warm/slightly Pungent | helps Liver Energy | upset digestion |
| Lettuce | Neutral | helps sleep, increases Fluid, promotes lactation | insomnia, mild dehydration, breast-feeding |
| Lotus root | Cool/slightly Sweet | stops bleeding, benefits Yin Energy | bleeding, dry cough |
| Mustard green | Warm/slightly Pungent | benefits Lung Energy | cough, chest congestion |
| Onion | Warm/Pungent | lowers blood pressure, clears congestion | hypertension, allergies to inhaled substances |
| Parsley | slightly Warm/ Pungent | detoxifies | meat or fish poisoning |
| Pea | Neutral | harmonizes digestion | constipation, spasms, boils |
| Potato | Cool | neutralizes acids | ulcers, hypertension |
| Pumpkin | Cool | helps blood sugar balance | diabetes, hypoglycemia |
| Romaine lettuce | Cool | benefits circulation, urination | hemorrhoids, difficult urination |
| Scallion | Hot/Pungent | benefits heart, opens airway | chest pain, congestion, arthritis |

# Vegetables (cont'd)

| Vegetable | Temperature/ Flavor | Action | Good for |
|-----------|---------------------|--------|----------|
| Seaweed | Cold/Salty | softens masses | lumps, swollen lymph glands, radiation exposure, metal poisoning |
| Soybean sprout | Cool | clears Heat | arthritis, spasms, cough |
| Spinach | Cool/Sweet | builds and nourishes Blood, moistens Dryness | anemia, night blindness, skin diseases, diabetic thirst |
| Squash | Cool/slightly Sweet | alleviates pain | inflammation |
| String bean | Neutral/ slightly Sweet | benefits Yin and Fluid | diabetes, frequent urination |
| Sweet potato | Neutral/Sweet | promotes Energy | fatigue, night blindness |
| Taro root | Neutral | harmonizes Liver Energy | irritability, anxiety |
| Turnip | Cool/slightly Pungent | removes mucus | asthma, sinus problems |
| Water chestnut | Cold | promotes urination | diabetes, hypertension, swelling |
| Watercress | Cool | reduces growth | cancer, facial blemishes |

# Vegetables (cont'd)

| Vegetable | Temperature/ Flavor | Action | Good for |
|---|---|---|---|
| Yam | Neutral/ slightly Sweet | increases milk, Qi and Yin | breast-feeding, menopause |
| Zucchini | Cool | promotes urination | edema |

# Grains

| Grain | Temperature/ Flavor | Action | Good for |
|---|---|---|---|
| Brown rice | Neutral/Sweet | strengthens Stomach Energy | morning sickness |
| Buckwheat | Neutral | eliminates Internal Heat | Internal Heat, painful diarrhea, cerebral hemorrhage |
| Corn | Neutral | promotes urination | difficult urination |
| Millet | Cool/Sweet | clears Heat | skin rashes, diarrhea |
| Oats | slightly Warm/ Sweet | balances nervous system | diabetes, high cholesterol |
| Pearl barley | Cool/Bland/ slightly Sweet | clears Dampness, benefits Qi | tumors, diarrhea, swelling |
| Rice | Neutral/Sweet | strengthens Stomach Energy | weakness, digestive discomfort |
| Sweet rice | slightly Warm/ Sweet | promotes lactation | lack of milk |

| Grain | Temperature/ Flavor | Action | Good for |
|---|---|---|---|
| Wheat | Cool | strengthens Kidney Energy | insomnia, irritability |
| Wheat germ | slightly Warm/ Sweet | strengthens Heart Energy | sadness, depression |

## Animal Products

| Animal Product | Temperature/ Flavor | Action | Good for |
|---|---|---|---|
| Beef | Warm/Sweet | strengthens Spleen Energy | general weakness |
| Chicken | slightly Warm/ Sweet | benefits Qi and nourishes Blood, aids lactation | recovery from childbirth or illness, breast-feeding |
| Chicken egg | Cool/Sweet | builds and nourishes Blood | helping to prevent miscarriage |
| Clam | Cool/Salty | reduces Dampness, softens nodules | hemorrhoids, goiter |
| Crab | Cool/Salty/ slightly Sweet | moistens Dryness | burns, poison ivy reaction |
| Dairy products | Neutral/Sweet | increases Fluid and body weight | gaining weight |
| Fish (freshwater) | Neutral/Sweet | promotes Fluid distribution | improving appetite |
| Fish (ocean) | Neutral/Sweet/ slightly Salty | dries Dampness | rheumatism |

# Animal Products (cont'd)

| Animal Product | Temperature/ Flavor | Action | Good for |
| --- | --- | --- | --- |
| Gelatin | Neutral/Sweet | stops bleeding | uterine bleeding |
| Lamb | Warm/Sweet | increases Internal Warmth | low back pain, anemia |
| Oyster | Neutral/Sweet/ slightly Salty | benefits Blood and Kidney Energies | insomnia, nervousness |
| Pork | Cool/Sweet | moistens Dryness | dry cough, constipation |
| Shrimp | Warm/Sweet | enhances Yang | decreased libido, weak lactation |
| Turkey | Neutral/Sweet | improves digestion | sensitive stomach |

## Fruits

| Fruit | Temperature/ Flavor | Action | Good for |
| --- | --- | --- | --- |
| Apple | Cool/Sweet/ slightly Sour | reduces Heat | protecting lungs from cigarette smoke |
| Apricot | Cool/Sweet/ slightly Sour | moistens Lung Energy | dry throat, asthma |
| Asian Pear | Cool/Sweet | moistens Dryness | dry cough, sore throat |
| Banana | Cold/Sweet | lubricates intestines | constipation, ulcers |
| Cantaloupe | Cold/Sweet | clears Heat | fever, sinus discharge |

# Fruits (cont'd)

| Fruit | Temperature/ Flavor | Action | Good for |
|---|---|---|---|
| Cherry | Warm/Sweet | improves and nourishes Blood | arthritis, cold limbs |
| Chinese black plum | Neutral/Sour | moistens Dryness, antiparasite | chronic cough, diabetes, parasite |
| Chinese date | Neutral/Sweet | builds Blood | anemia, dizziness |
| Fig | Neutral/Sweet | detoxifies skin, cleanses colon, alkalinizes body | skin diseases, boils, constipation |
| Grapes | Neutral/Sweet/ slightly Sour | purifies Blood, benefits Liver Energy | edema, painful urination, hepatitis, jaundice |
| Grapefruit | Cool/Sweet/ slightly Sour | relieves intoxication, clears Heat | hangover, fever, belching |
| Hawthorn berry | slightly Warm/ Sour | lowers blood pressure, dissolves fats | hypertension, high blood cholesterol, weight control |
| Lemon | Cool/Sour | clears mucus, regulates Liver Energy | indigestion, diabetes, Liver stagnation |
| Loquat | Neutral/slightly Sweet | moistens Lung and Colon Energies | cough, constipation |
| Lycii berry | Neutral/Sweet | tonifies Liver Energy and Kidney Yin | fatigue, anemia, dry skin |
| Lycium fruit | Warm/slightly Sweet | clears mucus | asthma, diarrhea |

| Fruit | Temperature/ Flavor | Action | Good for |
|---|---|---|---|
| Mango | Neutral/slightly Sweet | strengthens Stomach Energy | indigestion |
| Mulberry | Cold/Sweet | tonifies Blood, reduces fever | anemia, rheumatoid arthritis, neuralgia |
| Olive | Neutral | clears obstruction | alcoholism, sore throats |
| Orange | Cool/slightly Sweet | balances Qi | cough, common cold |
| Papaya | Warm/slightly Sweet | aids digestion | bloating, indigestion, GI parasites |
| Peach | Cool/slightly Sweet | promotes blood circulation | hernia pain, cough |
| Pear | Cool/slightly Sweet | increases Fluid | cough, constipation |
| Persimmon | Cool/slightly Stringent | cools Lung Heat | cough, hypertension, diarrhea |
| Pineapple | Warm/slightly Sour | heals swelling | edema, vomiting, diarrhea |
| Plum | Neutral/ slightly Sour | increases Fluid, promotes urination and digestion | diabetes, liver disease, swelling |
| Raspberry | slightly Warm/ Sweet/Sour | strengthens Kidney and Liver Energies | frequent urination, diarrhea |

| Fruit | Temperature/ Flavor | Action | Good for |
|---|---|---|---|
| Strawberry | Cool/slightly Sweet | moistens Lung Energy | dry cough, hangover |
| Tangerine | Cool/Sweet/ Sour | promotes Qi circulation | chest congestion, hiccups, vomiting |
| Tomato | Cool/slightly Sour | produces fluids | hypertension, constipation, prostate problems |
| Watermelon | Cold/Sweet | promotes urination, benefits Fluid | sore throat, canker sores, dehydration |

## Seeds, Nuts and Legumes

| Seed, Nut, Legume | Temperature/ Flavor | Action | Good for |
|---|---|---|---|
| Adzuki beans | Neutral | clears Heat and Toxin | mumps, carbuncles, hot diarrhea |
| Almond | slightly Warm/ slightly Bitter | clears Lung, moistens Colon Energy | cough, constipation |
| Black bean | Warm | benefits reproductive functions | infertility, hot flashes |
| Black sesame seeds | Neutral/Sweet | tonifies Blood, moistens Colon Energy | gray hair, constipation, rheumatism |
| Chestnut | Warm | benefits Kidney Energy and digestion | decreased libido |

## Seeds, Nuts and Legumes (cont'd)

| Seed, Nut, Legume | Temperature/ Flavor | Action | Good for |
|---|---|---|---|
| Filbert (hazelnut) | Neutral | harmonizes digestive Energy | stomach discomfort |
| Flaxseed | Neutral | relieves pain, moistens Colon Energy | degenerative disorders, constipation |
| Hyacinth bean | slightly Warm/ Sweet | strengthens Spleen Energy, dissolves excessive Dampness | weak digestion, diarrhea, vaginal discharge |
| Kidney bean | Neutral/Bland | promotes urination | swelling |
| Lentil | Warm | benefits Heart | lack of vitality |
| Lotus seed | Neutral/ Stringent | benefits Heart and Kidney Energies | chronic diarrhea, restlessness, insomnia |
| Mung bean | Cold/Sweet | detoxifies, clears Heat | food or plant poisoning, diarrhea |
| Pea | Neutral | produces fluids, lubricates dryness, eliminates mucus | promoting lactation |
| Peanut | Neutral/Sweet | lubricates joints | arthritis |
| Pine nut | slightly Warm/ slightly Sweet | lubricates intestines | constipation |
| Pumpkin seed | Cool/slightly Sweet | strengthens Kidney Energy, antiparasite | prostate inflammation, gastrointestinal tract parasites |

# Seeds, Nuts and Legumes (cont'd)

| Seed, Nut, Legume | Temperature/ Flavor | Action | Good for |
|---|---|---|---|
| Soybean | Cool/Sweet | strengthens digestive Energy | diarrhea, menopause |
| Sunflower seed | slightly Warm/ slightly Pungent | repairs intestinal wall | constipation, blood in stool |
| Walnut | Warm/Sweet | benefits Kidney, Lung Energies | miscarriage, cough, constipation |
| White sesame seed | Warm/slightly Sweet | benefits Colon Energy | constipation |
| Winter melon seed | Cool | eliminates mucus | coughing with mucus |

# Herbs and Spices

| Herb or Spice | Temperature/ Flavor | Action | Good for |
|---|---|---|---|
| American ginseng | Cool/Sweet/ slightly Bitter | tonifies Lung, Spleen and Liver Energies | general weakness, alcoholism |
| Astragalus | Warm/Sweet | strengthens Qi and immunity | general weakness, poor immunity |
| Basil | Warm/slightly Pungent | strengthens Stomach Energy | stomach pain |
| Black pepper | Hot/Pungent | warms Stomach Energy | stomachache |
| Cardamom seed | Warm/Pungent | dissolves Dampness, moves Qi | poor digestion and appetite, vomiting |

| Herb or Spice | Temperature/ Flavor | Action | Good for |
|---|---|---|---|
| Chili pepper | Hot/Pungent | promotes Qi and Blood circulation | stagnated Qi or Blood |
| Chrysanthemum | slightly Cold/ Bitter/Sweet | clears Wind and Heat | eye irritation, cold or flu, cough |
| Cilantro | Cool/slightly Pungent | clears Heat, aids digestion | fever, indigestion |
| Cinnamon bark | Hot/Sweet/ Pungent | warms Kidney, Spleen, Liver Energies | weakness with aversion to cold, poor circulation, arthritis, pain |
| Citrus peels | Warm/ Pungent/ Bitter | regulates Qi movement | gas, bloating, indigestion |
| Clove | Warm/Pungent | warms Spleen, Stomach, Liver Energies | indigestion, stomachache, hernia pain |
| Curry | Hot/Pungent | promotes Qi and Blood movement | arthritis, pain |
| Dang Qui | Warm/Sweet/ Pungent | regulates female hormones, tonifies and moves Blood | irregular menses, menstrual anemia, menstrual cramps, constipation |
| Dried ginger | Hot/Pungent | warms Kidney and Spleen Energies | cold low back, stomachache, arthritis |

# Herbs and Spices (cont'd)

| Herb or Spice | Temperature/ Flavor | Action | Good for |
|---|---|---|---|
| Fennel seed | Warm/Pungent | warms Kidney, Liver, Spleen Energies | pains in abdomen, lack of appetite |
| Fresh ginger | Warm/Pungent | expels cold, warms Stomach and Lung Energies | common cold, nausea and vomiting, stomach pain, arthritis, cough |
| Goldenseal root | Cold/Bitter | cools Liver Heat, detoxifies | red eyes, flank pain, onset of common cold |
| Honeysuckle flower | Cold/Sweet | clears Lung Heat and Toxin | common cold or flu, other infections |
| Licorice root | Neutral/Sweet | benefits and harmonizes Qi, detoxifies food | weakness, inflammation, drug or plant poisoning, cough, muscle cramps |
| Mint leaf | Cool/Pungent | clears Heat, soothes throat | common cold or flu, sore throat |
| Mulberry leaf | Cold/Bitter/ Sweet | clears Wind and Heat | common cold or flu, cough |
| Nutmeg seed | Warm/Pungent | warms and moves Spleen Qi | chronic diarrhea, poor digestion |

| Herb or Spice | Temperature/ Flavor | Action | Good for |
|---|---|---|---|
| Oriental ginseng | Warm/Sweet/ slightly Bitter | strengthens Qi | general weakness or fatigue |
| Parsley | Cool/slightly Sweet | promotes urination, helps Kidney Energy | edema, kidney disease |
| Perilla leaf | Warm/Pungent | expels cold, aids Qi movement | common cold, chest congestion, fish poisoning, morning sickness |

## Mushrooms

| Mushroom | Temperature/ Flavor | Action | Good for |
|---|---|---|---|
| Button | Cool | decreases fat levels in blood | high tryglycerides |
| Poria | Neutral/ Sweet/ Bland | reduces Dampness, tonifies Qi | diarrhea, edema, digestive weakness |
| Reishi | slightly Warm/ Sweet | strengthens immunity, anticancer | cancer, weakened immune system |
| Shiitake | Neutral/Sweet | benefits immune system | cancer, chronic viral infections |
| White | slightly Cold/ Sweet | benefits Stomach Energy | weak digestion |
| Wood ear | Neutral/Sweet | thins blood, raises WBC | blood stagnation or coagulation |

# Miscellaneous

| Miscellaneous | Temperature/ Flavor | Action | Good for |
|---|---|---|---|
| Bamboo | Cold/Sweet/ Bland | clears Heat, drains Dampness | fever, chest congestion, swelling |
| Barley malt | Neutral/Sweet | soothes cramps | stomach cramps, diarrhea |
| Brown sugar | Warm/Sweet | helps Energy flow | common cold, mood swings |
| Corn silk | Neutral/Sweet | promotes urination, clears Liver Energy | difficult and painful urination, edema, chronic kidney disease |
| Green tea | Cool/slightly Bitter | promotes Blood circulation | high cholesterol, cancer |
| Honey | Neutral/Sweet | lubricates intestines, repairs tissues | constipation, burns |
| Kudzu root | Cool/Sweet/ slightly Pungent | relaxes muscles, detoxifies | common cold or flu, stiff neck, thirst, abnormal blood sugar, diabetes, alcohol hangover |
| Lily bulb | slightly Cold/ Sweet | calms mind, moistens Lung Energy | restlessness, irritability, dry cough |
| Lily palm | Neutral/ slightly Stringent | clears summer Heat/Dampness | summer Heat, weight control |
| Molasses | Neutral/Sweet | stimulates Energy flow | depression |

# Miscellaneous (cont'd)

| Miscellaneous | Temperature/ Flavor | Action | Good for |
|---|---|---|---|
| Oyster shell | slightly Cold/ Salty | calms mind, regulates Liver Energy | restlessness, hypertension, tumor |
| Reed root | Cool/Sweet | generates fluid, clears Heat | dry throat, fever, cough, restlessness |
| Rice malt | Neutral/Sweet | builds strength | general weakness |
| Rice vinegar | Neutral/Sour | stimulates Energy flow | anxiety, preventing infection |
| Salt | Cold/Salty | promotes bowel action | constipation, inflammation |
| Tofu | Cool/slightly Sweet | benefits Fluids and Kidney Yin | menopause, diabetes, sulfur poisoning |

# 21

Recipes Using
Chinese Medicinal Herbs

The following recipes are organized by chapter and condition. Many of the recipes in this chapter contain herbal ingredients with multiple healing properties that are good for many different conditions. To avoid potentially harmful interactions, if you are taking Western drugs, talk to your Western M.D. before preparing any recipes using Chinese herbs.

When cooking rice, you can reduce the carbohydrate content by preparing "twice-washed" rice: Use 1 $^1/_2$ times the amount of water the recipe calls for. As you simmer the pot of rice, prepare a duplicate pot of water and simmer at the same time. Two-thirds through the cooking time, pour the starch-containing water off the rice, pour in clean water, and continue cooking.

## Chapter 6

### Recipes for GERD

**Congees:** Congee is a slow-cooked, grain-based porridge that is easily digested. Congees are a gentle way to deliver nutrition and medicinal elements to the very ill or people with weakened or sensitive digestion. Add appropriate foods to target a particular therapeutic goal. Congee—also called Jook—is popular in China as a breakfast food and as part of other meals.

*The benefits of grains*

> Barley: *is Cooling, soothing, builds Yin, helps reduce tumors and swellings, corrects diarrhea, is good for Kidney, Spleen, Pancreas and Gall Bladder*

Brown rice: *expels toxins and is beneficial for the nervous system or stress, increases Qi, has more nutrients than white rice*

Buckwheat: *strengthens blood vessels, improves appetite, corrects diarrhea, reduces blood pressure, removes radiation from the body*

Millet: *is silicon-rich and antifungal, stops vomiting, relieves diarrhea, clears Heat, is a diuretic, soothes morning sickness, alkalinizes*

White rice: *has the same qualities in lesser amounts, is easier to digest than brown rice*

To prepare a congee, use $1/2$ cup grain to 8 cups of water. Simmer for 2 to 3 hours on the stove—or use a crockpot on low for 6 hours. Add any of the following near the end of the cooking time for flavor and medicinal benefits.

Adzuki bean: *is a diuretic, used to treat edema and gout*

Asparagus: *is a diuretic and Yin tonic, cleanses arteries, is good for hypertension and arteriosclerosis*

Beet: *strengthens the heart, is sedative, promotes circulation*

Broccoli: *is good for hyperthyroidism (avoid for hypothyroidism)*

Cabbage: *eases depression and irritability, is good for arthritis.*

Celery: *is cooling, cleansing, high in silicon to build joints and bones (arthritis), lowers blood pressure*

Chicken: *builds strength*

Cucumber: *soothes bladder infections, is a skin purifier, counteracts toxins, lifts depression*

Dandelion: *highly nutritious, cleanses the liver, helps correct diabetes*

Ginger: *Warms and promotes digestive Energy, is good for joints*

Mushroom: *has dramatic immune-boosting and cancer-fighting properties*

Onion: *reduces hypertension and cough and promotes lung health, is good for insomnia*

Purslane: *detoxifies and is high in nutrients*

Spinach: *sedates*

# Soothing Sweet Rice Congee

*This congee is energetically neutral and Balanced. It is soothing in nature and will calm even the touchiest stomach. It functions by coating the esophagus and stomach. The porridge can be eaten by any type of GERD sufferer and can be eaten often to treat this condition.*

2- to 3-inch piece of lotus root
1 cup white rice
$^1/_4$ cup sweet rice
$^1/_4$ cup rice protein

dash baking soda *(moisten fingertip and touch baking soda, brush into water and rice)*
12 cups water
$^1/_4$ cup water

To make lotus puree, grind lotus root in a food mill or food processor.
In a medium saucepan over medium-low heat, bring white rice, sweet rice, rice protein and baking soda to a boil in 12 cups water. Reduce heat and simmer covered for 45 minutes to 1 hour. Two minutes before removing rice from heat, dissolve lotus powder into $^1/_4$ cup water and stir into rice.

*Makes 4 servings.*

# Clove Baked Potato Soup

*This soup is pleasantly warming and tingly, especially designed for the Spleen and Stomach Yang deficiency type, but the other types (with the exception of Stomach Yin deficiency with Heat) will also benefit from this recipe. Clove Baked Potato Soup has multiple functions: coating the esophagus and stomach, regulating motility and descending Stomach Energy,*

*invigorating Yang Energy and dispelling Cold and stagnation
in the stomach and promoting digestion.*

4 garlic cloves

2-inch piece ginger root, *peeled
and minced*

5 stalks fresh green onion, *cut into
1-inch pieces*

1 teaspoon ground fennel

1 tablespoon chopped basil

1 teaspoon dried and grated
tangerine peel *(optional)*

$^1/_2$ teaspoon minced fresh
turmeric *(optional)*

pinch of each: pepper, clove and
cardamom *(optional)*

pinch sea salt

15 cups water

1 pound potatoes, *baked or
roasted, then peeled and mashed*

Heat a small saucepan and roast garlic cloves for 2 minutes, stirring constantly. In a large saucepan, over medium-high heat, boil all ingredients except potatoes in water for 5 to 10 minutes. Strain and reserve stock. In the same pan, stir the mashed potatoes into the stock and cook over medium heat until the soup begins to have a creamy consistency.

*Makes 4 servings.*

# Emerald Pudding

*Emerald Pudding is Cooling and soothing and designed to
nourish Stomach Yin. It is particularly good for Stomach
Yin deficiency with Heat.*

4 ounces mung beans

$^1/_4$ ounce lily bulb *(optional)*

2 to 3 clusters white wood ear
mushroom *(optional)*

2 ounces sweet rice

6 cups water

1 pound fresh lotus root, *chopped
into 1-inch pieces and pureed in a
blender, or* $^3/_4$ pound fresh lotus
seeds, *or* $^1/_2$ pound dried lotus
seed, *soaked in water overnight
and then mashed*

3 tablespoons honey

Soak mung beans, lily bulb and mushrooms in water overnight, strain, then puree in a blender. Set aside. In a medium saucepan over medium-high heat, bring sweet rice in 6 cups water to a boil, reduce heat and simmer for 30 minutes. Add all ingredients except honey, stirring continuously until the mixture turns to a medium-thick consistency. Add honey and mix well. Remove from heat and cool. Chill in refrigerator before eating.

*Makes 4 servings.*

## Pearl Rice

*This congee is designed to strengthen digestive energy. It is neutral and gentle, and particularly appropriate for Spleen and Stomach Qi deficiency, although other types can benefit too.*

$1/2$ pound pearl barley *(whole grain)*

1 ounce Chinese yam, *crushed*

1 ounce poria mushroom, *crushed*

1 sheet fresh or dehydrated lotus leaf, *crushed into large pieces (optional)*

8 cups water

$1/4$ pound sweet rice

Soak the pearl barley, Chinese yam and poria mushroom in water for at least two hours or overnight. Strain and discard water. Set soaked ingredients aside. In a medium saucepan over medium-high heat, boil lotus leaf in water for 5 minutes. Strain, discard lotus leaf and reserve liquid. Put liquid, soaked ingredients and sweet rice into a rice steamer and cook until done.

*Makes 4 servings.*

Recipes for All Types of Chronic and Recurrent Illnesses

## Stuffed Shiitake Mushrooms

*This immune-boosting dish makes a wonderful appetizer or a
main dish with salad or vegetables.*

12 to 15 large, fresh shiitake
mushrooms

expeller-pressed extra-virgin olive
oil, *as needed*

1 parsnip, *peeled and very finely
cubed*

3 bulbs shallots, *finely minced
(about 2 tablespoons)*

4 cloves garlic, *minced finely*

1 small bunch spinach

12 dried shiitake mushrooms

1/3 cup grated Parmesan cheese (*a
crumbled block of smoked tofu
can be substituted to make recipe
dairy free*)

2 tablespoons minced parsley

1/2 teaspoon sea salt, *or to taste*

1/4 teaspoon freshly ground black
pepper, *or to taste*

Preheat oven to 400 degrees.

Use care with the fresh shiitake mushrooms when purchasing, storing
and handling, as they are brittle when fresh and the caps must be whole and
intact for this recipe. Remove the stems from the shiitakes and save for making stock in another recipe. Brush tops with olive oil on both sides and set
on baking sheet. Roast 7 minutes. Turn caps over and roast another 7 minutes. Roasting will release water and turn caps golden brown. Remove, drain
and dry well with paper towels.

Blanch spinach in boiling water for 30 seconds. Drain and squeeze out
all water until dry. Chop and reserve.

Toss finely cubed parsnip in 2 teaspoons olive oil. Place on a nonstick
baking sheet and roast for 10 to 12 minutes, shaking the pan a few times to
stir and turn the parsnip "croutons."

Soak the dried shiitakes in 1/2 cup hot water for 20 minutes. Drain,
squeeze dry and finely chop.

Mix shallots, garlic, roasted parsnip croutons, spinach, shiitakes, Parmesan cheese, parsley, salt and pepper in a small mixing bowl. Drizzle with one
teaspoon olive oil and toss again. Place the shiitake caps tops down on a

sheet tray and fill the bowl of the caps with stuffing mix by squeezing a small mound in your hand and pressing it gently into the caps.

Roast for 8 to 10 minutes and serve.

*Makes 6 to 8 appetizers or 4 entree servings.*

# Chapter 7

Recipes for Chronic Illnesses Such as Acne, Eczema, Herpes, Psoriasis, Shingles, Irritable Bowel Syndrome

# Cool Cucumber Green Soup

*A smooth summertime soup that is beneficial to anyone with skin concerns. It also soothes bladder infections.*

5 cucumbers, *lightly peeled, cut open lengthwise, pulp and seeds removed and diced*

1 bunch spinach, *washed, stemmed and lightly chopped*

1 small bunch dandelion greens, *washed, stemmed and lightly chopped (optional; use to taste, as dandelion greens can be bitter)*

2 leeks, *all but several inches of green stalks removed, washed well and finely sliced*

1 small bunch parsley, *stemmed*

1 large unpeeled brown potato, *boiled until soft, peeled and diced*

9 cups Immune Broth, *page 359, or Veggie Detox Broth, page 345, or use organic store-bought broth*

1 teaspoon sea salt, *or to taste*

1/2 teaspoon freshly ground black pepper, *or to taste*

1/2 cup heavy whipping cream or rice milk

For garnish: any combination of nasturtiums, pansies or violets, borage flowers, red clover blossoms, calendula petals, minced yarrow leaves *(use sparingly—this herb has an intense flavor)*, minced horehound leaves *(use sparingly—this herb has an intense flavor)*, or purslane *(chickweed)*

Place all ingredients except cream and garnishes in a large, heavy non-aluminum soup pot. Over a high heat, bring to a boil. Reduce heat and simmer 15 minutes.

Remove from heat and blend till very smooth with a hand-held immersion blender. If using a regular blender, *cool completely before blending.* (If soup is hot when blending, to prevent the hot soup from popping off the top of your blender, blend one cup at a time. Drape a dish towel over the top and hold firmly as you blend each batch.)

Chill soup completely in refrigerator. Add cream or rice milk for a smooth, rich texture.

If desired, any or all of the following ingredients can be added after cooking to add to the healing properties of this recipe: **1 tablespoon aloe vera juice; 1 tablespoon blue-green microalgae powder or spirulina powder; 2 teaspoons slippery elm powder.**

*Makes 8 servings.*

## Irritable Bowel Tea

*A refreshing fresh herbal brew that soothes and heals the bowels.*

3 quarts water

1 cup loosely packed fresh peppermint *(leaves and stems)*

1/2 cup loosely packed lemon balm *(Melissa) (leaves and stems)*

two 4-inch sprigs of fresh rosemary

3-inch piece ginger, *thinly sliced*

1/4 cup dry green tea leaves

12 tablespoons aloe vera juice

Boil water and pour over herbs. Let steep and cool 2 hours. Strain. Add 1 tablespoon aloe vera juice to each cup of tea to intensify healing properties.

*Makes 12 cups.*

# Lotus Porridge

*To ease chronic diarrhea and digestive weakness.*

1 sheet lily palms

1 teaspoon dried and grated orange or tangerine peel *(or zest)*

10 cups water

1/2 cup lotus seed

1 cup pearl barley

1 cup Chinese yam

1/2 cup poria mushroom

Dash royal jelly or stevia

Cut lily palms into 1-inch pieces. In a medium pot, over medium heat, simmer lily palms and grated tangerine peel in 10 cups water for 30 minutes. Strain off lily palms and discard. Reserve liquid in the same pot. Add lotus seed, pearl barley, Chinese yam and poria mushroom to the reserved liquid and simmer over medium heat for 1 hour. Stir occasionally. Add royal jelly or stevia to sweeten before serving. Serve hot.

*Makes 6 servings.*

# Chapter 8

## Recipes for Common Colds and Flu

# Duck Soup

*This is a nourishing, digestible, immune-boosting soup, rich in phytonutrients and minerals. This recipe is also good for common colds and flu.*

3 pounds, whole duck *(muscovy if available)*

1 1/2 quarts water

1 1/2 quarts Immune Broth, *page 359 or Veggie Detox Broth, page 345, or use organic store-bought broth*

1/4 cup soy sauce

1 garlic head, *unpeeled and cut in half sideways*

1 yellow onion, *unpeeled and quartered*

2 carrots, *unpeeled and roughly chopped*

1 cup coarsely chopped celery stalks or tops

2-inch piece sliced ginger root, *unpeeled*

1 serrano or jalapeño chili, *cut in half, or* 3 dried hot red chilies

10 dried shiitake mushrooms, *rinsed*

1/2 dried reishi mushroom

4 star anise spice, *whole (optional)*

1 teaspoon peppercorns

1 teaspoon sea salt

1/2 cup rice wine vinegar

To "white-cook" the duck (a traditional Chinese method of cooking a duck or chicken that leaves the meat very tender): In a large, heavy nonaluminum soup pot with a tight-fitting lid, cover duck with a few inches of cold water. Add remaining ingredients. Turn heat to medium-high until water boils. Boil for one to two minutes only, skimming off foam. Turn off heat, cover tightly and leave on stovetop for 1 1/2 to 2 hours—the residual heat will perfectly cook the bird. *Do not lift lid.*

Remove the duck from the stock. Remove all the meat from the duck—the meat may still be slightly pink at the bone—and chill. Return the bones and skin to the pot. Remove the shiitake caps, slice and reserve. Slowly simmer the stock again for 1 hour, uncovered. Carefully strain the stock. Discard the stock ingredients.

2 yellow onions, *thinly sliced*

3 medium carrots, *thinly sliced*

1/2 cup turnips, parsnips or daikon radish, *thinly sliced*

2 medium tomatoes, *seeded and coarsely chopped*

2 cups loosely shredded napa cabbage

1/2 cup chopped cilantro

Rinse pot and return the stock to it. Add the rest of the vegetables, except for cilantro, and the reserved duck meat and shiitake mushrooms. Over a low heat, simmer for 10 minutes. Add cilantro and serve.

*Makes 6 to 8 servings.*

# Chicken Soup

*In 2000, a team of scientists at the University of Nebraska Medical Center found that grandmother's chicken soup has anti-inflammatory properties and is good for your immune system. The team found that chicken soup helped stop the movement of neutrophils—cells that are released in great numbers by viral infections such as colds and flu. Neutrophil activity stimulates the release of mucus, which causes or exacerbates coughs and stuffy noses in upper respiratory infections such as colds.*

1 whole stewing chicken, about 4 pounds, *skin removed and discarded*

10 cups Immune Broth, *page 359, or Veggie Detox Broth, page 345, or use organic store-bought broth*

3 carrots, *coarsely chopped*

2 turnips, parsnips or daikon radish, *coarsely chopped*

10 dried shiitake mushrooms, *rinsed*

$^1/_2$ dried reishi mushroom

4 celery stalks with leaves, *coarsely chopped*

1 bunch fresh parsley, *coarsely chopped*

3 bay leaves

sea salt, *to taste*

freshly ground black pepper, *to taste*

In a large, heavy nonaluminum soup pot, bring chicken and broth to a boil. Skim off foam from the surface. When no more foam appears, add remaining ingredients. Reduce heat to low and simmer, covered, for 1 hour. Remove chicken. Remove meat from the bones and return to pot. Remove the shiitake caps, slice and return to pot. Remove the reishi and discard. Season with salt and pepper and serve.

*Makes 6 servings.*

## Mucous-Membrane-Cleansing Congee

*A barley congee that will help heal and soothe all mucous membranes, especially the mucous membranes of the lungs, stomach, throat, mouth and gastrointestinal tract.*

1 cup barley

8 cups water

2 tablespoons fennel seed

2 tablespoons fenugreek seed

2 teaspoons powdered licorice root

2 teaspoons dried and grated orange or tangerine peel (or zest)

$1/4$ cup honey

2 tablespoons flaxseed oil

Place all ingredients, except for flaxseed oil, in a large, heavy nonaluminum soup pot and mix well. Over low heat, simmer, covered for 2 $1/2$ hours, stirring occasionally. You can use a crockpot, on low, for 6 hours. Add flaxseed oil at the end and serve.

*Makes 6 to 8 servings.*

## Chapter 9

### A Recipe to Treat Anxiety

## Anxiety Salad

*The ingredients in this salad have soothing, Cooling, calming, sedative and antidepressant qualities. Lacturium, in lettuce and spinach, is a sedative. Cabbage helps mental depression and irritability. Cucumber helps lift depression. Beets have sedative properties. Onions and tomatoes lower blood pressure.*

## Dressing

2 cloves garlic, *finely minced*

1 tablespoon fresh thyme or 1 teaspoon dried thyme

2 tablespoons minced chives and/or parsley

$1/4$ cup lemon juice

$1/3$ cup expeller-pressed extra-virgin olive oil

Sea salt, *to taste*

Freshly ground black pepper, *to taste*

Mix the garlic, thyme and chives or parsley into the lemon juice and blend in olive oil. Add salt and pepper to taste.

## Salad

1 large head Romaine or dark loose-leafed lettuce, *washed and dried*

$3/4$ cup shredded purple cabbage

2 small handfuls spinach

1 medium cucumber, *peeled and sliced*

1 raw beet root peeled and sliced very thin

1 large tomato, *sliced,* or 12 cherry tomatoes

Mix lettuce, cabbage and spinach with a few tablespoons dressing. Arrange on two plates. Arrange the rest of the vegetables on top and drizzle with dressing.

Garnish with minced parsley and chives and serve.

*Makes 2 servings.*

## Chapter 10

Recipes to Treat the Symptoms of Adrenal Burnout

## Wheat Berry Congee

*To ease the symptoms of headache, tension, irritability, low
energy and mood swings, insomnia and restlessness.*

1 cup wheat berries

8 cups Immune Broth, *page 359,*
   *or Veggie Detox Broth, page 345,*
   *or use organic store-bought broth*

two 3-inch pieces of Dang Qui

1 teaspoon sea salt

1 pinch saffron threads

1 teaspoon royal jelly

1 tablespoon aloe vera juice

2 teaspoons butter or ghee

In a large, heavy nonaluminum soup pot on high, bring wheat berries,
broth, Dang Qui and salt to a boil, reduce heat to low and simmer for 2 to 3
hours—or 6 hours if using a crockpot.

With a slotted spoon, remove the softened Dang Qui pieces. Mince
Dang Qui and return to pot. Add the saffron, royal jelly, aloe vera and butter
and stir. Heat through for one minute and serve.

*Makes 6 servings.*

## Chapter 11

Recipes to Treat Allergies, Asthma, Chronic Fatigue
and Autoimmune Conditions

## Clear Heat Stir-fry

*A Chinese stir-fry meal that will benefit Heat conditions in the
heart, liver, gastrointestinal tract and gall bladder. This recipe*

*Cools the body and is good for inflammations,
fevers and detoxification.*

2 tablespoons expeller-pressed extra-virgin olive oil

1 box firm-style tofu, *drained and diced*

6-inch piece daikon radish, *peeled and diced*

1 large cucumber, *peeled, seeded and diced*

1 large burdock root, *peeled and diced*

3 stalks celery, *sliced thin*

2 large carrots, *peeled and diced*

2 large leeks, *cleaned and sliced*

3 tablespoons soy sauce

3 tablespoons cilantro leaves, *chopped*

In a wok or large sauté pan on high heat, heat olive oil. Add all ingredients except cilantro and stir-fry for about 6 minutes, until vegetables are soft. Garnish with cilantro and serve with rice.

*Makes 4 servings.*

# Braised Lily Bud Chicken

*The savory medicinal ingredients in this traditional Chinese dish can be helpful for those suffering from allergies, asthma, nasal congestion or chronic fatigue.*

10 dried shiitake mushrooms or 5 black mushrooms

15 to 20 small dried lily flower buds

4 chicken breasts, *split, boned*

few pinches sea salt

few pinches freshly ground black pepper

3 tablespoons expeller-pressed extra-virgin olive oil or peanut oil

2-inch piece ginger, *finely minced*

6 garlic cloves

1 teaspoon tangerine or citrus peel

1/4 teaspoon red chili flakes

4 tablespoons soy sauce

2 tablespoons rice wine or sherry

1 cup Immune Broth, *page 359, or Veggie Detox Broth, page 345, or use organic store-bought broth, with 1 tablespoon well-dissolved cornstarch*

$^1/_2$ cup slivered celery          $^1/_4$ cup slivered scallions
$^1/_2$ large onion, *sliced*

Soak shiitake mushrooms in 1 cup warm water for 20 minutes. Drain, slice and reserve. Discard woody bits. Soak lily flower buds in $^1/_2$ cup warm water for 20 minutes. Drain and reserve.

Rinse chicken pieces and pat dry with paper towels. Sprinkle with salt and pepper. In a wok or large sauté pan, over high heat, heat 3 tablespoons oil. Add chicken and brown on both sides, about 10 minutes.

Combine remaining ingredients except scallions and pour over chicken. Bring to a boil, reduce to simmer and cover. Cook 20 minutes, until chicken is done. Remove chicken to a platter, pour sauce over and garnish with scallions.

*Makes 4 to 6 servings.*

# Green Broth

*A broth to cleanse and purify. This broth can be eaten between meals as a tonic. It is helpful for weight loss, for detoxification and to treat arthritis and autoimmune conditions.*

10 cups Immune Broth, *page 359,*
   *or Veggie Detox Broth, page 345,*
   *or use organic store-bought broth*
$^1/_3$ cup loose fresh green tea
   leaves
1 fresh burdock root, *chopped*
$^1/_2$ cup alfalfa sprouts
1 bunch dandelion greens, *washed*
   *and coarsely chopped*

1 bunch parsley, *washed and*
   *coarsely chopped*
1 small bunch purslane, *washed*
   *and coarsely chopped*
3-inch piece Chai Hu Small
   (Bupleurum root)
two 3-inch pieces Huang Yao Zi
   (Dioscorea tuber)

In a large, heavy nonaluminum soup pot, over medium-low heat, simmer all ingredients for 30 to 40 minutes. Strain through sieve, pressing to extract essences.

*Makes 8 servings.*

# Immune-Building Roast Chicken

*The seasonings for this recipe have strong antifungal, candida-killing properties. This recipe benefits those with chronic fatigue and autoimmune conditions. The seasoning paste can also be used on roast potatoes or vegetables.*

3 ¹/₂ pound whole chicken or 3 ¹/₂ pounds chicken parts, *skin removed and discarded*

1 whole head garlic—about 12 cloves (more if desired), *cloves separated and peeled*

3-inch piece ginger, *peeled and coarsely chopped*

2 rounded tablespoons fresh chopped thyme

two 3-inch pieces of fresh rosemary, *stripped from stem, about 1 scant tablespoon*

2 teaspoons sea salt, *or to taste*

1 tablespoon crushed peppercorns

2 teaspoons lemon zest, *fresh or dried*

3 tablespoons lemon juice

2 tablespoons expeller-pressed extra-virgin olive oil

Preheat oven to 425 degrees. Rinse and pat chicken dry with paper towels. In a food processor or using a mortar and pestle, grind all remaining ingredients to a rough-textured paste. Rub the paste well into the chicken, inside and out.

Place chicken on wire rack over baking tray and let sit 15 minutes. Roast in center of oven for 12 to 15 minutes. Reduce heat to 350 degrees. Roast 25 minutes longer for chicken parts and 40 minutes for whole chicken.

*Makes 4 to 6 servings.*

# Green Goddess Cupcakes

*For strengthening Yin Energy and for detoxification.*

1 cup mung bean flour

1 cup small Chinese red bean flour

1 cup pearl barley flour

1 ¹/₂ cups water

<sup>1</sup>/<sub>2</sub> ounce white wood ear
mushroom

1 piece lotus root

<sup>1</sup>/<sub>2</sub> cup lily bulbs

2 tablespoons honey

1 teaspoon fresh aloe vera gel

Preheat the oven to 350 degrees. Soak white wood ear mushroom and lily bulbs in 2 cups hot water for 1 hour.

In a medium bowl, mix mung bean flour, Chinese red bean flour, barley flour and water. Strain mushroom and lily bulbs. Puree mushroom, lotus root and lily bulbs in a blender until smooth. Add the purée to the mixture and stir well. Fold in honey and aloe vera gel. Pour mixture into paper-lined cupcake tins and bake for 25 to 30 minutes.

*Makes 6 servings.*

# Chapters 12, 13, 14 and 15

## Recipes for Cancer, Hepatitis, Heart Disease, Type II Diabetes, Arthritis, Osteoporosis, HIV and AIDS

# Allium Power Soup

*An onion soup, using four kinds of alliums (members of the onion family). This soup is good for conditions such as cancer, AIDS and heart trouble. It is also good for common colds and flu.*

5 large yellow onions, *peeled and
sliced*

3 tablespoons expeller-pressed
extra-virgin olive oil

10 cloves minced garlic

5 large leeks, *cleaned well and
finely chopped*

1 bunch scallions, *cleaned and
finely chopped*

<sup>1</sup>/<sub>4</sub> cup soy sauce

1 whole chili pepper, *sliced
lengthwise*

10 cups Immune Broth, *page 359,
or Veggie Detox Broth, page 345
(or use organic store-bought broth)*

1-inch piece ginger, *peeled and
minced*

$^1/_2$ cup fresh parsley, *minced*

sea salt, *to taste*

freshly ground black pepper, *to taste*

In a large, heavy nonaluminum soup pot, over medium heat, heat olive oil. When hot, sauté onions for 20 to 30 minutes, until golden brown and very soft. Add garlic during the last 5 minutes. Make sure it does not burn.

Add remaining ingredients except parsley and simmer, uncovered, 25 minutes. Add parsley and season with salt and pepper to taste.

*Makes 8 servings.*

## Veggie Detox Broths

*Two veggie broths with antiviral and immune-enhancing properties, plus antioxidants and minerals. For detoxification, cancer, colds and flu. These broths can also be used as part of a weight-loss program.*

## Heavy Veggie Detox Broth 1

$^1/_2$ cup barley

1 brown potato, *peeled and diced*

5 stalks celery, *coarsely chopped*

2 beets, *coarsely chopped*

$^1/_2$ head garlic, *unpeeled, crushed or cut*

1 large yellow onion, *unpeeled, coarsely chopped*

1 small bunch parsley, *whole with stems, rinsed*

6 dried red dates

1-inch piece Ren Shen (*ginseng root*)

two 3-inch slices Huang Yao Zi (*Dioscorea tuber*)

1-inch piece ginger, *chopped or crushed*

12 dried shiitake mushrooms

1 teaspoon sea salt

10 cups water

In a large, heavy nonaluminum soup pot, over high heat, bring all ingredients to a boil. Reduce heat and simmer, uncovered, about 1 $^1/_2$ hours.

Strain and press through sieve to release all essences from vegetables. Reserve shiitake mushrooms for another use or chop and add to broth.

*Makes 8 servings.*

## Light Veggie Detox Broth 2

2 large yellow onions, *unpeeled, coarsely chopped*

4 large carrots, *unpeeled, coarsely chopped*

5 stalks celery, *coarsely chopped*

5 cloves garlic, *unpeeled, crushed*

1/2 small bunch parsley, *whole with stems, rinsed*

four 5-inch slices Huang Qi *(Astragalus root)*

4 dried lily flowers

6 dried shiitake mushrooms

1 teaspoon sea salt, *or to taste*

1/2 teaspoon peppercorns

10 cups water

In a large, heavy nonaluminum soup pot, simmer all ingredients, uncovered, about 1 1/2 hours. Strain and press through sieve to release all essences from vegetables. Reserve shiitake mushrooms for another use or chop and add to broth.

*Makes 8 servings.*

## Super Stamina Congee

*Super Stamina Congee delivers exceptional immune-building and -strengthening nutrients in a delicious and easily digestible way. This congee is good for people with chronic fatigue, AIDS and cancer. It is also nutritious for those pursuing endurance sports.*

10 cups water, Immune Broth, *page 359, or Veggie Detox Broth, page 345, or use organic store-bought broth*

2-inch piece dried Xi Yang Shen *(American ginseng root)*

four 5-inch slices dried Huang Qi
(Astragalus root)

three 3-inch slices dried Huang
Yao Zi (Dioscorea tuber)

1 cup brown rice

1/2 cup dried lotus seeds

10 shiitake mushrooms, soaked in
warm water for 15 minutes,
drained and slivered

5 garlic cloves, minced

2 carrots, diced small

1 cup yellow onions, chopped

2 tablespoons soy sauce

1/2 teaspoon red chili flakes

1 cup kale, chard or collard
greens, chopped

In a large, heavy nonaluminum soup pot, over medium-high heat, add the water or broth, ginseng, Astragalus, Dioscorea, brown rice, lotus seeds and shiitake mushrooms. Bring to a boil. Reduce heat to very low and simmer for two hours.

Add remaining ingredients and simmer 20 minutes more. The softened roots may be removed or eaten with the congee.

*Makes 8 servings.*

# Radiation Remedy

*A buckwheat, ginseng and seaweed congee to help remove the toxins from environmental and medicinal radiation from the body. This congee is good for people going through cancer treatments. It also contains antiaging properties.*

1 1/2 cups buckwheat

10 cups water

3-inch piece Xi Yang Shen
(American ginseng root)

2 green apples, peeled, seeded and
finely chopped

1 tablespoon French green clay

1 tablespoon aloe vera juice

1 tablespoon dried kelp, crumbled

1 tablespoon miso

In a large, heavy nonaluminum soup pot, over medium-high heat, bring buckwheat, water and ginseng to a boil. Simmer 2 hours, covered.

Add apple, clay, aloe vera, kelp and miso. Stir well. Simmer 10 minutes more, uncovered.

*Makes 8 servings.*

# Shiitake Reishi Barley Stew

*A nutritious mineral- and antioxidant-rich, digestible, immune-building, substantial stew for those with cancer, AIDS or arthritis.*

3 quarts **Immune Broth**, *page 359, or Veggie Detox Broth, page 345, or use organic store-bought broth*

1 ¹/2 cups **barley**

15 dried **shiitake mushrooms**

¹/2 large, dried **reishi mushroom**

1 large **yellow onion**, *chopped*

4 **carrots**, *sliced*

5 large stalks **celery**, *sliced*

6 **garlic cloves**, *minced*

1 bunch **parsley**, *minced*

2 cups **kale or spinach**, *shredded*

1 tablespoon **soy sauce**

¹/4 teaspoon **freshly ground black pepper**, *or to taste*

1 teaspoon **expeller-pressed toasted sesame oil**

In a large, heavy nonaluminum soup pot, over medium-high heat, bring stock, barley and shiitake mushrooms to a boil. Reduce heat and simmer uncovered for 1 hour. Remove shiitakes and slice. Discard woody stems and return the sliced shiitakes to the pot. Press all the juice from the reishi mushroom into the stew and discard mushroom. Add onion, carrot, celery and garlic and cook 30 minutes more. Add parsley, greens, soy sauce and pepper and cook 5 minutes more (a little longer if using kale). Stir in sesame oil and serve.

*Makes 6 servings.*

# Seafood Swimming in Seaweed

*This recipe is good for cancer, AIDS,
hypothyroidism and heart health.*

1 cup dulse seaweed

2 or 3 sheets kelp

2 large cloud ear mushrooms

15 shiitake mushrooms

2 pounds shark fillets, *cut into 2-inch pieces*

1/2 pound calamari tubes and tentacles, *washed and sliced*

1/2 pound raw medium-sized shrimp, *shelled*

2 tablespoons expeller-pressed extra-virgin olive oil

6 cloves garlic, *minced*

1 medium yellow onion, *peeled and sliced*

2 cups green cabbage

2 sheets nori seaweed, *cut into strips with scissors*

2 tablespoons soy sauce

1/2 teaspoon red pepper flakes

1 tablespoon cornstarch, *dissolved in 1/2 cup Immune Broth, page 359, or Veggie Detox Broth, page 345, or use organic store-bought broth*

2 tablespoons cilantro leaves, *chopped*

Soak dulse, kelp, cloud ear and shiitake mushrooms in 2 cups warm water for 30 minutes and drain. Slice the seaweed and mushrooms, discarding any tough bits, and set aside.

In a wok or large sauté pan, over medium-high heat, heat oil until hot. Stir-fry the shark for 2 minutes, then add the calamari and shrimp and stir-fry for 2 or 3 more minutes. *Do not overcook.* Remove with a slotted spoon and reserve close to stove to keep warm.

Add garlic and onion to the hot pan and stir-fry for 1 minute. Add cabbage, nori, red pepper and soy sauce and stir-fry for about 5 minutes to wilt the cabbage. Add the reserved soaked mushrooms, seaweeds, cornstarch and stock mixture. Stir 3 to 4 minutes more until thickened.

Place the seafood on top and heat through for 1 minute. Garnish with cilantro and serve.

*Makes 6 servings.*

## Mushrooms in Miso Sauce

*A mix of fresh and dried mushrooms in a garlic miso sauce to serve over rice or grains, this recipe is an immune builder for people with cancer or AIDS. It also benefits those with chronic fatigue.*

12 to 14 shiitake mushrooms

1/4 cup dried cloud ear mushrooms

1/2 large dried reishi mushroom

1 cup Immune Broth, *page 359, or Veggie Detox Broth, page 345, or use organic store-bought broth*

2 tablespoons olive oil

10 garlic cloves, *minced*

2 cups fresh mushrooms of your choice

3 stalks celery, *thinly sliced on the bias*

1 small yellow onion, *peeled and sliced*

3 tablespoons miso, *thinned with 1 tablespoon water, 1 tablespoon rice wine and 1 teaspoon nam pla (fish sauce)*

1 teaspoon expeller-pressed toasted sesame oil

1/4 teaspoon red chili flakes

2 tablespoons cornstarch, *dissolved in 1/4 cup water*

1 big bunch scallions, *washed and slivered*

2 tablespoons cilantro, *minced*

In a large saucepan, simmer the dried shiitake, cloud ear and reishi mushrooms with 1 1/2 cups water, uncovered, for 20 minutes. Strain and reserve liquid—about 1 cup. Discard the reishi (or use in another recipe). Slice the other mushrooms, discarding any woody bits. Add the cooked mushrooms back to the pot and add stock. You should have about 2 cups total.

In a wok or large sauté pan, over medium-high heat, heat olive oil to just hot. Add half of the garlic and half of the fresh mushrooms and lightly brown, about 2 to 3 minutes, stirring. Remove and repeat with the remaining garlic and mushrooms.

Add all the mushrooms back to the pan. Add celery and onion and stir-fry for 2 minutes. Add the mushroom and stock and continue to cook 8 minutes to reduce liquid, stirring.

Add miso, sesame oil and chili flakes and stir-fry for 1 minute. Add cornstarch mixture and scallions and stir till thickened, 3 to 5 minutes. Garnish with cilantro and serve.

*Makes 4 servings.*

# Smooth Jade Green Soup

*A delicious smooth jade green soup. Artichokes (and all thistles) benefit the liver. Dandelion greens contain Bitter properties that are a super liver-cleansing and -support herb for those with hepatitis. Artichokes have a unique effect on the taste buds that makes the other ingredients taste even better. This is a perfect first course; it is medicinal, with a gourmet flavor. It is also useful for the treatment of dermatological problems, and for detoxification and weight loss.*

8 large artichokes

1 teaspoon sea salt

1/2 teaspoon peppercorns

3 quarts Immune Broth, *page 359, or Veggie Dextox Broth, page 345, or use organic store-bought broth*

2 large yellow onions, *sliced*

2 tablespoons expeller-pressed extra-virgin olive oil

10 to 12 garlic cloves, *peeled and cut in half*

2 medium-sized brown potatoes, *diced*

1 small bunch dandelion greens, *washed and thinly chopped*

1 small bunch parsley, *washed and chopped*

juice of 1 lemon

sea salt, *to taste*

freshly ground black pepper, *to taste*

1/2 cup heavy whipping cream or sour cream

Preheat oven to 350 degrees.

In a large pot, add water to cover artichokes, 1 teaspoon salt and peppercorns. Over high heat, bring to boil, reduce to simmer and cover. Cook 45 minutes, until tender. Or place artichokes in a steamer basket over water and steam, covered, about 1 hour. Remove and reserve the soft edible pulp of the stems and choke and scrape the base of the leaves with a spoon. Dice the pulp, season with salt and pepper and reserve.

On a nonstick sheet pan, drizzle onions with olive oil and slow-roast in oven for 25 minutes. Add garlic to onions halfway through roasting.

In a large, heavy nonaluminum soup pot, put stock, artichokes, roasted onions and garlic and potato and simmer about 20 minutes until potato is soft.

Remove from heat and blend till very smooth with a hand-held immersion blender. If using a regular blender, *cool completely before blending.* If soup is hot when blending, to prevent the hot soup from popping off the top of your blender, blend one cup at a time. Drape a dish towel over the top and hold firmly as you blend each batch.

Return to heat. Add dandelion, parsley, lemon, salt and pepper to taste. Cook 6 minutes, till greens are wilted. Add a streak of cream or sour cream as a garnish to each bowl.

*Makes 8 servings.*

# Roasted Roots

*This recipe is helpful for those suffering from diabetes, cancer or arthritis. The root vegetables in this recipe were selected to balance insulin levels. You can serve roasted roots as a side dish, as a quick addition to a broth or grain dish or cold as a salad.*

4 tablespoons expeller-pressed extra-virgin olive oil

1 tablespoon lemon juice

5 garlic cloves, *peeled and finely minced*

2 tablespoons parsley, *finely minced*

1 1/2 teaspoons sea salt

1/2 teaspoon freshly ground black pepper

2 large beets, *peeled and diced*

5 Jerusalem artichokes, *peeled and diced*

2 kohlrabi roots, *scrubbed and diced*

1 large yam or sweet potato, *scrubbed and diced*

1 large brown potato, *peeled and diced*

3 large carrots, *peeled and coarsely chopped*

2 yellow onions, *peeled and quartered*

Heat oven to 375 degrees.

In a medium bowl, mix oil, lemon juice, garlic, parsley, salt and pepper. Remove 1 tablespoon of this mixture and place in a smaller bowl with the beets, which will help prevent the color from bleeding onto the other vegetables. Toss the rest of the vegetables with the marinade.

Using as many nonstick baking sheets as needed, spread the roots in one layer with space between. Roast in oven for 35 to 45 minutes, until soft and golden brown. Shake pan or turn vegetables with a spatula several times when cooking to brown evenly and keep from sticking.

*Makes 6 side-dish servings.*

# Bitter Melon Soup

*This recipe is good for people suffering from diabetes. Bitter melon is available at Chinese markets. Chinese bitter melon has a strong flavor and should be soaked in a light brine (salt water), then squeezed to draw out some of the bitterness.*

5-inch piece Chinese bitter melon

6 cups water

1 tablespoon sea salt

8 cups Immune Broth, *page 359, or Veggie Detox Broth, page 345, or use organic store-bought broth*

3 stalks celery, *cut into slivers*

1 small onion, *peeled and sliced thin*

1 cup kale or chard leaves, *slivered*

1 cup fresh shiitake or other mushrooms, *wiped clean and slivered*

1 cup soft-style tofu, *drained and diced*

2 teaspoons minced garlic

2 teaspoons minced ginger

1 teaspoon powdered turmeric

1 teaspoon powdered fenugreek

$^1$/2 teaspoon freshly ground black pepper

$^1$/2 teaspoon red pepper flakes

1 teaspoon sea salt

3 tablespoons slivered scallions

2 sheets nori seaweed, *cut to slivers with scissors (or torn)*

1 teaspoon expeller-pressed toasted sesame oil

Lightly peel the bitter melon and slice thinly. Soak slices in 6 cups of water and 1 tablespoon salt for 1 to 1 $^1$/2 hours. Drain well, pressing to release liquid. Reserve melon and discard water.

In a large, nonaluminum soup pot, over medium heat, bring to a boil broth, celery, onion, kale or chard, mushrooms, tofu, garlic, ginger, turmeric, fenugreek, black pepper, red pepper flakes and salt. Reduce heat and simmer 15 minutes. Add scallions, nori and sesame oil and simmer 5 more minutes.

*Makes 6 servings.*

# Ginger Cabbage Soup

*A silicon-rich, cartilage-building recipe for easing and healing joint pain from arthritis and fibromyalgia.*

10 cups Immune Broth, *page 359, or Veggie Detox Broth, page 345, or use organic store-bought broth*

4 cups loosely packed shredded green cabbage

1 yellow onion, *peeled and thinly sliced*

2 carrots, *peeled and thinly sliced*

6 stalks celery, *sliced*

2-inch piece ginger, *peeled and minced*

1/4 cup rice wine or apple cider vinegar

sea salt, *to taste*

freshly ground black pepper, *to taste*

1/4 cup parsley, *minced*

In a large, heavy nonaluminum soup pot, on high heat, bring all ingredients except salt, pepper and parsley to a boil. Reduce heat and simmer, uncovered, for 25 minutes. Season with salt and pepper to taste. Add parsley and serve.

*Makes 8 servings.*

# Happy Heart Beet Salad

*A delicious ginger-flavored roasted beet salad for heart health. In Chinese medicine, beets are important for heart health. Onions and garlic lower cholesterol, prevent blood clots and are antihypertensive. Expeller-pressed olive oil is a healthy cholesterol-lowering oil. Parsley is a powerhouse of vitamins, minerals and antioxidants.*

6 large beets, *unpeeled, scrubbed and trimmed*

2-inch piece ginger, *peeled and grated (about 1 tablespoon)*

6 garlic cloves, *peeled and minced*

1/3 cup seasoned rice wine vinegar

1/4 cup expeller-pressed extra-virgin olive oil *(or substitute other heart-healthy oils such as flaxseed, avocado or borage oil)*

1/2 cup parsley, *chopped*

sea salt, *to taste*

freshly ground black pepper, *to taste*

Preheat oven to 375 degrees. Roast beets on nonstick baking sheet 45 to 55 minutes, until tender when pierced. Cool to lukewarm. Using your fingers, rub off skins and dice. In a medium-sized mixing bowl, soak garlic and ginger in rice wine vinegar about 15 minutes. Toss in beets and parsley. Drizzle on oils and gently toss. Season to taste with salt and pepper.

*Makes 6 servings.*

## Super Berry Fruit Salad

*This recipe is good for hemorrhoids, varicose veins, arthritis and osteoporosis. Proanthocyanidins and anthocyanidins in berries strengthen vein and collagen structure. All berries— especially blueberries—have an exceptionally high antioxidant content. Pectin in apples and pears supply additional support.*

1/2 cup whole plain yogurt or whole sour cream

1 tablespoon honey

1 tablespoon lemon juice

1 tablespoon fresh minced mint leaves

1 teaspoon grated ginger

1 pint basket blueberries, *rinsed and drained*

1 pint basket strawberries, *rinsed and drained*

1 pint basket raspberries, *rinsed and drained*

1 pint basket blackberries, *rinsed and drained*

2 green apples, *unpeeled, seeded and diced*

2 ripe pears, *seeded and diced*

In a medium mixing bowl, mix yogurt, honey, lemon juice, mint leaves and ginger. Gently toss in fruits.

*Makes 4 to 6 servings.*

# Gallstone Flush Salad

*A Waldorf-style salad with an Asian touch that promotes gall bladder health and gallstone softening. Also good for AIDS and for gentle detoxification. Apples and daikon radishes help dissolve and flush out gallstones. Parsley is detoxifying.*

## Dressing

1 garlic clove, *minced*

1 teaspoon grated fresh ginger

1/4 cup seasoned rice wine vinegar

2 tablespoons apple juice

2 teaspoons honey

4 tablespoons sour cream

1 tablespoon expeller-pressed extra-virgin olive oil

In a large salad bowl, blend all dressing ingredients.

## Salad

6 to 8 Chinese red dates, *chopped (use 1/4 cup raisins if dates are unavailable)*

3 to 4 green organic apples, *seeded*

4-inch piece daikon radish, *peeled and diced small*

2 carrots, *peeled and grated*

1/4 cup parsley, *minced*

1/4 cup almonds

1 cup loosely packed shredded green cabbage

1 cup loosely packed shredded red cabbage

In the salad bowl with dressing, mix dates or raisins, apples, daikon, carrots, parsley and almonds together. Toss salad with dressing.

Arrange a bed of cabbage on plates. Scoop the salad on top and serve.

*Makes 4 servings.*

# Mushroom
# Immune-Building Stew

*This stew is a nutritious, digestible, immune-building substantial meal for people with weak immune systems or those with cancer, HIV or AIDS. Barley boosts immunity and helps reduce swelling. Mushrooms are known to boost immunity.*

3 quarts Immune Broth, *page 359, or Veggie Detox Broth, page 345, or use organic store-bought broth*

1 $^{1}/_{2}$ cups barley

pinch sea salt

1 cup dried shiitake mushrooms

1 large dried reishi mushroom

$^{1}/_{2}$ cup poria mushrooms

1 large yellow onion, *sliced*

5 medium carrots, *chopped*

5 large stalks celery, *chopped*

5 cloves garlic, *minced*

large bunch parsley, *minced*

2 cups green kale, *shredded*

1 tablespoon soy sauce

sea salt, *to taste*

freshly ground black pepper, *to taste*

1 teaspoon expeller-pressed toasted sesame oil

In a large, heavy nonaluminum soup pot, over medium-low heat, add stock or broth, barley and salt. Simmer about 1 hour. Add mushrooms, onion, carrots, celery, garlic and parsley and simmer 25 minutes. Add kale, soy sauce, salt, pepper, sesame oil and simmer 10 more minutes.

*Makes 8 servings.*

# Bean and Barley Detox Soup

1 ounce mung beans

1 ounce small Chinese red beans

1 ounce pearl barley

8 cups water

2 cups Immune Broth, *page 359,*
  *or Veggie Detox Broth, page 345,*
  *or use organic store-bought broth*

3 tablespoons honey

Soak dry ingredients in 3 cups water for 1 $1/2$ hours. Rinse and drain. In a medium pot over low heat combine beans, barley, broth and honey and simmer for one hour.

*Makes 4 to 6 servings.*

## Tofu, Shiitakes and Greens

*This is a substantial, nourishing meal that is rich in phytonutrients and antioxidants to boost your immune system and fight disease.*

1 box firm-style tofu, *drained and cubed*

2 tablespoons expeller-pressed extra-virgin olive oil

1 $1/2$-inch piece ginger, *finely minced*

6 or more garlic cloves, *peeled and finely minced*

1 teaspoon red chili flakes

1 medium yellow onion, *peeled and sliced*

3 carrots, *peeled and sliced thin*

12 to 20 shiitake mushrooms, *soaked and sliced*

3 to 4 cups kale, collard greens, chard or green cabbage, *chopped*

3 tablespoons soy sauce

2 tablespoons rice wine

In a large wok or sauté pan, over medium-high heat, heat olive oil. When hot add tofu, ginger, garlic and chili flakes and stir-fry 1 to 2 minutes, until golden. Add carrots, onions and shiitake mushrooms and continue stir-frying another 3 to 5 minutes. Add the greens, reduce heat to medium-low, cover and cook for 5 minutes, until greens were wilted. Remove cover, increase heat to high, add soy sauce and rice wine and stir-fry for 1 minute. Serve with rice.

*Makes 6 servings.*

# Immune Broths

*These broths have immune-enhancing and -regulating ingredients and are excellent for the treatment of autoimmune conditions. They can also be used for frequent colds, cancer, AIDS and degenerative diseases. Some ingredients also have antiaging properties. Either can be used as a delicious clear broth or as a stock base for recipes. The first is strongly flavored with mushrooms and the second is lighter and more suitable for use in recipes that call for a lighter flavor.*

# Immune Broth 1

3 pounds chicken bones or pieces *(backs, wings, neck)* or **one whole chicken**, *skin removed and discarded*

3 quarts water

1 or 2 large onions, *with skin, quartered or coarsely chopped*

3 large carrots, *unpeeled, coarsely chopped*

5 large stalks celery, *coarsely chopped*

small bunch parsley, *whole*

2 garlic cloves, *unpeeled, coarsely chopped*

one 3-inch piece of fresh ginseng root, *crushed (or substitute powdered, about 1 teaspoon)*

three 4-inch slices of Huang Qi (Astragalus), *crushed (or substitute powdered, about 2 teaspoons)*

three 3-inch slices of Huang Yao Zi *(Dioscorea tuber)*

1 whole large reishi mushroom

1 cup dried shiitake mushrooms

1 teaspoon sea salt, *or to taste*

$^1/_2$ teaspoon freshly ground black pepper, *or to taste*

In a large, heavy nonaluminum soup pot, over medium-low heat, cover all ingredients with water. Bring to a boil, reduce heat, and simmer 30 minutes. Lift the chicken from the broth and remove all meat. Reserve meat and return bones to pot. Continue simmering, partially covered, for 2 hours.

Strain well, pressing with a fork to extract essences. Shiitake may be saved for another use. Discard other ingredients.

*Makes about 2 ¹/2 quarts.*

## Immune Broth 2

3 pounds chicken bones or pieces *(backs, wings, neck) or one* whole chicken, *skin removed and discarded*

3 quarts water

1 or 2 large onions, *with skin, quartered or coarsely chopped*

3 large carrots, *unpeeled, coarsely chopped*

5 large stalks celery, *coarsely chopped*

2 garlic cloves, *unpeeled, coarsely chopped*

1 small turnip, *unpeeled, quartered*

10 dried lily flowers

¹/4 cup dried lily seeds

3-inch piece Ren Shen *(ginseng root)*

1 teaspoon sea salt, *or to taste*

¹/2 teaspoon freshly ground black pepper, *or to taste*

In a large, heavy nonaluminum soup pot, over medium-low heat, cover all ingredients with water. Bring to a boil, reduce heat, and simmer 30 minutes. Lift the chicken from the broth and remove all meat. Reserve meat and return bones to pot. Continue simmering, partially covered, for 2 hours. Strain well, pressing with a fork to extract essences. Discard ingredients.

*Makes about 2 ¹/2 quarts.*

## Sweet Almond Soup

*Almond Soup is a traditional Chinese recipe that is delicious and soothing for those suffering from AIDS. It is also helpful for those with asthma and constipation.*

8 cups water

3 cups fresh raw almonds

8 cups rice milk

1 teaspoon vanilla

$^1/_2$ teaspoon sea salt

3 tablespoons cornstarch, *well dissolved in ¼ cup water*

2 tablespoons Chinese red dates, *finely diced*

2 tablespoons dried apricots, *finely slivered*

2 teaspoons lemon peel, *finely slivered*

1 teaspoon cinnamon

Preheat oven to 250 degrees.

In a medium-sized pot, over high heat, bring the water to a boil and add almonds. Remove from heat and let sit uncovered until cool. Drain and discard water. Using your fingers, rub the skins off the almonds and dry on a paper towel. Spread almonds on a nonstick baking sheet and bake for 5 to 6 minutes. Stir several times while cooking. Make sure the almonds do not brown. Cool for 5 to 10 minutes. In a food processor, or using a mortar and pestle, grind almonds to a fine powder.

In a medium-sized soup pot, over medium heat, heat rice milk to a simmer. Add the almond powder and whisk until smooth. Add vanilla, salt and cornstarch water and mix well. Continue whisking a few more minutes until thickened.

Serve hot or chilled, garnished with the dates, apricots, lemon peel and cinnamon.

*Makes 6 servings.*

# Chapter 17

## Recipes for Women's Health

## Angelica Sweet Congee

*A sweet rice congee for women that is nourishing, digestible and soothing. Good for PMS, menopause and menstrual problems such as abdominal cramps, bloating, backache, headache, tension, irritability, low energy and mood swings.*

six 3-inch pieces Dang Qui

six 3-inch slices Huang Qi *(Astragalus)*

six 3-inch slices Huang Yao Zi *(Dioscorea tuber)*

four 3-inch cinnamon sticks

3-inch piece ginger, *sliced*

12 cardamom pods, *crushed*

4 cups water

5 cups rice or soy milk

1 cup white or brown rice

1 cup red Chinese dates, *chopped*

1 tablespoon dried and grated
    tangerine peel *(or zest)*

grated cinnamon *(optional)*

borage flowers *(optional)*

In a large, heavy nonaluminum soup pot on high heat, bring all ingredients to a boil. Reduce heat and simmer about 2 $^1/_2$ hours, stirring every half hour—or simmer 6 hours if using a crockpot.

Serve hot or cold, garnished with cinnamon powder and borage flowers if desired.

*Makes 8 servings.*

## Women's Salad

*This is a beautiful and colorful salad made with ingredients that contain properties that promote women's health. Lettuce has sedative properties, and dark greens are rich in calcium. Beets and carrots balance female sex hormones. Asparagus Clears Heat, corrects constipation, promotes blood circulation and is highly diuretic. Jerusalem artichokes balance insulin levels. Seaweed has iodine and minerals for thyroid health. Sesame seeds Tonify Yin, are antiaging and reduce graying of hair.*

### Salad

1 cake firm-style tofu, *cut in* $^1/_2$-*inch strips*

$^1/_4$ cup soy sauce

1 tablespoon expeller-pressed
    toasted sesame oil

4 asparagus spears

4 cups total of a combination of
    romaine, kale, spinach and

radicchio leaves, *well washed,
    dried and torn into bite-sized
    pieces*

$^1/_2$ cup grated beets

$^1/_2$ cup grated carrots

$^1/_2$ cup grated Jerusalem artichoke
    *(or daikon radish or jicama)*

## Dressing

1 minced garlic clove

$^1/_4$ cup rice wine vinegar

$^1/_3$ cup expeller-pressed extra-virgin olive oil

1 tablespoon soy sauce

1 teaspoon expeller-pressed toasted sesame oil

$^1/_4$ teaspoon chili oil or flakes

## Garnish

1 sheet nori seaweed

$^1/_4$ cup minced parsley

$^1/_4$ cup minced cilantro

1 tablespoon black sesame seeds

Preheat oven to 350 degrees.

In a medium-sized bowl, marinate tofu in soy sauce and sesame oil for at least 15 minutes. Place on a nonstick baking pan or oiled pan and bake 15 minutes.

Blanch asparagus in boiling water for 1 minute only. Drain and reserve.

In a small bowl, mix garlic, vinegar and soy sauce. Blend in olive oil, sesame oil, and chili oil or flakes.

Arrange torn greens on a large serving platter or on individual plates. Place separate mounds of beets (red), carrots (orange) and Jerusalem artichoke (white) on top. Alternate tofu strips and asparagus spears in a wheel around each salad. Sprinkle with parsley and cilantro.

Holding nori with tongs, pass over flame or electric burner for a few seconds to toast. Crumble toasted nori. Drizzle salad with dressing and garnish with nori and sesame seeds.

*Makes 2 large or 4 small salads.*

# Ginger Eggplant

*A spicy Chinese eggplant stir-fry dish. Promotes circulation, treats Blood stagnation, eases menstrual cramps, detoxifies liver.*

3 tablespoons expeller-pressed, extra-virgin olive oil

2 cups diced eggplant

1 small yellow onion, *peeled and sliced*

2 small leeks, *cleaned and sliced*

6 garlic cloves, *peeled and minced*

3-inch piece ginger, *peeled and minced*

1/4 teaspoon red pepper flakes

1/2 teaspoon turmeric

1 tablespoon soy sauce

1 tablespoon cornstarch, *well dissolved in 1 cup of Immune Broth, page 359, or Veggie Detox Broth, page 345, or use organic store-bought broth*

1 tablespoon chopped cilantro

In a wok or large sauté pan over high heat, heat oil until hot. Add eggplant, onion, leeks garlic, ginger, red pepper flakes and turmeric and stir-fry about 4 minutes. Reduce heat to medium, add soy sauce and cornstarch and simmer another 5 minutes. Garnish with cilantro. Serve with rice.

*Makes 4 servings.*

## Calcium Soup

*A hearty barley, seaweed and greens soup that has a very high absorbable calcium content along with other valuable nutrients and properties. Good for osteoporosis and to promote strong bones.*

2 cups barley

8 cups water

3 to 4 pounds skinless chicken parts with bones or carcasses

3 1/2 quarts water

1 yellow onion, *unpeeled, quartered*

10 garlic cloves, *unpeeled, crushed*

2 dried bay leaves

1/4 cup rice wine vinegar or apple cider vinegar

2 dried cloud ear mushrooms

3 cups loosely packed, stemmed, chopped kale

3 sheets nori seaweed *(or any other seaweed)*, crumbled

2 tablespoons soy sauce

1/4 teaspoon freshly ground black pepper

In a medium bowl, soak the barley in 8 cups water for 8 hours or overnight. Drain and discard water.

In a large, heavy nonaluminum soup pot on high heat bring chicken, water, onion, garlic, bay leaf and vinegar to a boil. Skim foam from the stock the first few minutes, then reduce heat to simmer and cook $1 \frac{1}{2}$ to 2 hours, uncovered. Strain stock and discard the stock ingredients. Rinse and wipe pot and return stock to it and place back on low heat to simmer. You may choose to skim some of the fat off the top. Calcium must be eaten with fat to be absorbed, so do not skim all fat. Add barley and cloud ear mushrooms into the simmering stock and cook about $1 \frac{1}{2}$ hours. Remove the cloud ears and slice them, discarding the woody stems. Return the sliced mushrooms to the pot. Add the kale, seaweed, soy sauce and pepper and simmer 15 minutes more.

*Makes 6 to 8 servings.*

# Chapter 18

Recipes Based on Coach Ma's Philosophy of Using Chinese Herbs' Energetic Properties to Enhance Athletic Performance

# Golden Soup

*Enhances athletic performance, builds strength and endurance*

1 small whole chicken

1 tablespoon Dong Chong Xia Cao *(Cordyceps)*

1 ounce Huang Qi *(Astragalus)*

1 teaspoon Ren Shen *(ginseng)*

1 teaspoon crushed Lu Rong *(Deer Velvet Antler)*

1 tablespoon grated ginger

3 stalks green onion

1 teaspoon salt

$\frac{1}{2}$ teaspoon pepper

8 cups water

Completely skin the chicken. Stuff Cordyceps and Astragalus into the cavity of the chicken and close with poultry pins.

In a large, heavy nonaluminum soup pot on high heat bring chicken, ginseng, Deer Velvet Antler, ginger, onion, salt and pepper to a boil. Skim foam from the stock the first few minutes, then reduce heat to simmer and cook 1 hour, uncovered. Remove chicken from the pot, cool, shred meat and reserve. Strain stock and discard the stock ingredients. Return chicken meat to the broth. Serve hot.

*Makes 6 servings.*

# Honey Yam Pudding

*Enhances athletic performance, builds strength and endurance.*

2 ounces Chinese yam

2 ounces pearl barley

1 ounce poria mushroom

4 cups water

3 tablespoons honey

2 tablespoons kudzu starch

1 tablespoon bee pollen

1 tablespoon lycium fruit

1/2 teaspoon American ginseng powder

In a large pot, soak Chinese yam, pearl barley and poria mushroom in 4 cups water overnight. In the same pot, over medium heat, cook for 40 minutes. Let cool. Blend in batches until pureed. Return pureed mixture to the same pot and cook over medium heat until it begins to boil. Stir in honey, kudzu starch, bee pollen, lycium fruit and ginseng powder until the mixture begins to gel. Remove from heat and divide into 6 pudding cups. Let cool to room temperature, then refrigerate for at least 2 hours. Serve cold.

*Makes 6 servings.*

# Qi-Strengthening Gingerbread

1/4 cup lotus powder *(To make lotus powder grind lotus seeds in a food mill or coffee grinder)*

1 1/2 cups whole-wheat flour

1/2 cup Huang Yao Zi *(Dioscorea tuber)* powder

1/4 cup poria mushroom powder

1 cup oat or bran flour

4 tablespoons grated ginger

2 teaspoons cinnamon

1/4 teaspoon powdered cloves

2 teaspoons baking powder

1 teaspoon sea salt

3/4 cup apple or orange juice

1/2 cup molasses

1/2 cup honey

4 eggs, separated

Preheat oven to 350 degrees. Grease a bread tin.

In a large mixing bowl, mix all dry ingredients until thoroughly blended.

In a medium bowl, mix orange juice, molasses, honey and egg yolks. In a small bowl, using electric beater, beat egg whites until stiff. Fold orange juice and honey mixture into dry mixture until blended. Gently fold in egg whites.

Pour into bread tin. Bake for 40 to 50 minutes, until knife comes out clean.

*Makes 8 servings.*

# Qi-Strengthening
# Banana Coconut Lotus Cake

1 ¹/2 cups whole-wheat flour

1 cup fine cornmeal

1 cup lotus powder

1 teaspoon baking powder

2 ripe bananas

1 egg

one 8-ounce can pineapple chunks

1 ¹/2 cups coconut milk

1 ¹/4 cup chopped red dates or raisins *(or a combination of the two)*

1 cup fresh grated coconut *(or dry shredded)*

Preheat oven to 350 degrees. Grease a bread tin.

In a large mixing bowl, mix dry ingredients. Puree banana and egg in a blender and add to dry mixture along with pineapple, coconut milk and dates or raisins. Stir in coconut.

Bake for 50 to 60 minutes until a knife inserted comes out clean.

*Makes 8 servings.*

# Chinese Honey Pecan Spice Sweets

*Keep a bag of Honey Pecan Sweets in the freezer to use as a garnish on salads, serve with cocktails, bake into cookies or to eat when out on a long hike or bike ride.*

<sup></sup>

1/2 cup water

1 teaspoon expeller-pressed extra-virgin olive oil

2 star anise seed pods, *broken*

1 small piece of whole cinnamon bark, *about 1 tablespoon*

2-inch piece of vanilla pod

1/2 cup evaporated cane juice crystals (sugar)

1/2 cup honey

1 pound fresh whole raw pecans

Preheat oven to 350 degrees.

In a small bowl, place water, olive oil, star anise seed pods, cinnamon and vanilla pod in a warm place for an hour.

Heat a large, heavy saucepan over medium-high heat. Add the spice mixture.

Add sugar and honey and stir briskly, allowing mixture to reach a boil. Boil 1 minute, stirring constantly. Add pecans to the very hot syrup and stir constantly, 5 to 9 minutes—depending on atmospheric conditions—until the water evaporates. Listen for a rustling dry sound.

Arrange nuts, with space in between, on nonstick baking sheets. Roast nuts about 10 minutes. Set timer and watch carefully—do not let brown or burn. Remove and spread apart on a platter and cool. Store in an airtight container.

*Makes about 1 1/4 pounds.*

# Chapter 19

## Antiaging Recipes

## Omega-3 Cold Noodle Salad

*The dressing on this popular pan-Asian dish is an easy way to incorporate the omega-3-rich oils into your meals. Lecithin-rich soybeans reduce cholesterol and saturated fats in the body, and the vitamin C and antioxidants in the vegetables contribute to the healthy properties of this recipe. Good for heart health, immune boosting and antiaging.*

### Dressing

3 garlic cloves, *minced*

1-inch piece ginger, *minced*

$1/4$ teaspoon red pepper flakes

$1/2$ teaspoon sea salt

$1/4$ cup seasoned rice wine vinegar

2 tablespoons soy sauce

3 tablespoons flaxseed oil

1 tablespoon expeller-pressed toasted sesame oil

### Salad

1 package thin or thick rice noodles, or high-protein pasta

1 $1/2$ cups separated broccoli flowerets

3 carrots, *peeled and thinly sliced*

1 large bunch scallions, *slivered*

3 stalks celery, *thinly sliced*

1 red bell pepper, *seeded and slivered*

1 green bell pepper, *seeded and slivered*

$1/4$ cup cilantro leaves, *loosely packed, lightly chopped*

1 cup roasted soybeans

1 sheet nori seaweed, *cut into slivers with scissors*

leftover cold chicken or fish, *cut into bite-sized pieces (optional)*

In a small bowl, mix together all dressing ingredients except the oils. Drizzle in oils while whisking to emulsify.

Prepare rice noodles or pasta according to package directions. You want the noodles/pasta to be al dente, so do not overcook. Rinse under cold water and drain.

Bring a medium-sized saucepan of water to a boil and add broccoli and carrots to blanch for 2 minutes. Drain and rinse with cold water to stop the cooking.

In a large salad bowl mix cold noodles, broccoli, carrots, scallions, celery, red and green bell peppers, cilantro, soybeans and seaweed. Pour dressing over the salad and gently mix. Cold cooked chicken or fish may be added to the salad if desired.

*Makes 6 to 8 servings.*

# Long Life Hot-and-Sour Soup

*A classic thickened Chinese soup with the super antiaging properties of several mushrooms, seaweed, ginseng, Astragalus and Deer Velvet Antler.*

## Stock

3 pounds chicken parts *(back, neck and wings)* or one small whole chicken

12 cups water

1/2 cup onion, *unpeeled and coarsely chopped*

1 unpeeled carrot, *coarsely chopped*

1 stalk celery, *coarsely chopped*

12 dried shiitake mushrooms

2 dried cloud ear mushrooms

1 large piece wakame seaweed, *broken into bits*

1 gram sliced Deer Velvet Antler

3-inch piece Ren Shen *(ginseng)*, *broken*

four 4-inch slices dried Huang Qi *(Astragalus root)*

3-inch piece ginger, *sliced*

6 large garlic cloves, *unpeeled and crushed*

1 teaspoon sea salt

2 teaspoons peppercorns

2 dried red chilis, *broken into bits*

1/2 cup rice wine vinegar

## Soup

1 carrot, *peeled and grated*

1 bunch scallions, *slivered*

4-inch piece daikon radish, *slivered*

1 cup bean sprouts

1 cup slivered spinach leaves

2 sheets nori seaweed, *slivered with scissors (or torn)*

1 teaspoon expeller-pressed toasted sesame oil

1 teaspoon chili oil

2 tablespoons soy sauce

1 tablespoon cornstarch, *well dissolved in $1/4$ cup warm water*

3 beaten eggs

$1/2$ cup cilantro leaves

Shredded cooked chicken meat *(optional)*

In a large, heavy nonaluminum soup pot, bring stock ingredients to a boil, then reduce heat. Skim foam the first 10 minutes of cooking. Simmer for 1 $1/2$ hours. Strain stock, pressing though sieve to extract essences. Remove shiitake, cloud ear and wakame and sliver mushrooms into strips, discarding any tough bits and replace them into stock.

Rinse and wipe pot. To the pot add the stock, carrot, scallions, daikon radish, bean sprouts, spinach leaves and nori and simmer on low heat for 5 minutes.

Add sesame oil, chili oil, soy sauce and cornstarch in water. Add eggs by whisking into soup quickly to break into threads. Cook 2 minutes more. Add cilantro and serve. Shredded cooked chicken meat can also be added if desired.

*Makes 8 servings.*

# Braised Fish with Red Dates

*This traditional Chinese recipe has the healthful qualities of the good oils in fish along with heart-healthy, cell-renewing vegetables, mushrooms and Chinese dates. It is good for heart health and antiaging.*

12 dried shiitake or black mushrooms

8 to 10 dried Chinese red dates

2 $1/2$ to 3 pounds cold-water fish such as tuna, halibut, snapper or swordfish

4 tablespoons white flour or fine cornmeal

4-inch piece of the thick part of a daikon radish, *peeled and sliced into half moons*

3 garlic cloves, *minced*

2-inch piece of ginger, *peeled and sliced thin*

$1/2$ teaspoon dried and grated orange or tangerine peel *(or zest)*

1/2 bunch scallions, *cleaned and slivered*

1 1/2 cups Immune Broth, *page 359, or Veggie Detox Broth, page 345, or use organic store-bought broth, with 1 tablespoon well-dissolved cornstarch*

3 tablespoons rice wine or sherry

2 tablespoons soy sauce

1 teaspoon expeller-pressed toasted sesame oil

1/4 teaspoon red pepper flakes

3 to 4 tablespoons expeller-pressed extra-virgin olive oil or peanut oil

1/4 cup cilantro, *loosely packed, lightly chopped*

In a small bowl, soak shiitake mushrooms in 1/2 cup water for 20 minutes, drain, slice and reserve. Discard tough stems. In another bowl, soak red dates in 1/2 cup water for 20 minutes, drain and reserve.

Dust fish pieces lightly with flour or very fine cornmeal.

In a medium-sized bowl, combine mushrooms, dates, daikon radish, garlic, ginger, tangerine peel, scallions, broth and cornstarch mixture, rice wine, soy sauce, sesame oil and red pepper flakes and let soak while you brown the fish.

In wok or large sauté pan, over medium-high heat, heat olive oil until just hot. Fry fish one minute on each side to lightly brown, turning carefully. Reduce heat to medium. Pour off oil, leaving about 1 tablespoon. Pour broth mixture over the fish. Turn heat to high and bring back to a boil. Reduce heat to simmer and cook, covered, 10 to 12 minutes more for whole fish, 6 to 8 minutes more for steaks. Remove lid during last few minutes of cooking.

Remove fish carefully to a platter. Pour sauce—which can be reduced a few minutes more to thicken if desired—over fish. Garnish with cilantro.

*Makes 6 servings.*

# Glossary of Chinese Medical Terms

*Acupressure:* Based on the same principles as acupuncture, though the pressure of touch is used instead of needles.

*Acupuncture:* A Chinese medical technique that has been developed and refined for over three thousand years. Acupuncture consists of inserting a number of very fine steel needles into the skin at specific Meridian points to reestablish harmony within your Energetic systems.

*An Mo:* A massage therapy working primarily with soft tissues. An Mo is based on Chinese medical theory and focuses on acupuncture points and Meridians to achieve its effects.

*Ancestral (Zong Qi):* Originates from within the region of your chest (lungs and heart), and is closely connected to the air you breathe. Its main function is to support breathing and blood circulation.

*Ascending:* One of the basic tendencies of Energetic movement of herbs. Any herb that is Energetically uplifting, dispersing, opening up orifices, or inducing vomit, is considered Ascending in its property of Energetic movement.

*Ascending Qi:* Qi distributes and spreads nutrients and oxygen throughout your body as it ascends.

*Assistant Herb:* The herb or herbs in an herbal formula that assist and enhance the effects of the Primary and Secondary Herbs. Can also directly address the secondary disharmony or illness or secondary symptom, or be used as a buffer to moderate the harshness of the Primary and Secondary Herbs.

*Auricular (Ear) Acupuncture:* A branch of acupuncture that treats disharmonies or illnesses by needling acupuncture points exclusively on the ear.

*Balance/Harmony:* Normal or healthy state where all the components or aspects of the body come into optimal equilibrium.

*Bitter:* One of the Five Flavors. Any property that is Clearing or Drying is considered Bitter.

*Bland:* One of the Five Flavors. Any property that is draining (Dampness) or promoting urination is considered Bland.

*Blood (Xue):* One of the Four Vital Substances. The primary function of Blood is to nourish. Blood has an intimate connection with Qi. Blood circulation is powered and carried by the movement of Qi. Blood is the substance that circulates throughout the blood vessels. During this circulation all Five Major Energetic systems—Heart, Lung, Spleen, Liver and Kidney—are involved in maintaining Blood's movement and distribution.

*Blood Stasis/Stagnation:* Slowed or bogged-down circulation of Blood. It also refers to the Blood that is congealed, leaked or accumulated outside of the blood vessels/Meridians.

*Chinese herbs:* There are well over eight thousand herbs known to have medicinal qualities. Only about five hundred are commonly used. Herbal formulas contain combinations of roots, seeds, grains, flowers, berries, fruit peel, bark, leaves, stems, kernels, wood, shells, nuts, minerals, pollen, resin, seaweed, clay, fossilized bones and occasionally animal parts or proteins, depending on your condition.

*Circulating Qi:* Energy or Life Force circulating within your body.

*Clearing:* One of the principal treatment strategies or methods in herbal therapy. The herbal treatment strategy to eliminate Heat or Toxin. Any herb that has this type of effect is considered a Clearing Heat or Clearing Toxin herb.

*Cold/Cold disharmony:* Cold is both the name of one of the External Causes and also an Energetic property of herbs as well as an Energetic characterization of certain disharmony. Any pattern of disharmony that is Cooling, contracting, degenerative and decreasing or damaging Yang is considered Cold disharmony.

*Cold:* An External Cause. Associated with degeneration and a decrease in metabolism. Congealing, contracting and damaging or decreasing Yang Energy. Any External Cause that creates the patterns of disharmony or illnesses displaying these characters is considered Cold in nature. One of the basic Energetic temperatures of herbs. Similar to Cool but stronger or more extreme.

*Constitutional Factors:* Each individual has a unique configuration of Yin and Yang balance. This defines your Energetic individuality. Everyone has his or her own unique constitution. Some of us run Hot, others Cold. A Chinese doctor can predict which direction your health is heading in the future based on your constitutional tendency, and can take steps to prevent illness from occurring.

*Cool:* One of the basic Energetic temperatures of herbs. Any herb that can counteract or decrease Heat disharmony is considered Cool in its Energetic temperature.

*Cun:* A standardized unit of measure for locating the correct acupuncture point(s).

*Cupping:* A modality of treatment where a vacuum is created inside glass or bamboo jars placed upon certain locations of the body to stimulate the movement of Qi or Blood, or draw the stagnated Qi or Blood to the body surface away from the Meridians.

*Dampness:* An External Cause. Connected with properties such as abnormal accumulation of Fluid or moisture, swelling, sluggishness and a stubborn and protracted illness. Heavy, clinging, stagnating and sinking. Any External Cause that causes the patterns of disharmony or illnesses displaying these characters is considered Damp in nature.

*Dan Tian:* Energy centers upon which to focus the mind or consciousness in Qigong.

*Dao/Tao:* Often translated as "the Way." According to Daoism/Taoism, it is the essence or the ideal of existence—a state of complete harmony with nature, unspoiled by any intellectual evaluations.

*Daoism/Taoism:* The philosophy of Taoism is a philosophical system derived chiefly from the *Tao-te-ching,* a book traditionally ascribed to Chinese philosopher Lao-tze but believed to have been written in the sixth century B.C. Taoism, a central influence of Chinese medicine, states that "the heaven and the human are one" and describes an ideal human condition of freedom from desire and of effortless simplicity, achieved by following the Tao (path)—the spontaneous, creative, effortless path taken by natural events in the universe.

*Decoction:* Dried herbal formulas are brewed into a concentrated tea called a decoction to extract the medicinal qualities.

*Deficiency:* Basic pattern of disharmony or imbalance where one or more combination of Yin, Yang, Qi, Blood, Jing, Jin Ye or Shen becomes weakened or lacking.

*Deficient Cold:* The complex of Cold symptoms created when the body's Warming Energy (Yang) is not enough to balance the Cooling Energy (Yin) in the situation of Yang deficiency.

*Deficient Heat:* The complex of Heat symptoms created when the body's Cooling Energy (Yin) is not enough to balance the Warming Energy (Yang) in the situation of Yin deficiency.

*Deqi:* Literally "gaining the Qi." A term used in acupuncture treatment to describe the sensations of the physician and patient upon the insertion of the needle when the Qi can be felt. The patient experiences sensations of numbness, heaviness, distension or radiating tingles. The acupuncturist, on the other hand, experiences a subtle heaviness or pulling beneath the tip of the needle when deqi occurs.

*Descending:* One of the basic tendencies of Energetic movement of herbs. Any herb that is Energetically purging, draining, clearing, calming, dissolving, or constricting is considered Descending in its property of Energetic movement.

*Descending Qi:* Qi passes down metabolic waste and toxins for elimination, and can also deliver nutrients as it descends.

*Diagnosis:* Diagnosis in Chinese medicine includes an assessment of the basic substances that make up the human body: Yin, Yang, Qi, Jing (Essence), Blood, Fluid and Shen. The traditional Chinese medical diagnostic procedure follows what is called the Four Examinations: inquiring, looking, listening/smelling and touching. The Four Examinations determine the pattern of harmony and disharmony.

*Differentiation of Patterns of Disharmony (Bian Zheng):* Recognizing and identifying the patterns of imbalance or disharmony. It is the most important process and method of diagnosis in Chinese medicine, during which doctors collect information and weave it into a meaningful pattern, and upon which the treatment is targeted.

*Dissolving:* One of the principal treatment strategies or methods in herbal therapy. The herbal treatment strategy to disperse certain stagnations, soften hardness or masses, or assist digestion of old, undigested foods. It is usually used for abnormally accumulated Qi, Blood, Phlegm, Fluid and foods that cannot be eliminated through Clearing or Purging. Any herb that has this type of effect is considered a Dissolver.

*D.O.M.:* Doctor of Oriental Medicine.

*Draining:* One of the principal treatment strategies or methods in herbal therapy. The herbal treatment strategy to promote urination. It is usually used for edema (abnormal Fluid accumulation) or certain types of Dampness. Any herb that has this type of effect is considered a diuretic.

*Dryness:* An External Cause. Dryness mainly damages your body's Fluid—such as symptoms that can be seen in certain types of bronchitis where the patient has dry cough, accompanied by pronounced dry mouth, throat, lips and nostrils.

*Eight Principal Differentiations:* The most fundamental system of diagnosis or differentiation of Patterns of disharmony in Chinese medicine. The eight principles are Yin, Yang, deficiency, excess, Cold, Hot, Exterior and Interior.

*Eight Strategies/Methods:* Principal treatment strategies or methods in herbal therapy. They are Clearing, Dissolving, Harmonizing, Inducing Vomiting, Purging, Sweating/Releasing Exterior, Tonifying, Warming. Additional strategies include Draining and Moving.

*Electroacupuncture:* Acupuncture using a high-frequency stimulator that sends an electronic pulsation through electric wires connected to the acupuncture needles.

*Essence (Jing):* One of the Four Vital Substances. An entirely inherited specific part of Kidney Energy, which governs reproduction and development. It can be strengthened or depleted during the course of life. It is confined within the Kidney Energy system.

*Evaluation of body language, posture and self-presentation:* Part of the Four Examinations. Whether you are thin or heavy, slouched over or erect, pointed in your speech or mumbling, strong or weak, physically fit or out of shape, hyper or sedate are all factors that will give your Chinese doctor an impression of you as a whole.

*Excess:* Basic pattern of disharmony or imbalance where one or any combination of Yin, Yang, Qi, Blood, Jing, Jin Ye or Shen becomes accumulated or excessive. It can also result from abnormal settlement or accumulation in the body of External Causes or mucus, Phlegm, stagnated Blood, food, urine and fecal matter.

*Excess Cold:* The complex of Cold symptoms due to abnormal accumulation of certain Causes in the body such as Cold in the situation of Yin excess.

*Excess Heat:* The complex of Heat symptoms due to abnormal accumulation of certain Causes in the body such as Heat or Fire in the situation of Yang excess.

*Exterior/Exterior disharmony:* Exterior is the part of the body that is relatively superficial or closer to the body surface. Any pattern of disharmony that occurs in this part of the body is considered Exterior disharmony.

*External Causes:* Anything that can cause disharmony or illness by invading our body from the environment. They are labeled Wind, Cold, Summer Heat, Dampness, Dryness, Fire and Toxins.

*External Causes and Internal Causes:* When identifying the causes of illnesses, Chinese medicine refers to External Causes: Wind, Cold, Summer Heat, Dampness, Dryness and Fire or Internal Causes: imbalanced emotions and other Lifestyle Factors. A disease is typically caused by a combination of several Causes.

*External Toxins:* Chemical and biological toxins such as environmental pollutants, viruses and bacteria.

*Fire/Heat:* Consuming Fluid and Yin, ascending, stirring and accelerating. Any External Cause that causes the patterns of disharmony or illnesses displaying these characters is considered Fire/Heat in nature.

*Five Element Theory:* First formed in China at about the time of the Zhou dynasty (867 to 255 B.C.). Historically, it arose from observations of the natural world made in early times by people in the course of their lives and productive labor. Wood, fire, earth, metal and water were considered to be five indispensible materials for the maintenance of life and production, as well as representing five important states that initiated normal changes in the natural world. In other words, all phenomena in the universe correspond in nature either to wood, fire, earth, metal or water, and these are in a state of constant motion and change. Chinese medicine uses the properties associated with them to explain the makeup and dynamics of the world, including our bodies, as well as to organize the clinical data and provide guidance for treatments.

*Five Flavors:* Basic Energetic properties used to characterize herbs in Chinese herbal medicine. They are Sour, Bitter, Sweet, Acrid, Salty. Bland and Stringent were added later to the list.

*Floating:* One of the basic tendencies of Energetic movement of herbs. Similar to Ascending but primarily affects the upper part of the body.

*Fluid (Jin Ye):* One of the Four Vital Substances. Encompasses all of your bodily fluids (except Blood), including secretions such as gastric juices, tears, saliva and perspiration. Fluid contains many other nourishing substances that are important to your body.

*Four Energetic Tendencies/Movements:* Four basic tendencies of Energetic movement of herbs. They are Ascending, Descending, Floating and Sinking.

*Four Examinations:* Inquiring, Looking, Listening/Smelling and Touching.

*Four Temperatures:* Basic Energetic Temperatures (different from physical temperature) used in Chinese herbal medicine to characterize properties of herbs. They are Cool, Cold, Warm and Hot. Neutral was later added to the list.

*Four Vital Substances:* Blood (Xue), Fluid (Jin Ye), Essence (Jing) and Shen.

*Fu:* The (Yang) minor Energetic systems: Gall Bladder, Small Intestine, Stomach, Large Intestine and Urinary Bladder.

*Gall Bladder:* A Yang organ, one of the Fu/Six Minor Energetic Systems. Its main functions are storing and releasing bile. The Gall Bladder underlies one's ability in decision-making. Closely associated with Liver Energy, Gall Bladder Energy also assists in digestion, which is similar to the function in Western medicine perspective.

*Harmonizing:* One of the principal treatment strategies or methods in herbal therapy. The herbal treatment strategy to regulate or balance certain relationships or disharmony. It is usually used in the situations where neither simply eliminating nor strengthening is appropriate. Any herb that has this type of effect is considered a Harmonizer.

*Harmonizing Herb:* The herb in a formula that regulates or adjusts a Vital Substance or an Energetic System toward its normal level or balance, or that facilitates the synergy of the whole formula. It makes all the herbs of the formula work better together.

*Heart:* A Yin organ, one of the Zang/Five Major Energetic Systems. It provides the dynamic source for the Qi and Blood circulations. It governs Shen or Spirit and dictates much of the mind's cognitive activities. It has particularly close connections to tongue, blood vessels and sweats, and its predominant associating emotion is happiness.

*Heat/Heat disharmony:* One of the External Causes and also an Energetic characterization of certain disharmony. Any pattern of disharmony that is Warming, accelerating, inflammatory, consuming or damaging Yin is considered Heat disharmony.

*Herbal transdermal ionization (HTI):* The use of an electric ionizing device along with topical herbs. HTI delivers concentrated herbs deep into the affected sites by converting the herbs into electrically charged particles, then, through polarity, expelling or pulling the herbal application deep into the body.

*Hot:* One of the basic Energetic temperatures of herbs. Similar to Warm but stronger or more extreme.

*Imbalance/Disharmony:* Abnormal or suboptimal or diseased state where the balance is off or upset.

*Inducing Vomiting:* One of the principal treatment strategies or methods in herbal therapy. The herbal treatment strategy to induce vomiting. It is usually used for helping the body to expel Toxins or abnormally accumulated Foods and Phlegm or Mucus. Any herb that has this type of effect is considered an emetic (vomiting inducer).

*Inquiring/Questioning:* Part of the Four Examinations: In-depth questions about yourself, your history, your current complaints and symptoms or anything else related to your condition.

*Interior/Interior Disharmony:* Interior is the part of the body that is relatively deep or closer to the body center. Any pattern of disharmony that occurs in this part of the body is considered Interior disharmony.

*Intermediate Causes:* At various stages, some diseases can create or generate disease-causing substances such as stagnation of Blood and Phlegm that cause other illnesses (imbalances). Others are Internal Toxins, which are mostly due to abnormally accumulated metabolic waste.

*Internal Causes:* Some are psychological in nature. The Seven Emotions are Anger, Joy, Sadness, Grief, Pensiveness, Fear and Fright. These emotions represent a wide range of emotional states. They are, by themselves, neither good nor bad. But when excessive or out of control, they can lead to imbalances and illness. Other Internal Causes include imbalanced behavioral patterns such as physical, mental or sexual overexertion or stress, lack of activity and improper diet.

*Inward/Outward Qi:* Qi supports and strengthens your body through inward movement. Qi disperses nutrients and expels toxins through outward movement.

*Kidney:* A Yin Organ, one of the Zang/Five Major Energetic Systems. It stores Jing and supplies the body with the most important life force or vitality. It governs the development and reproduction, and also regulates fluid and helps deep breathing. It generates bone marrow and is important for certain cognitive functions. It has particularly close connections to ears and bones, and its predominant associated emotion is fear.

*Large Intestine:* A Yang organ, one of the Fu/Six Minor Energetic Systems. It receives the impurity of foods and extracts moisture from them, then excretes the rest as waste. Associated with Lung Energy, the main function of Large Intestine Energy is the transportation and elimination of digestive waste.

*Lic. Ac.:* Licensed Acupuncturist.

*Lifestyle Factors:* Includes dietary patterns, stress levels and management, excessiveness and/or indulgence due to lack of moderation and discipline.

*Listening:* One of the Four Examinations. Some people have big voices, some quiet, some bright, some hoarse. Some people articulate and are clear, others are scattered and inarticulate. The strength of your breathing, rhythm and rate are all important, as are obstructions or wheezing and the sound of coughing. Listening also includes the sounds of your digestive track, heartbeat, hiccups, burping, sniffling, sneezing or coughing.

*Liver:* A Yin Organ, one of the Zang/Five Major Energetic Systems. It is the great regulator of the body. It regulates the Energy flow and circulation, digestion, emotions and menstruation; it has particularly close connections to eyes, connective tissues and tears; its predominant associating emotion is anger.

*Looking/Inspecting:* One of the Four Examinations. The Chinese doctor learns about you by observing your body build and body language, movement, appearance and complexion, behavior, tongue, eyes, ears, palms, hair, fingernails, tears, sweat, phlegm, nasal discharge, vaginal discharge, vomit, urine and feces.

*Lung:* A Yin Organ, one of the Zang/Five Major Energetic Systems. It is chiefly responsible for breathing, especially for intake of Qing Qi; also involved in regulating fluid, Qi movement and assisting the heart to govern the blood circulation. It has particularly close connections to the skin, nose and nasal mucus, and its predominant associating emotion is grief.

*Meridian Affinities:* Basic property of herbs that tend to selectively affect a particular part of the body or Meridian. An herb that enters the Heart Meridian would be said to be a Heart herb. Most herbs have multiple Meridian Affinities.

*Meridian (Jin)Qi:* This is the Qi that circulates within the Meridians. It connects all of the Energetic systems and parts of your body into an integrated whole. It nourishes, regulates and detoxifies. This is the Qi that acupuncture primarily works through.

*Meridians (channels):* Meridians are invisible channels in your body in which Qi flows. Meridians connect most of the acupuncture points and weave the various parts of the body into an integrated whole.

*Moving:* One of the principal treatment strategies or methods in herbal therapy. The herbal treatment strategy to promote or invigorate the movement of Qi, Blood, Fluid and Foods. It is usually used for stagnation. Any herb that has this type of effect is considered a Mover.

*Moxa/Moxabustion:* Moxa is the dried and pulverized herb Mugwort (Ai Ye) prepared and used for moxabustion treatment. Moxabustion treatment involves burning the moxa in certain forms and with certain methods, and directing the heat toward the site of treatment, usually acupuncture points. It is often used for stagnated Qi or Blood, or deficient and Cold Disharmony.

*Neutral:* One of the basic Energetic temperatures of herbs. Even, or neither Warm nor Cool in temperature. Appropriate to be used for disharmonies other than Heat or Cold in nature.

*Non-Internal, Non-External Causes:* Constitutional Factors, Lifestyle Factors, Intermediate Causes and Unforeseen Events.

*Nutritive (Ying Qi):* This is the Qi most intimately associated with the Vital Substance of Blood. It circulates along blood vessels. Its primary function is to deliver nutrients to and throughout the body.

*O.M.D.:* Oriental Medical Doctor.

*Organ (Zang Fu) Qi:* This Qi belongs to and carries the functions of each individual major and minor Energetic system.

*Patent formulas:* Herbal formulas that are processed into standardized over-the-counter medications in the form of pills, tablets, capsules, tinctures, powders, plasters.

*Phlegm:* Concentrated and sticky bodily fluid created from abnormal accumulation of Fluid or moisture. It can cause a wide range of disharmonies or illnesses.

*Primary herb:* The most important and essential herb in an herbal formula. It is the chief therapeutic agent targeting the main disharmony or illness, or the main symptom.

*Primordial (Yuan) Qi:* The most fundamental and important Qi. It is primarily inherited (genetic). It can be strengthened or depleted throughout the course of life. It provides the most important part of vitality. It nourishes and supports all the other specific Energetic systems. It dictates growth, development and aging.

*Protective (Wei) Qi:* The Qi created from nutrients by Spleen Energy, supported and enhanced by Kidney Energy, and distributed by Lung Energy. It is active and circulates primarily along the exterior of your body to protect against the invasion of External Causes.

*Pulse:* Part of the Four Examinations. Aside from the pulse rate, the Chinese doctor feels for the depth, strength, width, shape, rhythm and length of the pulse.

*Purging:* One of the principal treatment strategies or methods in herbal therapy. The herbal treatment strategy to cleanse Stomach and Intestines or induce diarrhea. It is usually used to eliminate stagnation that settled in the digestive tracts such as abnormally accumulated foods, fecal matter, Blood, Phlegm and Fluid. Any herb that has this type of effect is considered a Purgative.

*Qi (Vital Energy, Life Force):* The basic substance (mass or matter), as well as the Energy necessary to create the physical world, which includes all living things. Qi is the singular common bond that connects all existence, thereby being able to pass back and forth and interact. Qi cannot be created or destroyed; it can only be transformed from one form to another. Qi is the most basic Vital Energy that provides all the actual physical building blocks that make up the human body. Qi supports and sustains your body's life functions such as breathing, metabolism, thoughts and feelings, but it is also the life function itself.

*Qi Level:* The second level in the evolution of disease. Qi level involvement is experienced as high fever, profuse sweating, thirst and strong pulse. Your body is actively fighting the invading Cause. In other words, both the Cause and your Qi are strong.

*Qigong:* Energy work of Chinese medicine for promoting health and treating disharmonies. It involves cultivating and guiding the movement of Qi through meditation. Certain poses or gentle movements are sometimes employed as well to assist the process.

*Salty:* One of the Five Flavors. Any property that is softening (hardness or any mass) or purging is considered Salty.

*San Jiao (Triple Warmer):* A Yang organ, one of the Fu/Six Minor Energetic Systems encompassing Upper (Heart and Lung), Middle (Spleen, Stomach, Liver and Gall Bladder), and Lower (Kidney, Small Intestine, Large Intestine and Urinary Bladder) Jiao. It especially refers to the functional connections of these parts of the body in the process of transforming and transporting Qi and Fluid.

*Secondary herb:* The herb or herbs in an herbal formula that enhance the effect of the primary herb, or act as the chief therapeutic agent for the secondary disharmony or illness, or the secondary symptom.

*Seeds:* The seeds of the Wang Bu Liu Xing plant (Vaccaria), or stainless-steel beads that are attached to surgical tape and adhered to certain specific acupuncture points on the ear. Stimulating the seeds with the tips of your fingers can provide relief from anxiety, stress or cravings, among other conditions.

**Seven Emotions:** Joy, Anger, Sadness, Pensiveness, Grief, Fear and Fright. They represent the full range of normal emotional response of life, but when extreme they can cause disharmonies or illnesses.

**Shen:** One of the Four Vital Substances. Spirit without a religious affiliation. Shen is all of the mental and psychological functions and activities of an individual.

**Shen Nong:** The divine husbandman. Believed to have lived around five thousand years ago. Shen Nong is mentioned in dozens of books dating as far back as 607 B.C. He is said to have discovered the medicinal properties of herbs by systematically trying herbs himself, sometimes with toxic or adverse reactions, compelling him to quickly find an antidote.

**Shen Nong's Herbal Material Medica:** Three volumes, attributed to Shen Nong, containing 365 medicinal substances. More than 60 percent of these 365 medicinal substances are still in use today. *Shen Nong's Herbal Material Medica* established the basic theory of herbology.

**Sinking:** One of the basic tendencies of Energetic movement of herbs. Similar to Descending but primarily affects lower part of the body.

**Small Intestine:** A Yang organ, one of the Fu/Six Minor Energetic Systems. It receives preliminarily digested foods from the Stomach and extracts the Purity (nutrients) from the Impurity (indigestible portion of the foods). Associated with Heart Energy.

**Smelling:** Part of the Four Examinations. Smelling includes the detection of unusual odor not only from bodily discharge, but from the patient's breath and overall body scent as well.

**Sour:** One of the Five Flavors. Any property that is contracting, holding or pulling back is considered Sour.

**Spicy/Acrid/Pungent:** One of the Five Flavors. Any property that disperses or promotes Qi movement is considered Spicy/Acrid, Pungent.

**Spleen:** A Yin Organ, one of the Zang/Five Major Energetic Systems. It represents much of the digestive functions and also participates in the regulation of Fluid and Blood. Its Energy is the primary supporter of the limbs and muscles. It has particularly close connections to the mouth and saliva, and its predominant associating emotion is pensiveness.

**Stagnation:** Lack of normal movement. It can involve Qi, Blood, Fluid or Food.

**Stomach:** A Yang organ, one of the Fu/Six Minor Energetic Systems. It stores and performs preliminary digestion of the foods. The descending energy of Stomach ensures the foods get passed along the digestive tract. Associated with

Spleen Energy, Stomach Energy stores, transports and assists in the digestion of food. After food has left the stomach, Stomach Energy moves Purities downward through your gastrointestinal tract to the small intestines and, ultimately, the large intestine. As Stomach Energy pushes downward, the Purities are extracted by Spleen Energy, which moves these Purities upward and distributes them to nourish your body.

*Stringent:* One of the Five Flavors. Any property that is contracting, holding or pulling back, yet stronger than Sour, is considered Stringent.

*Summer Heat:* An External Cause. Hot, extremely dispersing, strictly seasonal (only occurring in Summer), and often combining with Dampness. Any External Cause that causes the patterns of disharmony or illnesses displaying these characters are considered Summer Heat in nature.

*Sweating/Releasing Exterior:* One of the principal treatment strategies or methods in herbal therapy. The herbal treatment strategy to create or induce perspiration. Any herb that has this type of effect is considered an Exterior Releaser.

*Sweet:* One of the Five Flavors. Any property that is Tonifying, Harmonizing or soothing urgency is considered Sweet.

*Tai Chi:* A Chinese exercise integrating energy work and physical movement. Known as "the meditation in motion," it involves slow, fluid, dancelike sequences of movements with deep breathing, and can be of great value in promoting health and treating certain illnesses.

*Three Treasures:* Refers to Jing, Qi and Shen.

*Tian Kui:* A special type of Kidney Jing.

*Tincture:* A form of herbal preparation where a medicinal substance is soaked in alcohol for a certain length of time to produce an alcohol-based extract.

*Tongue Diagnosis:* Part of the Four Examinations. Observing the tongue is one of the most important diagnostic methods of Chinese medicine. The doctor looks at the form, including the size and shape, color, texture, movement, coating and moisture.

*Tonifying:* Part of the principal treatment strategies or methods in herbal therapy. The herbal treatment strategy to strengthen or support Vital Substance. It is usually used for conditions of deficiency. Any herb that has this type of effect is considered a Tonifier or Tonic.

*Touching/Palpating:* Part of the Four Examinations. Touching as a means of diagnosing involves two methods. One method is to palpate the body. Certain information about the nature of the imbalance can be acquired through feeling the patient's temperature (hot or cold), muscle tone (hard or flaccid), moisture (clammy or dry), pain (physical pressure helps or aggravates pain), abnormal mass and around certain acupuncture points or along the fourteen Meridians. The other method is to palpate the pulse.

*Toxin:* Contagious or poisonous substance causing deterioration or abnormal proliferation. Any External Cause that causes the patterns of disharmony or illnesses displaying these characters is considered Toxin in nature. Internal Toxin refers mostly to metabolic waste.

*Tui Na:* A type of bodywork in Chinese medicine. Tui Na employs hands-on techniques such as massage, acupressure, adjustment, even orthopedic manipulation. Often used for musculoskeletal problems, it can also be used to treat many disharmonies or illnesses. While An Mo works mostly with soft tissues, Tui Na integrates the work of muscles, connective tissues and bones.

*Unforeseen Events:* Illnesses caused by unforeseen events such as accidents and injuries cause severe damage to the structure and Energy of a healthy person. Therefore they are considered one of the causes of illnesses, and can be treated based on exactly what is damaged.

*Urinary Bladder:* A Yang organ, one of the Fu/Six Minor Energetic Systems. It stores and controls the excretion of urine. Associated with Kidney Energy, Urinary Bladder Energy stores and eliminates urine, which is similar to the function in Western medical perspective.

*Warm:* One of the basic Energetic temperatures of herbs. Any herb that can counteract or decrease Cold Disharmony is considered Warm in its Energetic temperature.

*Warming:* One of the principal treatment strategies or methods in herbal therapy. The herbal treatment strategy to counteract Cold disharmonies or some types of stagnation. Any herb that has this type of effect is considered a Yang Warmer, or Yang Tonic.

*Wei (Level):* Wei is the protective energy that circulates at the very surface/exterior of your body. Wei level is the first protective barrier against External Causes. At this level, the cause is not yet very strong and the Qi is strong and intact.

*Wen Yi:* An External Cause. Any External Cause may also be considered Li Qi if, aside from exhibiting typical properties of other External Causes, it also is highly contagious, rapidly evolving and causes the same or very similar pattern of severe symptoms among different patients. Smallpox, typhus, tuberculosis and HIV would all be considered caused by Li Qi.

*Wholeness:* Chinese medicine's philosophical concept that life always functions or malfunctions in its entirety. There is an essential indivisibility among different parts of the body, between the body and mind, and between life and the environment it exists within.

*Wind:* An External Cause. In nature, wind is swift, mobile, changeable and strikes suddenly. Any External Cause that causes the patterns of disharmony or illnesses displaying these characters are considered Wind in nature.

*Xue level:* The last, or final, level, in the evolution of certain infectious diseases, which is critical and potentially fatal. Often, the earmark of the Xue level is the presence of multiorgan failure. The patient's blood coagulation factors are exhausted, which results in internal coagulation and extensive bleeding simultaneously. At this stage, Qi has become depleted.

*Yang:* Opposed and complementary to Yin. Yang represents everything that is positive, aggressive, vigorous, hot, bright, masculine, upward, functional, external, of day and summer.

*Yang Deficiency and Yin Excess:* Pattern of imbalance or disharmony where the Yang level becomes weakened; in the meantime the Yin level becomes accumulated or excessive.

*Yang deficiency, also known as deficient Cold imbalance:* Pattern of imbalance or disharmony where Yin is normal yet the person exhibits some Yin symptoms because there is not enough Yang Energy to balance the Yin.

*Yang excess, also known as excess Heat imbalance:* Pattern of disharmony that displays a Yang character such as hot, inflammatory, agitating, overstimulating or hyperfunctional. Pronounced Yang symptoms but without any weakness.

*Yang organs—the Fu—the Six Minor Energetic Systems:* Small Intestine Energy, Large Intestine Energy, Gall Bladder Energy, Urinary Bladder Energy, Stomach Energy and San Jiao (Triple Warmer). The Six Minor Energetic Systems actually come closer to relating to the organ of similar name, in terms of their functional similarities, than do the Five Major Energetic Systems.

*Yin:* Opposed and complementary to Yang. Yin represents everything negative, passive, dormant, cold, dark, still, feminine, downward, substantive, internal, of night and winter.

*Yin and Yang deficiency:* Pattern of imbalance or disharmony where both the Yin and Yang levels become weakened.

*Yin and Yang excess:* Pattern of imbalance or disharmony where both Yin and Yang level become accentuated or excessive. Exhibiting Heat and Cold symptoms at the same time or alternately without any discernible weakness. This is demonstrated in certain types of common cold or flu or malaria, when the person can fluctuate between having both fever and chills.

*Yin deficiency/Yang excess:* Imbalance or disharmony where the Yin level becomes weakened; in the meantime the Yang level becomes accumulated or excessive. Pronounced Heat symptoms along with Yin weakness.

*Yin deficiency, also known as deficient Heat imbalance:* Pattern of imbalance or disharmony when Yang is normal but the person can exhibit some Yang symptoms because there is not enough Yin Energy to balance the Yang.

*Yin deficiency:* Pattern of imbalance or disharmony where the Yin level has become weakened, whereas Yang remains relatively normal.

*Yin excess, also known as excess Cold imbalance:* Pattern of imbalance or disharmony where the person shows pronounced Yin symptoms but without any weakness.

*Ying Level:* The third level in the evolution of certain infectious diseases. When the External Cause pierces through your Qi level and enters the Ying level, which is evident in the development of pneumonia, endocarditis and myocarditis, to name a few problems. At this level the Qi begins to be overwhelmed, or worn down, by the Cause.

*Yin Organs—the Zang—The Five Major Energetic Systems:* Comprised of Kidney, Heart, Lungs, Spleen and Liver Energies.

*Yin/Yang:* Yin and Yang are the most basic concepts used by Chinese philosophy to characterize the world and life. To ancient Chinese sages, Yin and Yang were the essence of existence and changes. Everything embodies Ying and Yang, and the interactions and movement between Yin and Yang provide the dynamic source for occurrence, development and shifting of all things. Optimal health is achieved through a state of balance and harmony of your body, mind and environment. Harmony is determined by the balance between Yin and Yang.

*Zangfu:* A collective name for the solid Yin organ systems: Lung, Heart, Spleen, Liver and Kidneys, and the hollow Yang organ systems: Small Intestine, Large Intestine, Gall Bladder, Urinary Bladder, Stomach and San Jiao (Triple Warmer).

*Zangfu System:* The general term for all five major and six minor Energetic systems and their associations to other aspects of the body and its functions. These are Energetic organs, different from their physical counterparts of the same names. Zang refers to the (Yin) Five Major Energetic systems: Liver, Heart, Spleen, Lung and Kidney. Fu refers to the Six Minor Energetic systems: Gall Bladder, Small Intestine, Stomach, Large Intestine, Urinary Bladder and Triple Warmer.

*Zang Xiang System/Theory:* Zang means "organ" (in an Energetic sense), and Xiang means "sign" or "manifestation." The Zang Xiang system is the functional connection of an Energetic system in its entirety. It is the Energetic web that weaves together a major Energetic system with its associated minor

Energetic system. Zang Xiang Theory is the study of how the harmony or disharmony of internal Energetic systems reflects or expresses itself outwardly.

*Zheng:* The result of a comprehensive assessment of the nature of the patient's condition that weaves together all the relevant information about the condition into a meaningful pattern. It is the most important objective in Chinese medicine.

# Glossary of Chinese Herbs

| Chinese Name | Latin Name | English Name |
|---|---|---|
| Ba Ji Tian | *Radix Morindae Officianalis* | Morinda root |

Tonifies Kidney Yang. Expels Wind-Damp Cold. Used for impotence and infertility, back pain and muscular atrophy and urinary incontinence.

| | | |
|---|---|---|
| Bai Bu | *Radix Stemonae* | Stemona root |

Moistens the Lungs and stops cough, expels parasites and kills lice. Treats both chronic and acute cough.

| | | |
|---|---|---|
| Bai Dou Kou | *Fructus Amomi Kravanh* | Cardamom seed |

An aromatic herb often used to resolve Dampness. Dampness from a Western point of view could be diarrhea, loose stools, obesity with fluid retention, poor digestion, chronic mucus, candida, fatigue or cloudy-headedness.

| | | |
|---|---|---|
| Bai He | *Bulbus Lilii* | Lily bulb |

Moistens Lung Energy, stops cough, clears Heat and calms the Spirit. Used for chronic dry cough and sore throat. Also treats insomnia, restlessness and irritability.

| | | |
|---|---|---|
| Bai Hua She She Cao | *Herba Hedyotidis Diffusae* | Hedyotis |

Relieves Fire Toxicity, clears Heat and resolves Dampness through promoting urination. Used to treat esophageal, colon and stomach cancer, as well as snakebite, boils, intestinal abscess, painful urination and jaundice.

| Chinese Name | Latin Name | English Name |
|---|---|---|
| Bai Ji | *Rhizoma Bletillae Striatae* | Bletilla rhizome |

Stops bleeding, reduces swelling and promotes tissue growth. Bai Ji is an astringent for leaking blood such as hemorrhage from traumatic injury, ulcers, coughing of blood and nosebleeds.

| Bai Jiang Cao | *Herba cum Radice Patriniae* | Thiaspi |
|---|---|---|

Clears Heat and Toxicity, stops pain (in the chest and abdomen) and dispels Blood stasis. Used to treat intestinal infection or abscess and abdominal pain. Used for postpartum and postoperative pain.

| Bai Mao Gen | *Rhizoma Imperatae Cylindricae* | Imperata |
|---|---|---|

Cools the Blood to stop bleeding, promotes urination and clears Heat from the Stomach and Lungs. Treats bleeding anywhere in the body, blood in the urine, painful urination, edema, acute nephritis, nausea and wheezing.

| Bai Shao | *Radix Paeoniae Lactiflorae* | White Peony root |
|---|---|---|

Nourishes the Blood and soothes muscle tension. Pacifies the Liver and alleviates pain. Retains the Yin. Treats gynecological disorders, abdominal, flank and chest pain, headache, dizziness, cramping and muscle spasms, spermatorrhea and sweating disorders.

| Bai Xian Pi | *Cortex Dictamni Dasycarpi Radicis* | Cortex of Dictamnus |
|---|---|---|

Clears Heat Toxins, expels Wind and dries Dampness. Treats sores with pus, scabies, hives, eczema, carbuncles, itchy rashes and jaundice.

| Bai Zhi | *Radix Angelicae Dahuricae* | Chinese Angelica root |
|---|---|---|

Expels Wind, Damp and Cold. Alleviates swelling, pain and vaginal discharge. Opens up congested nasal passages. Useful for colds with headaches and nasal congestion. Effective in treating toothache, headache and trigeminal neuralgia (facial nerve pain).

| Bai Zhu | *Rhizoma Atractylodis Macrocephalae* | Atractylodes (white) |
|---|---|---|

Tonifies the Spleen and Qi and dries Dampness. Treats diarrhea with fatigue, lack of appetite, vomiting and edema.

| Chinese Name | Latin Name | English Name |
| --- | --- | --- |
| Ban Lan Gen | Radix Isathidis Tinctoria | Isatis root |

Drains Heat and Fire Toxicity and Cools the Blood. Treats sore throat, mumps and jaundice. Ban Lan Gen has potent antiviral properties, particularly for flu and sore throat. Also acts as an antiviral for the liver (in cases of hepatitis B and C).

| Ban Xia | Pinelliae Tematae Rhizoma | Pinellia |
| --- | --- | --- |

Important herb for dissolving Phlegm and drying Dampness. Often used to reduce nausea.

| Bei Mu (Zhe) | Bulbus Fritillariae Thunbergii | Thunberg Fritillaria bulb |
| --- | --- | --- |

Clears Lung Heat and Phlegm. Treats an acute phlegmy cough. Bei Mu also reduces swellings, abscesses and nodules in the neck, lung and breasts.

| Bian Xu | Herba Polygoni Avicularis | Polygonum aviculare |
| --- | --- | --- |

Clears Damp Heat from the Bladder, kills parasites and stops itching. For painful urination and intestinal parasites.

| Bie Jia | Carapax Amydae Sinensis | Turtle shell |
| --- | --- | --- |

Nourishes Yin, anchors Yang, Invigorates the Blood, promotes menstruation and reduces lumps or nodules. Used to treat a fever with night sweats and amennorhea (ceased menstruation).

| Bing Lang | Semen Arecae Catechu | Betel nut |
| --- | --- | --- |

Kills parasites (especially tapeworms) and expels the parasites' bodies downward and out. This herb also promotes both bowel movement and urination. Bing Lang is also indicated for malarial disorders.

| Bing Pian | Borneol | Borneol |
| --- | --- | --- |

This aromatic herb is used to open the orifices and revive the spirit during fainting or convulsions. Bing Pian also clears Heat and is applied topically to treat a swollen throat, skin sores and scabies, excessive tearing of the eyes.

| Bo He | Herba Menthae Haplocalycis | Mint |
| --- | --- | --- |

Clears Wind-Heat, clears the head and eyes, benefits the throat, vents rashes and frees Liver Qi. Used for colds or flu with fever, sore throat and cough and early-stage measles.

| Chinese Name | Latin Name | English Name |
|---|---|---|
| Bu Gu Zhi | *Fructus Psoraleae Corylifoliae* | Psoralea fruit |

Tonifies the Kidneys, Spleen, Essence and Yang. It reserves the urine and aids the Kidneys in grasping the Lung Qi. Used for impotence, premature ejaculation, low back pain, urinary problems including incontinence, digestive difficulties including diarrhea, and wheezing. It has been used recently as a topical application for psoriasis, vitiligo and alopecia.

| | | |
|---|---|---|
| Cang Er Zi | *Fructus Xanthii Sibirici* | Cocklebur fruit |

Clears Wind and Damp to treat body ache and itchy skin, opens the nasal passages to treat congestion, treats severe headaches that accompany colds.

| | | |
|---|---|---|
| Cang Zhu | *Rhizoma Atractylodis* | Actractylodes rhizome |

An aromatic herb that dries Dampness and strengthens the Spleen to treat diarrhea, poor appetite, stomachache, nausea, vomiting and fatigue. Also treats pain in the arms and legs and eye disorders (night blindness, cataracts and glaucoma.)

| | | |
|---|---|---|
| Cao Jiao Ci | *Spina Gleditsiae Sinensis* | Gleditsia spine |

Used to encourage swollen sores to form and burst. It kills parasites and treats leprosy.

| | | |
|---|---|---|
| Chai Hu | *Radix Bupleuri* | Bupleurum |

Reduces fever during illness characterized by alternating fever and chills. Also frees Liver Qi and treats dizziness, vertigo, menstrual disorders and emotional instability. Also treats hemorrhoids, prolapse of the uterus, indigestion and diarrhea.

| | | |
|---|---|---|
| Chan Tui | *Periostracum Cicadae* | Cicada molting |

Clears Wind and Heat, vents rashes, stops spasms and benefits the eyes. Treats itchy red eyes, hoarseness of the throat, measles and convulsions or night terrors.

| | | |
|---|---|---|
| Chen Pi | *Percarpium Citri Reticulatae* | Tangerine peel |

Strengthens Spleen Qi to improve digestion and to treat abdominal bloating and distention, nausea, belching and vomiting. Also dries Damp to treat cough with Phlegm.

| Chinese Name | Latin Name | English Name |
|---|---|---|
| Chen Xiang | Lignum Aquilariae | Aquilaria |

Moves Qi, directs rebellious Qi downward and aids the Kidneys in grasping the Qi. It alleviates pain, especially abdominal, treats belching, hiccups, vomiting and wheezing.

| Chi Shao | Radix Paeoniae Rubrae | Red Peony root |
|---|---|---|

Invigorates the Blood to treat Blood Stasis, Cools the Blood and clears Heat and Liver Fire. Treats menstrual and eye disorders.

| Chuan Lian Zi | Meliae Toosendan Fructus | Melia |
|---|---|---|

Moves Qi, Clears Heat and dries Damp, kills parasites and alleviates pain. This herb relieves the pain associated with hernia and parasitic infection. Treats abdominal, epigastric (the base of the sternum/upper abdominal region), rib and flank pain.

| Chuan Xiong | Radix Ligustici Chuanxiong | Cnidium |
|---|---|---|

Invigorates the Blood, moves Qi, expels Wind and alleviates headache and pain. Treats colds with headache, body ache and dizziness. Also treats gynecological disorders and soreness in the chest or flanks.

| Da Suan | Bulbus Alli Sativi | Garlic |
|---|---|---|

Warm and Spicy herb that stimulates the Energy flow and circulation. Garlic's Qi moving and circulating properties can be seen in its acknowledgment by Western doctors and researchers for cardiovascular benefits. It is also a premier antiviral, antibacterial and most of all antifungal.

| Dang Gui | Corpus Radicis Angelicae Sinensis | Angelica root |
|---|---|---|

The body of the root of Angelica strongly Tonifies Blood and regulates menses. It Harmonizes Blood, clears cold, moistens the intestines and treats sores and abscesses. Is commonly used to treat menstrual disorders such as irregular or painful menstruation. Also treats constipation, traumatic injury and sores.

| Dang Gui Wei | Extremitas Radicis Angelicae Sinensis | Angelica tails |
|---|---|---|

Strongly moves the Blood, disperses Cold, alleviates pain, generates flesh, reduces swelling and pus and promotes bowel movement. Treats abdominal pain, traumatic injury and carbuncles. Also treats constipation and sores.

| Chinese Name | Latin Name | English Name |
| --- | --- | --- |
| Dang Qui (Dong Quai) | *Corpus Radicis Angelicae Sinensis* | Angelica root |

Strongly Tonifies Blood and regulates menses. Harmonizes Blood, clears Cold, moistens the Intestines and treats sores and abscesses. A member of the celery family, it is known as the female ginseng. Dang Qui has a balancing effect on the female reproductive system and helps to ease menopausal symptoms, fibrocystic breasts, PMS and painful menstruation.

| Dang Shen | *Radix Codonopsitis Pilosulae* | Codonopsis root |

Tonifies Qi and the Lungs and nourishes Fluids. Is useful for reduced appetite, fatigue, vomiting and diarrhea. Is also used to treat diabetes and chronic cough.

| Dan Nan Xing | *Pulvis Arisaemae cum Felle Bovis* | Arisaema Pulvis and bovine bile |

Clears Phlegm, Heat and Wind and stops tremors of the body. Is often used in pediatrics for seizures and tremors. Also treats stroke.

| Dan Qing Ye | *Folium Isatidis Tinctoria* | Woad leaf |

Dan Qing Ye is the leaf of the Ban Lan Gen plant. Clears Heat, relieves Toxicity, Cools the Blood and reduces blotches. Is used to treat epidemic outbreaks, mumps, sore throat or tonsilitis, severe fever and blotchy skin.

| Dan Shen | *Radix Salviae Miltiorrhizae* | Salvia root |

Invigorates the Blood, clears Heat and decreases irritability. Dan Shen treats menstrual and breast disorders, pain in the abdomen and chest, insomnia and irritability.

| Di Fu Zi | *Fructus Kochiae Scopariae* | Kochia fruit |

Drains Damp-Heat, promotes urination and stops itching. Is used to treat painful urination and itching skin disorders such as eczema or scabies.

| Di Long | *Lumbricus* | Earthworm |

Expels Wind and Heat, stops spasms and promotes urination. Is used to treat convulsions and seizures.

| Chinese Name | Latin Name | English Name |
|---|---|---|
| Di Yu | *Radix Sanguisorbae Officinalis* | Sanguisorba root |

Stops bleeding, Cools the Blood, clears Heat and heals flesh. Is used in ointments to treat burns and sores. Used for bleeding hemorrhoids, uterine bleeding or blood in the stool.

| Ding Xiang | *Flos Caryophylli* | Clove bud |
|---|---|---|

Qi mobilizer. Warming and slightly Spicy. Often used to treat stomachache caused by Cold External Cause.

| Dong Chong Xia Cao | *Cordyceps Sinensis* | Cordyceps carcass with fungus |
|---|---|---|

Tonifies the Yang and Kidney Energy. It increases Lung Yin, transforms phlegm and stops bleeding. Used to treat impotence, sore back and legs, chronic cough and wheezing.

| Du Huo | *Radix Angelicae Pubescentis* | Pubescent Angelica root |
|---|---|---|

Used to treat pain in the low back and legs, toothache, headache and flu or colds.

| Du Zhong | *Cortex Eucommiae Ulmoidis* | Eucommia bark |
|---|---|---|

Tonifies Liver and Kidney Energies, strengthens the sinews and bones, allows Qi and Blood to flow smoothly throughout the body and calms a restless fetus. Used for low back pain, frequent urination, hypertension and miscarriage.

| Fang Feng | *Radix Ledebouriella Divaricatae* | Siler root |
|---|---|---|

Expels Wind, treating headache, chills, body aches and pain, migraines, tetanus and painful, bloody diarrhea.

| Fu Ling | *Sclerotium Poriae Cocos* | Poria Cocos fungus |
|---|---|---|

An important Qi Tonic. Gentle in nature. Also has a diuretic property.

| Fu Zi | *Radix Aconiti Carmichaeli Praeparata* | Prepared aconite |
|---|---|---|

Strengthens and Tonifies the Yang Qi in general and specifically the Yang of the Heart, Kidney and Spleen. Also expels Cold and warms the channels to alleviate

| Chinese Name | Latin Name | English Name |
| --- | --- | --- |

pain in the body. Used to treat Yang deficiency with a weak pulse, cold extremities, diarrhea and chills.

| Gan Cao | *Radix Glycyrrhizae Uralensis* | Licorice root |

This commonly used herb Tonifies the Spleen and Qi, moistens the Lungs and clears Heat. Stops coughs, moderates spasms and alleviates pain. A frequent use of this herb is in formulas to moderate other herbs' properties and relieve toxicity. Used to treat heart palpitations, shortness of breath, fatigue, coughing, carbuncles, sore throat and painful spasms in the legs.

| Ge Gen | *Radix Puerariae* | Kudzu root |

Releases the muscles, clears Heat, nourishes the Fluids, alleviates thirst and diarrhea, lowers blood pressure and treats hypertension symptoms. Used for measles, hypertension, colds and flu where body aches predominate and there is fever, thirst, headache and stiff neck or back. Also treats diarrhea and alcohol hangover.

| Ge Jie | *Gecko* | Gecko |

Tonifies Kidney and Lung Yang. Used to treat difficulty breathing, consumptive cough, impotence, diarrhea and urinary frequency.

| Gou Ji | *Rhizoma Cibotii Barometz* | Cibotum |

Tonifies Blood and Kidneys. It strengthens the sinews and bones and expels Wind-Damp. Gou Ji treats back problems, pain, weakness and stiffness of the low back and legs, urinary incontinence and vaginal discharge.

| Gou Qi Zi | *Fructus Lycii* | Lycium fruit |

Tonifies the blood of the Kidneys and Liver. It benefits Jing, brightens the eyes and moistens the Lungs. Gou Qi Zi treats impotence, back and leg soreness and weakness, nocturnal emission, diabetes and consumption. Also treats eye problems.

| Gou Teng | *Ramulus Uncariae* | Gambier |

Slightly Cool. Commonly used to treat internal Wind conditions. Helps lower blood pressure. Treats headache.

| Chinese Name | Latin Name | English Name |
|---|---|---|

**Gu Sui Bu** — *Rhizoma Drynariae* — Drynaria

Tonifies the Kidneys, heals muscle and bone tissue and stimulates hair growth. Useful for treating alopecia, broken or fractured bones, torn ligaments, hearing loss, tinnitus, gum and tooth problems, weak back and knees and diarrhea.

**Gui Ban** — *Plastrum Testudinis* — Testudinis

Nourishes the Yin, Cools and nourishes the Blood, Tonifies the Heart and Kidneys, anchors the Yang, strengthens the bones, stops uterine bleeding and heals sores and ulcers. Treats night sweats, dizziness and tinnitus. Also treats tremors of the feet and hands, poor development in children, weak back or legs, uterine bleeding, anxiety and insomnia and nonhealing sores.

**Gui Zhi** — *Ramulus Cinnamomi Cassiae* — Cinnamon twigs

Warms the channels and the Yang Qi of the chest, expels Cold and allows the blood and Yang Qi to flow smoothly. Treats common cold where fever and chills with spontaneous sweating are predominant. Treats painful joints and limbs, gynecological problems, edema and palpitations.

**Han Fang Ji** — *Radix Stephaniae Tetrandrae* — Stephania root

Expels Wind-Damp, alleviates pain and promotes urination to reduce edema. Treats edema of the legs, ascites (fluid retention in abdominal cavities), abdominal distention and fever with painful, swollen joints.

**He Huan Hua** — *Flos Albizziae Julibrissin* — Albizzia flower

Allows Liver Qi to flow smoothly throughout the body and calms the Spirit. He Huan Hua treats the symptoms due to unexpressed emotions such as insomnia, poor memory, irritability and chest pain and pressure.

**He Shou Wu** — *Radix Polygoni Multiflori* — Fleeceflower root

Strengthens the Blood, Liver, Kidneys and Essence. It moistens the intestines to promote bowel movement, stops leakage and relieves Toxicity. Used to treat anemia, premature aging with symptoms such as premature graying of the hair, blurred vision, weak back, sore extremities and insomnia. Also treats nocturnal emission and spermatorrhea, vaginal discharge, carbuncles, goiter, constipation, skin rash and hair loss.

| Chinese Name | Latin Name | English Name |
|---|---|---|
| Hong Hua | *Flos Carthami Tinctorii* | Carthamus |

Unblocks Blood stasis, treats menstrual problems and alleviates pain. Treats amenorrhea (ceased menstration), chest and abdominal pain, carbuncles and sores, painful wounds, measles and postpartum lochioschesis (abnormal postpartum discharge).

| Hou Po | *Cortex Magnoliae Officinalis* | Magnolia bark |
|---|---|---|

Moves Qi and transforms Damp and Phlegm. Used to treat digestive problems with abdominal fullness and distention. Also treats wheezing and coughing with phlegm.

| Hu Zhang | *Radix et Rhizoma Polygoni Cuspidati* | Bushy Knotweed root and rhizome |
|---|---|---|

Invigorates the Blood, clears and drains Heat, resolves Phlegm and Damp and expels Toxins. Treats amenorrhea (ceased menstruation), traumatic injury, pain in the body, jaundice, cough, constipation, snakebite, burns and skin infections.

| Hua Shi | *Talcum* | Talcum |
|---|---|---|

Promotes urination, clears Heat and expels Damp through the urine. Treats urinary problems and fever and excess thirst. Also used topically for oozing skin lesions.

| Huang Bai | *Cortex Phellodendri* | Phellodendron |
|---|---|---|

Drains Damp-Heat and Kidney Fire and relieves Toxicity. Used to treat dysentery, diarrhea, vaginal discharge, pain and swelling of the legs, night sweats and skin lesions.

| Huang Lian | *Rhizoma Coptidis* | Coptis rhizome |
|---|---|---|

Drains Fire, clears Heat, relieves Toxicity, drains Damp, stops bleeding and clears Heat topically. Treats illness with high fever, severe irritability and delirium. Also treats insomnia, digestive problems, dysentery, bleeding problems (such as nosebleed) and mouth and tongue ulcers.

| Huang Qi | *Radix Astragali Membranaceus* | Astragalus root |
|---|---|---|

Important Qi Tonic that strengthens Wei Qi (Qi that assists in fighting off External Causes), Spleen and Stomach Qi, reduces edema and heals sores. It is for weak patients with immune disorders, leukemia, chronic illness or nonhealing

| Chinese Name | Latin Name | English Name |
| --- | --- | --- |

sores, or general debility. Treats fatigue, diarrhea, loss of appetite, prolapse of organs, frequent colds and diabetes.

| Huang Qin | *Radix Scutellariae Baicalensis* | Baical Skullcap root |

Clears Heat and Damp. Calms the fetus and stops bleeding. Used to treat high fever with irritability, thirst and cough. Also treats dysentery or diarrhea, vomiting or coughing up blood, nosebleed, restless kicking of a fetus and headache.

| Huo Ma Ren | *Semen Cannabis Sativae* | Linum, Hemp seeds |

This laxative moistens the Intestines and Yin to treat constipation, especially in postpartum women or the elderly.

| Huo Xiang | *Herba Agastaches seu Pogostemi* | Patchouli |

This aromatic herb transforms Damp and stops vomiting. Used for digestive problems including nausea and vomiting, abdominal bloating and a poor appetite. Also treats colds or flu with fever and accompanying digestive problems such as stomachache, nausea, vomiting and diarrhea.

| Ji Nei Jin | *Endothelium Corneum Gigeriae Galli* | Chicken Gizzard's internal lining |

Strengthens the Stomach's transportive function, stops enuresis and dissolves stones and hardness. Used for digestive problems, childhood malnutrition, bed-wetting and urinary or biliary tract stones.

| Ji Xue Teng | *Radix et Caulis Jixueteng* | Millettia root and vine |

Invigorates the Blood and channels, Tonifies the Blood and relaxes the sinews. Treats muscle and joint pain, menstrual disorders, paralysis and vertigo.

| Jiang Huang | *Rhizoma Curcumae Longae* | Turmeric rhizome |

Moves the Blood and Qi, relieves pain and allows the menses to flow. Used for painful menstrual problems, postpartum pain and pain in the abdomen, shoulders or any other injured area.

| Chinese Name | Latin Name | English Name |
|---|---|---|
| Jiang Xiang | *Lignum Dalbergiae Odoriferae* | Dalbergia heartwood |

Stops bleeding, invigorates the Blood, moves Qi and alleviates pain. Used for internal injuries, bleeding lacerations and for abdominal and chest pain.

| Jiao Gu Lan | *Herba Gynostemma Pentaphyllum* | Seven Leaf ginseng |
|---|---|---|

Known as the "herb of immortality," Jiao Gu Lan drains Damp, Tonifies Qi and Yin and relieves toxic swellings. Used to lower blood cholesterol levels, stress and blood pressure. Also used to increase resistance to infection, boost the immune system, treat diabetes and aid in cancer inhibition.

| Jie Geng | *Radix Platycodi Grandiflori* | Balloon Flower root |
|---|---|---|

Opens up and distributes the Lung Qi, expels Phlegm and pus, benefits the throat and guides other herbs in a formula to the upper body. Used mainly for cough and lung and throat infections that may contain pus.

| Jin Yin Hua | *Flos Lonicerae* | Japonicae/Honeysuckle flower |
|---|---|---|

Strongly Clears Heat and relieves toxicity. Releases Wind-Heat. Jin Yin Hua is used for inflamed, painful swellings and sores of the intestines, breasts, throat and eyes. Also treats fever with headache and sore throat.

| Jing Jie | *Herba seu Flos Schizonepetae Tenuifoliae* | Schizonepeta stem/bud |
|---|---|---|

Releases the Exterior, vents rashes and stops bleeding and itching. Treats chills and fever, initial-stage measles, skin eruptions and hemorrhage.

| Ju Hong | *Pars Rubra Epicarpii Citri Erythrocarpae* | Red Tangerine peel |
|---|---|---|

Dries Dampness, transforms Phlegm and prevents stagnation. Used primarily for stopping cough, vomiting and belching.

| Jue Ming Zi | *Semen Cassiae* | Cassia seed |
|---|---|---|

Drains Fire, clears the Liver, benefits the eyes, expels Wind-Heat, moistens the intestines, unblocks the bowels and prevents atherosclerosis (plaquing of the arteries). Primarily treats eye disorders such as red, itchy, painful, sensitive eyes.

| Chinese Name | Latin Name | English Name |
|---|---|---|

Treats headache, excessive tearing and constipation. This seed has been used recently to lower blood pressure and cholesterol.

| Ku Shen | Radix Sophorae Flavescentis | Sophora root |

Dries Damp, clears Heat and promotes urination. Also rids the body of Wind, parasites and itching. Treats Damp in the body that causes symptoms such as dysentery, excessive vaginal discharge, jaundice, itchy, seeping sores, genital itching, edema and painful urination.

| Lian Qiao | Fructus Forsythiae Suspensae | Forsythia fruit |

Clears Heat, Wind and Toxins and dissipates nodules to treat Hot sores, carbuncles and neck lumps. Used for fever and chills with sore throat and headache.

| Ling Zhi | Ganoderma Lucidum | Reishi mushroom |

Tonifies immunity and is used for cancer and tumors.

| Long Dan Cao | Radix Gentianae Longdancao | Gentiana |

Drains Damp-Heat and Fire from the Liver and Damp-Heat from the gallbladder. Used for painful, swollen throat, eyes, ears or genitals. Also treats sudden deafness, foul-smelling vaginal discharge and itching, convulsions, spasms, flank pain, headache, fever and red eyes.

| Lu Dou Yi | Cortex Semen Phaseoli Radiati | Mung Bean skin |

Used as an antidote to aconite poisoning. Treats and prevents a disorder called Summerheat, including the symptoms of thirst, irritability and fever.

| Lu Gen | Rhizoma Phragmitis Communis | Reed rhizome |

Clears Heat from the Lungs, Stomach and entire body. It generates fluids, promotes urination and clears rashes. Treats fever, irritability, thirst, cough, thick yellow sputum, rash, vomiting, belching and scant, dark or bloody urine.

| Lu Hui | Herba Aloes | Dried Aloe juice |

A purgative that drains Fire, kills parasites, strengthens the Stomach and Cools the Liver. Treats acute or chronic constipation, red eyes, irritability and dizziness. Also treats childhood malnutrition, roundworm and ringworm. It is useful for epigastric discomfort (the base of the sternum/upper abdominal region) headache,

| Chinese Name | *Latin Name* | English Name |
| --- | --- | --- |

ringing of the ears and fever. A tissue promoter that heals mucous membranes and treats burns.

| Lu Rong | *Cornu Cervi Parvum* | Deer Velvet Antler |
| --- | --- | --- |

Tonifies the Kidneys, Yang, Essence, Blood and Qi. Also strengthens the sinews and bones. Treats infertility, impotence, mental or physical developmental disorders, rickets, learning disabilities, fatigue, Cold extremities, weak back and legs, ringing of the ears and light-headedness. Also treats vaginal discharge, uterine bleeding and frequent urination.

| Luo Bu Ma | *Apocynum Venetum* | Dogbane |
| --- | --- | --- |

Clears Heat, lowers blood pressure, strengthens the Heart and promotes urination to treat heart disease, hypertension, nephritic edema, headache, insomnia, dizziness and irritability.

| Mang Xiao | *Mirabilitum* | Glauber's salt |
| --- | --- | --- |

This mineral eliminates stagnation, clears Heat and reduces swelling. Treats constipation with dry, hard stools, eye disorders, breast problems and mouth and throat ulcers.

| Mu Dan Pi | *Cortex Moutan Radicis* | Moutan bark |
| --- | --- | --- |

Cools and invigorates the Blood, clears Yin-deficient Fire and Liver Fire, dispels Blood stasis and reduces swelling and pus. Treats bleeding problems including nosebleed, bloody sputum or vomit, profuse menstruation or subcutaneous bleeding. Also treats amenorrhea (ceased menstruation), painful menstruation, masses or lumps in the abdomen, bruises from injury, headache, intestinal abscess and eye and flank pain. Mu Dan Pi is also used topically for skin sores with pus.

| Mu Gua | *Fructus Chaenomelis* | Chaenomeles |
| --- | --- | --- |

Relaxes the sinews, unblocks the Channels, Harmonizes the Stomach and transforms Damp. Primarily treats weak, cramping, tight, painful low back and extremities. Treats indigestion due to food stagnation, abdominal pain and cramping. Also treats edema and cramping of the leg or calves.

| Mu Li | *Concha Ostreae* | Oyster shell |
| --- | --- | --- |

Settles and calms the Spirit, anchors the Yang, prevents fluid leakage, softens and dissipates hard nodules and absorbs excess stomach acid. Used to treat anxi-

| Chinese Name | Latin Name | English Name |
|---|---|---|

ety, restlessness, insomnia, irritability, dizziness, blurred vision, headache, hot tempers and a flushed, red face. Used for sweating disorders, including continuous, spontaneous and night sweating. Also treats goiter, scrofula and neck lumps.

Niu Bang Zi          *Fructus Arctii Lappae*          Great burdock fruit

Clears Wind-Heat, benefits the throat, relieves toxicity and vents rashes. Treats fever, cough, sore throat, mumps, rashes, erythemas, carbuncles, early-stage measles and constipation.

Nu Zhen Zi          *Fructus Ligustri Lucidi*          Privet fruit

Tonifies, nourishes and augments the Liver and Kidneys. Also clears Yin-deficient Heat and improves vision. Used for dizziness, sore low back, premature graying, ringing of the ears, poor vision and spots before the eyes.

Pi Pa Ye          *Foliurn Eriobotryae Japonicae*          Loquat leaf

Relieves wheezing and coughing by transforming Phlegm, clearing Lung Heat and redirecting Lung Qi down. Also clears Stomach Heat to treat vomiting, nausea and belching.

Pu Gong Ying   *Herba Taraxaci Mongolici cum Radice*   Dandelion

Clears Heat, relieves Toxicity, dries Damp, promotes lactation and reduces nodules and abscesses. Used to treat red, swollen eyes, breast and intestinal abscesses, insufficient lactation and painful urination.

Pu Huang          *Pollen Typhae*          Cattail pollen

Used to stop bleeding, invigorate the Blood and dispel Blood stagnation. Treats various types of internal and external bleeding as well as chest, menstrual and postpartum pain.

Qian Nian Jian          *Rhizoma*          Homalomena rhizome
          *Homalomenae Occultae*

Dispels Wind-Damp and strengthens the sinews and bones. Used to treat painful obstructions in the body, especially in the elderly. It is useful for arthritis, low back pain, muscular spasms and numbness of the arms or legs.

| Chinese Name | Latin Name | English Name |
| --- | --- | --- |

**Qing Dai** — *Indigo Pulverata Levis* — Indigo

Clears Heat, relieves Toxicity, reduces swellings and Cools the Blood. Treats bleeding, childhood convulsions due to fever and cough. It is applied topically to treat mouth and throat inflammation.

**Qing Hao** — *Artemisiae Annuae Herba* — Artemisia Qing Hao

Clears Summer Heat—the Heat with Dampness that comes in summertime. Clears deficiency Heat—fever that lingers after an illness or from Yin deficiency. Cools Blood and stops bleeding, particularly for purpuric (characterized by hemorrhages) rashes or nosebleeds from Heat in the Blood. An antimalarial herb. Also effective in treating certain other tropical-born infections.

**Qu Mai** — *Herba Dianthi* — Dianthus

Qu Mai clears Damp-Heat, promotes urination and bowel movement and dispels Blood stagnation. Used to treat painful urinary problems, constipation and amenorrhea (ceased menstruation).

**Ren Dong Teng** — *Ramus Lonicerae Japonicae* — Lonicera vine

Clears Heat, Toxicity and Wind-Damp and is used to treat abscesses, sores and hot, painful joints that are difficult to move.

**Ren Shen** — *Radix Ginseng* — Ginseng root

Strongly Tonifies the Qi, Lungs, Spleen and Stomach. It benefits the Heart Qi, calms the Spirit, stops thirst and generates fluids. Treats shock, hollow respiration, Cold limbs, a weak pulse and profuse sweating. It is often used for weak digestion, lack of appetite, lethargy, chronic diarrhea, prolapse, bloating, wheezing, shortness of breath, diabetes, anxiety, insomnia and palpitations. Contraindicated in high blood pressure or Yin deficiency (except American ginseng, which is used for Yin deficiency). When using ginseng always consult an herbalist.

**Rou Cong Rong** — *Herba Cistanches Deserticolae* — Cistanche

Tonifies Yang and Kidneys. Also warms the womb and moistens the intestines. Treats impotence, infertility, spermatorrhea, urinary incontinence, weak and cold low back and knees, uterine bleeding and constipation.

| Chinese Name | Latin Name | English Name |
| --- | --- | --- |
| Rou Dou Kou | *Semen Myristicae Fragrantis* | Nutmeg seeds |

Stops diarrhea, warms the Middle Burner, moves Qi and alleviates pain. Used for diarrhea, poor digestion, vomiting and distention of the abdomen.

| Rou Gui | *Cortex Cinnamomi Cassiae* | Cinnamon bark |
| --- | --- | --- |

Warms the Kidneys and Yang, leads Fire back to its source, disperses Cold, warms and unblocks the Channels and Vessels, alleviates pain and encourages Qi and Blood formation. Used for a group of symptoms characteristic of Kidney Yang Deficiency including Cold limbs, weak back, impotence and frequent urination. Also treats reduced appetite, diarrhea, abdominal pain, wheezing, severe sweating, weak and Cold lower extremities, amenorrhea (absence or abnormal cessation of menses), dysmenorrhea (difficult and painful menstruation), pain in the body and nonhealing chronic sores.

| San Qi | *Radix Notoginseng* | Pseudoginseng root |
| --- | --- | --- |

Stops bleeding, reduces swelling, alleviates pain and breaks up Blood stasis. Used for internal and external bleeding, traumatic injuries, fractures, sprains, contusions and abdominal or chest pain.

| Sang Bai Pi | *Cortex Mori Albae Radicis* | Mulberry root bark |
| --- | --- | --- |

Clears Heat from the Lungs to stop coughing and wheezing, promotes urination and reduces edema. It has been used recently to treat hypertension.

| Sang Ji Sheng | *Ramulus Loranthus* | Loranthus |
| --- | --- | --- |

Tonifies Liver and Kidney, nourishes the blood, strengthens the sinews and bones, clears Wind-Damp, benefits the skin and calms the womb. Used to treat pain, stiffness, weakness and soreness of the back and legs. Also treats problems during pregnancy such as a restless fetus or uterine bleeding. Used for dry scaly skin. Has been used recently for hypertension.

| Sang Shen Zi | *Fructus Mori Albae* | Mulberry fruit |
| --- | --- | --- |

Tonifies the Blood and Yin to treat dizziness, insomnia, premature graying, constipation, diabetes and ringing of the ears.

| Chinese Name | Latin Name | English Name |
|---|---|---|
| Sha Ji Zi You | Semen Hippophae Rhamnoides | Seabuckthorn seed oil |

Invigorates the Blood, breaks up stagnation to promote blood circulation, alleviates pain, reduces inflammation and benefits the Heart. Used to delay aging, enhance the immune system and prevent atherosclerosis. Used for stomach ulcer, ulcers, gastrointestinal problems and cancer.

| | | |
|---|---|---|
| Sha Shen (Bei) | Radix Adenophorae seu Glehniae (North) | Glehnia root |

Tonifies Lung Yin, stops cough, nourishes the Stomach, generates fluids, clears Heat and moistens the skin. Used for consumptive cough with bloody sputum and hoarseness, dry mouth and throat, constipation and dry itchy skin.

| | | |
|---|---|---|
| Sha Yuan Zi | Semen Astragali Complanati | Astragalus seed |

Tonifies the Yang, Liver and Kidneys, secures the Essence and improves vision. Used for low back pain, ringing of the ears, impotence, urinary problems, premature ejaculation, vaginal discharge and problems with vision.

| | | |
|---|---|---|
| Shan Yao | Radix Dioscoreae Oppositae | Chinese yam |

Tonifies Spleen, Stomach, Lung Qi and Kidney Energy. Used for diarrhea, fatigue, spontaneous sweating, poor appetite, chronic cough, wheezing, diabetes, spermatorrhea, frequent urination and vaginal discharge.

| | | |
|---|---|---|
| Shan Zha | Fructose Crataegi | Hawthorn fruit |

Relieves food stagnation for symptoms of abdominal distention, abdominal pain and diarrhea. When charred, this herb treats dysentery and diarrhea. It has been used recently to treat hypertension, heart disease and serum cholesterol problems.

| | | |
|---|---|---|
| Shan Zhu Yu | Fructus Corni Officinalis | Cornus fruit |

Tonifies and binds the Essence and Kidney Energy. It stops excessive sweating, restores collapsed Yang or Qi, Tonifies the Liver and Kidney Energies and stops excessive uterine bleeding during menses. Used for fluids leaking from the body such as sweat, urine or sperm. Also treats prolonged or excessive menstruation, light-headedness, dizziness, impotence and sore low back or knees.

| Chinese Name | Latin Name | English Name |
|---|---|---|
| She Chuang Zi | *Fructus Cnidii Monnieri* | Cnidium seeds |

Dries Damp, stops itching, kills parasites, warms Kidney Energy and Yang and dispels Cold and Wind. Used topically for scabies, ringworm or any oozing, itchy rash. She Chuang Zi also treats impotence, infertility, vaginal discharge and low back pain.

| She Gan | *Rhizoma Belamcandae Chinensis* | Belamcanda rhizome |
|---|---|---|

Clears Heat, relieves Toxicity, benefits the throat and clears Phlegm in the Lungs. Used for sore throat, cough and wheezing.

| Shen Qu | *Massa Fermentata* | Medicated Leaven |
|---|---|---|

Relieves Food Stagnation and Harmonizes the stomach to treat abdominal and epigastric bloating (the base of the sternum/upper abdominal region), poor appetite, borborygmus and diarrhea. It is added to pills to aid in mineral digestion.

| Sheng Di Huang | *Radix Rehmanniae Glutinosae* | Chinese Foxglove root |
|---|---|---|

Clears Heat, Cools the Blood, generates fluids to nourish the Yin and Cools Heart Fire. Treats a severe fever with thirst, hemorrhage, dry mouth, constipation, continuous low-grade fever, mouth and tongue sores, insomnia, irritability and diabetes.

| Sheng Jiang | *Rhizoma Zingiberis Officinalis Recens* | Fresh Ginger |
|---|---|---|

Warms the body to dispel Cold. Alleviates nausea and vomiting, stops coughing and reduces toxicity of other herbs. Has anti-inflammatory, antiparasitic, antimicrobial, antioxidant, analgesic, antiarthritis, antiulcer, antinausea properties and digestive benefits, among others.

| Sheng Ma | *Rhizoma Cimicifugae* | Cimicifuga |
|---|---|---|

Releases the Exterior, vents rashes, clears Heat, relieves Toxicity and raises Yang. Used for colds, early-stage measles, sore teeth and gums, lip or gum ulcers, canker sores, sore throat, prolapse, fatigue and shortness of breath.

| Shi Chang Pu | *Rhizoma Acori Graminei* | Acorus |
|---|---|---|

Opens the Orifices, clears Phlegm, calms the Spirit and Harmonizes the Middle Burner. Used to open the sensory orifices to treat deafness, dizziness,

| Chinese Name | Latin Name | English Name |
| --- | --- | --- |

forgetfulness, dulled senses, seizures, coma. Also treats chest, epigastric (the base of the sternum/upper abdominal region) or abdominal pain, traumatic injury and sores.

| Shi Gao | *Gypsum* | Gypsum |
| --- | --- | --- |

Clears Heat and drains Fire, especially clearing Heat from the Lungs and Clearing Stomach Fire. Used for a high fever, thirst, irritability, sweating, cough, wheezing, headache, toothache, swollen gums, eczema, sores and burns.

| Shu Di Huang | *Radix Rehmanniae Glutinosae Conquitae* | Chinese Foxglove root |
| --- | --- | --- |

Strongly Tonifies the Blood, nourishes the Yin and builds the Essence. Used for insomnia, dizziness, palpitations, irregular menstruation, uterine or postpartum bleeding, night sweats, nocturnal emissions, diabetes, weak and painful low back, weak legs, light-headedness, tinnitis, loss of hearing and premature graying of the hair.

| Shui Zhi | *Hirudo seu Witmania* | Leech |
| --- | --- | --- |

Invigorates the Blood and reduces stasis and masses. Used for abdominal masses, amenorrhea (ceased menstruation) and traumatic injury.

| Si Gua Luo | *Luffae Fasciculus Vascularis* | Luffa fiber |
| --- | --- | --- |

Invigorates the Channels, expels Wind and Phlegm, promotes urination and benefits the breasts. Treats muscle soreness and stiff joints, breast abscess, traumatic injury, insufficient lactation and breast pain and swelling.

| Su Zi | *Fructus Perillae Frutesentis* | Perilla fruit |
| --- | --- | --- |

Stops cough and wheezing, directs Lung Qi down, dissolves Phlegm and moistens the intestines. Used for labored exhalation when breathing, stifling sensation in the chest and constipation.

| Suan Zao Ren | *Semen Zizyphi Spinosae* | Sour Jujube seed |
| --- | --- | --- |

Nourishes Heart Yin, increases Liver Blood, quiets the Spirit and stops sweating. Used for irritability, palpitations, insomnia, night sweating and spontaneous sweating.

| Chinese Name | Latin Name | English Name |
| --- | --- | --- |
| Suo Yang | *Herba Cynomorii Songarici* | Cynomorium |

Tonifies Yang, Kidney Energy, Blood and Essence. It strengthens the sinews, moistens the intestines and unblocks the bowels. Used for impotence, atrophy, premature ejaculation, spermatorrhea, paralysis or motor impairment, urinary frequency and constipation.

| Chinese Name | Latin Name | English Name |
| --- | --- | --- |
| Tao Ren | *Semen Persicae* | Peach kernel |

Dispels Blood stagnation, moistens the intestines and unblocks the bowels. Used for menstrual disorders, pain in the abdomen, lung and intestinal abscess and constipation.

| Chinese Name | Latin Name | English Name |
| --- | --- | --- |
| Tian Nan Xing | *Rhizoma Arisaematis* | Arisaema |

Dries Damp, expels Phlegm and Wind, stops spasms, reduces swellings and alleviates pain. Treats cough, spasms in the hands or feet, facial paralysis, stroke, seizures, lockjaw, numb limbs, dizziness and sores.

| Chinese Name | Latin Name | English Name |
| --- | --- | --- |
| Tou Gu Cao | *Speranskiae Herba* | Speranskia Herb |

Dispels Wind-Damp, relaxes the sinews, invigorates the Blood and alleviates pain. Used for muscle and joint pain or contracture, swelling and toxins in the body and pain or edema of the legs.

| Chinese Name | Latin Name | English Name |
| --- | --- | --- |
| Tu Fu Ling | *Rhizoma Smilacis Glabrae* | Smilax |

Relieves toxicity, clears Heat and Damp, especially from the skin. Treats joint pain, jaundice, painful urination, ulcers and skin lesions.

| Chinese Name | Latin Name | English Name |
| --- | --- | --- |
| Tu Si Zi | *Semen Cuscutae Chinensis* | Chinese Dodder seed |

Tonifies the Kidneys, Essence and Liver. Also benefits the Spleen, stops diarrhea, reserves the urine and calms a fetus. Used for impotence, urinary frequency, weak and sore back, nocturnal emission, premature ejaculation and vaginal discharge. Also treats spots in front of the eyes, ringing in the ears, dizziness and blurred vision. Used for diarrhea, poor appetite and a threatened miscarriage.

| Chinese Name | Latin Name | English Name |
|---|---|---|
| Wei Ling Xian | *Radix Clematidis* | Clematis |

Dispels Wind-Damp, alleviates pain, unblocks the channels and reduces Phlegm. Treats painful obstruction and abdominal distention. Used when fish bones have lodged in the throat.

| Wu Ling Zhi | *Excrementum Trogopteri seu Pteromi* | Excrementum Pteropus |
|---|---|---|

Breaks up Blood stasis, alleviates pain, stops bleeding and treats childhood nutritional impairment. Used for amenorrhea (absence or abnormal cessation of menses), dysmenorrhea (difficult and painful menstruation), postpartum or epigastric (the base of the sternum/upper abdominal region) pain, uterine bleeding and malnutrition.

| Wu Mei | *Fructus Pruni Mume* | Mume fruit |
|---|---|---|

Retains Lung Qi to stop cough, binds the intestines to stop diarrhea, generates fluids to alleviate thirst, expels roundworm and treats the accompanying pain and stops bleeding. Used for chronic cough, chronic diarrhea, vomiting and abdominal pain caused by roundworms and bloody stool or uterine bleeding with thirst and dry mouth. It is also applied topically as a plaster for corns and warts.

| Wu Wei Zi | *Fructus Schisandrae Chinensis* | Schisandra fruit |
|---|---|---|

Stabilizes and strengthens Lung Qi and Essence, stops coughing and diarrhea, Tonifies Kidney Energy, inhibits sweating, generates fluids and calms the Spirit and Heart. Used to treat chronic coughing and wheezing, daybreak diarrhea, urinary frequency, vaginal discharge and nocturnal emission. Treats sweating disorders including excessive sweating, thirst and dry mouth. Wu Wei Zi helps sleeping disorders, palpitations and irritability and recently has been used for skin allergies and hepatitis.

| Wu Zhu Yu | *Fructus Evodiae Rutaecarpae* | Evodia fruit |
|---|---|---|

Warms the Middle and Spleen Energy, disperses Cold and Damp, alleviates pain, stops vomiting and redirects rebellious Qi and Fire downward. Treats vomiting, epigastric (the base of the sternum/upper abdominal region) pain with drooling, nausea and lack of taste, regurgitation, headache, flank pain, diarrhea, pain in the legs and mouth or tongue sores.

| Chinese Name | Latin Name | English Name |
|---|---|---|
| Xian He Cao | *Herba Agrimoniae Pilosae* | Agrimony |

Stops bleeding and diarrhea. Also kills parasites. Used for bleeding anywhere in the body, chronic diarrhea and dysentery, trichomonas vaginitis and tapeworms.

| Chinese Name | Latin Name | English Name |
|---|---|---|
| Xiao Mai | *Fructus Tritici* | Wheat |

Is used to stop sweating and bed-wetting, calm the Spirit and nourish the Heart. Used for sweating disorders, bed-wetting in children, anxiety, insomnia and palpitations.

| Chinese Name | Latin Name | English Name |
|---|---|---|
| Xie Bai | *Bulbus Allii* | Bakeri |

Unblocks Yang Qi, disperses Cold Phlegm, alleviates pain, promotes Qi and Blood movement and directs Qi downward. Xie Bai is useful for chest, flank, upper back and abdominal pain. Treats dyspnea, coughing, wheezing, epigastric distention (the base of the sternum/upper abdominal region) and dysentery.

| Chinese Name | Latin Name | English Name |
|---|---|---|
| Xin Yi Hua | *Flos Magnoliae* | Magnolia flower |

Unblocks the nasal passages and dispels Wind-Cold for nasal congestion and sinus problems.

| Chinese Name | Latin Name | English Name |
|---|---|---|
| Xing Ren | *Semen Pruni Armeniacae* | Apricot seed |

Stops cough and wheezing, moistens the Lungs and intestines and unblocks the bowels. Apricot seed treats a broad range of coughs and constipation.

| Chinese Name | Latin Name | English Name |
|---|---|---|
| Xu Duan | *Radix Dipsaci Asperi* | Japanese Teasel root |

Tonifies the Liver and Kidneys, strengthens the sinews and bones, alleviates pain, generates flesh, promotes the movement of Blood, calms a restless fetus and stops uterine bleeding. Treats a sore and painful back, stiff joints, weak legs, threatened miscarriage, vaginal discharge and trauma.

| Chinese Name | Latin Name | English Name |
|---|---|---|
| Xuan Shen | *Radux Scrophulariae Ningpoensis* | Ningpo Figwort root |

Cools the Blood, nourishes the Yin, drains Fire, relieves Toxicity and softens nonmalignant growths. Used for fever with bleeding, dry mouth, constipation and irritability after a fever, swollen, red eyes, sore throat and neck lumps. Treats scrofula, goiter, ulcers and sores.

| Chinese Name | Latin Name | English Name |
|---|---|---|
| Xue Jie | *Sanguis Draconis* | Dragon's Blood |

Dispels stasis of the Blood, alleviates pain, stops bleeding and treats chronic nonhealing ulcers. Used for traumatic injury, fractures, sprains and contusions. It is applied topically to stop bleeding from injury.

| Chinese Name | Latin Name | English Name |
|---|---|---|
| Yan Hu Suo | *Rhizoma Corydalis Yanhusuo* | Corydalis rhizome |

Invigorates the Blood, alleviates pain and promotes the movement of Qi. Used to treat dysmenorrhea, traumatic injury, hernia, chest, abdominal, menstrual and epigastric (the base of the sternum/upper abdominal region) pain.

| Chinese Name | Latin Name | English Name |
|---|---|---|
| Ye Jiao Teng | *Caulis Polygoni Multiflori* | Polygonum vine |

Nourishes Heart Energy and Blood, calms the Spirit and unblocks the Channels. Used for insomnia, irritability, dream-disturbed sleep, weakness, soreness, numbness or pain. Used as an external wash to alleviate itching and rashes.

| Chinese Name | Latin Name | English Name |
|---|---|---|
| Ye Ju Hua | *Flos Chrysanthemi Indici* | Wild Chrysanthemum flower |

Drains Fire and relieves Toxicity. Treats sores, carbuncles, sore throat and red eyes.

| Chinese Name | Latin Name | English Name |
|---|---|---|
| Yi Mu Cao | *Herba Leonuri Heterophylli* | Leonurus |

Invigorates Blood and regulates the menses. It reduces masses and swelling. Also promotes urination. Treats gynecological disorders, abdominal masses and pain, acute systemic edema and bloody urine.

| Chinese Name | Latin Name | English Name |
|---|---|---|
| Yi Yi Ren | *Semen Coicis Lachryma-jobi* | Coix |

Drains Dampness, promotes urination, strengthens Spleen Energy to stop diarrhea and clears Damp, Wind and Pus. Treats edema accompanied by urinary difficulty, pustulated sores and abscesses, joint pain and immobility, digestive problems and plantar warts.

| Chinese Name | Latin Name | English Name |
|---|---|---|
| Yin Chen Hao | *Artemisiae Yinchenhao Herba* | Capillaris |

Clears Heat and Dampness. Used to treat such disorders as hepatitis A and B. Also contains some antibacterial properties.

| Chinese Name | Latin Name | English Name |
|---|---|---|
| Yin Guo Ye | *Folium Ginkgo Bilobae* | Ginkgo leaves |

Benefits Lung Energy, stops wheezing and alleviates pain. Used for cough, wheezing, hypertension, coronary artery disease, angina pectoris and cerebrovascular disease.

| | | |
|---|---|---|
| Yin Yang Huo | *Herba Epimedii* | Epimedium |

Tonifies Yang and Kidney Yang, expels Wind-Cold-Damp, sends ascending Liver Yang down. Treats impotence, spermatorrhea, forgetfulness, dizziness and menstrual irregularity. Also treats pain, numbness, Cold and cramping of the lower back, extremities, hands and feet, knees and joints.

| | | |
|---|---|---|
| Yu Jin | *Tuber Curcumae* | Turmeric tuber |

Invigorates the Blood, promotes the movement of Qi and Blood, clears the Heart, Cools the Blood and benefits the Gall Bladder. Treats traumatic injury, chronic sores, chest or menstrual pain, anxiety, seizures, mental derangement and jaundice.

| | | |
|---|---|---|
| Yu Xing Cao | *Herba cum Radice Houttuyniae Cordatae* | Houttuynia |

Clears Heat, Damp-Heat and Toxins. It reduces and relieves pus, swellings and abscesses. Also promotes urination. Treats Lung abscess, cough, sores, diarrhea and painful urinary dysfunction. A potent antiviral herb for the lung. Best used in combination with other herbs for upper respiratory tract infections.

| | | |
|---|---|---|
| Yu Zhu | *Rhizoma Polygonati Odorati* | Polygonatum |

Tonifies the Yin, moistens dryness and softens sinews. Used for cough, irritability, dry throat and thirst, diabetes with intense thirst, dizziness and pain and spasms in the sinews.

| | | |
|---|---|---|
| Yuan Zhi | *Radix Polygalae Tenuifoliae* | Polygala |

Calms the Spirit and Heart, expels Phlegm, Clears the orifices, reduces abscesses and dissipates swelling. Treats insomnia, palpitations, restlessness, mental disorientation, emotional problems, seizures, cough, boils, abscesses, sores and painful breasts.

| Chinese Name | Latin Name | English Name |
|---|---|---|
| Zao Jiao Ci | *Gleditsiae Sinensis Spina* | Gleditsia Spine |

Relieves swelling and abscesses, expels pus and invigorates the Blood. It encourages swollen sores to mature, kills parasites and treats ringworm and leprosy.

| | | |
|---|---|---|
| Ze Lan | *Herba Lycopi Lucidi* | Lycopus |

Promotes the movement of Blood, menstruation and urination. Used for menstrual or postpartum pain, internal injury or abscess and postpartum, facial or systemic edema.

| | | |
|---|---|---|
| Ze Xie | *Rhizoma Alismatis Orientalis* | Water Plantain rhizome |

Drains Damp and Kidney Energy Fire and promotes urination to treat difficult urination, edema, diarrhea, ringing in the ears and dizziness.

| | | |
|---|---|---|
| Zhen Zhu Mu | *Concha Margaritaferae* | Mother of Pearl |

Calms Liver Energy, anchors the Yang and benefits vision. Used for red eyes, blurry vision, ringing in the ears, dizziness, insomnia and seizures.

| | | |
|---|---|---|
| Zhen Zhu | *Margarita* | Pearl |

Calms Heart Energy, clears Liver Energy, stops tremors and spasms, clears the vision and heals and generates flesh. Used for seizures, childhood convulsions, palpitations, eye disorders and nonhealing ulcers.

| | | |
|---|---|---|
| Zhi Ke | *Fructus Citri Aurantii* | Bitter Orange fruit |

Moves Qi and reduces distention. Used for abdominal bloating, pressure and gas in a weak patient. Can be used for weight loss without the side effects of Ma Huang.

| | | |
|---|---|---|
| Zhi Mu | *Rhizoma Anemarrhenae Asphodeloidis* | Anemarrhena rhizome |

Clears Heat, drains Fire, increases Yin and fluids and moistens dryness. Used for high fever, thirst, night sweats, irritability, afternoon fever, bleeding gums, abnormally elevated sex drive with spermatorrhea or nocturnal emission, and oral ulcers.

| Chinese Name | Latin Name | English Name |
|---|---|---|

**Zhi Zi** — *Fructus Gardeniae Jasminoidis* — Gardenia

Clears Heat, drains Damp-Heat, Cools the Blood, eliminates irritability, stops bleeding and reduces swelling from trauma. Its primary use is for Heat in the body with irritability, restlessness, chest pressure and insomnia. Zhi Zi also treats painful urination, jaundice and mouth or face sores. Stops nosebleeds, bloody stools, vomiting blood and blood in the urine. It is applied topically with vinegar to reduce swelling in injuries.

**Zhu Ru** — *Caulis Bambussae in Taeniis* — Bamboo shavings

Clears Heat and Phlegm, Cools the Blood and stops bleeding and vomiting. Used for cough with thick sputum or blood, nausea and vomiting and nosebleed.

**Zi Cao Gen** — *Radix Arnebiae seu Lithospemi* — Lithospermum root

Clears Heat, Cools the Blood, relieves Fire Toxin to vent rashes, clears Damp-Heat from the skin, moistens the intestines and promotes bowel movement. Used for measles, chicken pox, rashes in their early stage, skin or vaginal itching and burns. Treats cold sores and constipation.

**Zi He Che** — *Hominis Placenta* — Placenta

Tonifies Kidney and Liver Energies, Essence, Qi, Blood and Lung Qi. Used for infertility, impotence, low back pain, spermatorrhea, ringing of the ears, light-headedness, insufficient lactation, seizures, chronic or acute coughing and wheezing and consumption with night sweats.

**Zi Su Ye** — *Folium Perillae Frutescentis* — Perilla leaf

Disperses Cold, moves Qi and alleviates congestion, seafood poisoning and morning sickness. Used for fever, chills, congestion, headache, cough, stifling sensation in the chest, nausea, vomiting, poor appetite, restless fetal movements, morning sickness and seafood poisoning.

**Zi Wan** — *Radix Asteris Tatarici* — Aster

Stops cough and clears Phlegm. Treats chronic cough that has difficulty expectorating, copious or blood-streaked sputum.

# Glossary of Chinese Mushrooms

| Chinese Name | Latin Name | English Name |
| --- | --- | --- |
| Dong Chong Xia Cao | *Cordyceps sinensis* | Winter Worm and Summer Grass |

Tonifies Kidney Yang and augments (a slightly milder form of Tonification) Lung Yin. Because it Tonfies Yin and Yang it is safe to use for long periods of time. Treats tuberculosis. Thought to extend the longevity of healthy cells, increase blood flow and lower cholesterol levels. Antitumor and immune stimulant used to treat lymphoma and other cancers. Shown to help prevent kidney disease and to have short-term curative effects on hepatitis B. Has been credited for enhanced performance in athletes. Improves sexual function in men.

| Hou Tou Jun | *Hericium erinaceus* | Monkey's Head, Yamabushiitake |
| --- | --- | --- |

Benefits Stomach Energy and immunity (Wei Qi of the Lung). Treats stomach ailments. Anticancer, immune stimulant, nerve regenerator, antimicrobial. Used for the treatment of atrophic gastritis. A nerve tonic, promotes good digestion and general vigor. Inhibits cancer, gastric and duodenal ulcers, nerve damage and is a nerve-growth stimulator.

| Jin Zhen Gu | *Flammulina velutipes* | Golden Needle Mushroom |
| --- | --- | --- |

Moves Blood stagnation and clears Heat. Isolated ingredients have been shown to stimulate antitumor responses. A possible treatment for Gardener's lymphoma, sarcoma 180, B-16 melanoma and prostate cancer. Also contains blood-pressure-lowering compounds.

| Chinese Name | Latin Name | English Name |
|---|---|---|
| Lian Hua Gu | *Grifola frondosa* | Hen-of-the-Woods, Maitake |

Benefits Stomach Energy and immunity (Wei Qi of the Lung). Antitumor, antidiabetic, antiviral. Has been shown to shrink cancer tumors. Possible treatment for diabetes by lowering and moderating glucose levels. Immune system support, normal blood pressure support, normal blood sugar metabolism and normal cholesterol support.

| | | |
|---|---|---|
| Ling Zhi | *Ganoderma lucidum* | Varnished Conk, Reishi |

Tonifies Qi, Blood, Yin and Jing. Used for recovery from prolonged illness and severe depletion of the entire system as in cancer and AIDS. Antitumor, immune-enhancing, antiviral, cholesterol-reducing, antifatigue, anti-inflammatory. Enhances endurance. May be useful in treating inflammation of the brain. Could be effective for treating atherosclerosis and diabetes. A blood-vessel dilator. Not to be taken before surgery or by women experiencing heavy menstrual flow.

| | | |
|---|---|---|
| Tan Zi Jun | *Agaricus blazei* | God's Mushroom, Himematsutake |

Benefits Stomach Energy and immunity (Wei Qi of the Lung). Antitumor, immune-enhancing, interferon- and interleukin-enhancing, antiviral, cholesterol-reducing and blood-sugar-modulating. Also known for bactericidal properties. Used to treat salmonella.

| | | |
|---|---|---|
| Xiang Gu | *Lentinula edodes* | Black Forest, Shiitake |

Benefits Stomach Energy and immunity (Wei Qi of the Lung). Immunomodulating, antibacterial, antiviral and liver-fortifying. An isolated ingredient called lentinan has been used as an anticancer drug in Asia. Studied for its cholesterol-reducing, immunostimulating and antiviral properties. Shown to be effective against type 1 Herpes Simplex virus. Has been found to limit HIV replication and stimulate the proliferation of bone marrow cells. Suggested as a treatment for chronic fatigue and as a tonic.

| | | |
|---|---|---|
| Yun Zhi | *Trametes versicolor* | Turkey Tail, Cloud Mushroom |

Clears Heat and Toxins. Tonifies Qi. Antitumor, immune enhancement, antiviral, antibacterial, antioxidant. Possible antiviral agents to inhibit HIV replication, for antitumor properties, as an immunomodulator, to bolster the immune sys-

| Chinese Name | Latin Name | English Name |
|---|---|---|

tem's natural killer cells, as well as treat breast, lung and colon cancer, sarcoma, carcinoma.

| Zhu Ling | *Polyporus umbellatus* | Chorei |
|---|---|---|

Promotes urination and drains Damp. Used for edema from fluid retention. Contains natural antibiotics. Antitumor (lung, bladder, liver), immune enhancement, antibiotic, anti-inflammatory, liver protectant, diuretic and effective in combating urinary-tract infections. Helps the immune system rebound after chemotherapy and radiation therapy. Effective in treatment of chronic hepatitis B.

# Resources

## Product Referrals

For further information about Chinese patent formulas, Chinese medicinal herbs for making the recipes in this book, Western supplements, super green food, vegetable pills, caffeine substitutes, juicers, air and water purifiers and continued updates on integrative medicine and current scientific research, log on to www.ancientherbsmodernmedicine.com.

## How to Find a Chinese Doctor in Your Area

Now that you have read this book and are excited about finding a doctor of Chinese medicine for yourself or for someone you love, the following will provide you with some helpful tips. Herbology is an art form, which some master better than others. The best recommendation is by word of mouth. Inquiring about other people's experiences with a particular herbalist will often tell you a lot about the herbalist's qualifications—more than just a diploma on the wall. There are generally three categories of training:

1. **Doctors trained in Chinese medicine in the Orient (mainland China, South Korea, Taiwan and Hong Kong):** Trained herbalists and acupuncturists are educated in certified Chinese medical schools in the Orient. To practice in the United States they must be licensed in the state where they are practicing, in accordance with that state's licensing criteria.
2. **Doctors originally trained in Western medicine in the Orient:** Many of these Western-trained doctors, who have immigrated to the United States

and set up practices in Chinese medicine here, have extended their training in Chinese medicine and have become qualified herbologists.

3. **Doctors trained in the United States:** There is a difference between an acupuncturist and a doctor of Chinese medicine who is trained in herbology. Some practitioners have had an education in acupuncture, but may not have been adequately trained in herbs. In California, most educational programs in Chinese medicine that are approved by the Acupuncture Board require students to study herbology even if a student is only interested in practicing acupuncture. In other states where the study of herbs is not required to practice acupuncture, more students are either choosing to study herbology or are pursuing postgraduate studies in herbology. For that reason, well-trained, experienced herbologists can be found in many communities, and the number is growing.

*The Top Seven Schools Within Mainland China Known for Producing Highly Trained Herbalists*

- Beijing University of Traditional Chinese Medicine (TCM)
- Shanghai University of TCM
- Guangzhou (the capital city of Canton province) University of TCM
- Chendu (the capital city of Szechuan province) University of TCM
- Nanjing (the capital city of Jiang Su province) College of TCM
- Shenyang (the capital city of Liao Ning province) College of TCM
- Hei Long Jiang University of TCM

*Questions to Ask an Herbalist*

- In what country were you trained?
- From what university did you graduate?
- How long have you been in practice?
- How many years of experience in the specific area of herbology do you have (not just acupuncture)?
- Do you have a full herbal pharmacy that is capable of filling customized herbal prescriptions, either in bulk or granulated form?
- Do you have an herbal pharmacist on staff?
- Are you able to effectively communicate in English, or do you have the necessary assistants who can communicate all of the critical information?

# Chinese Herbal/Acupuncture Clinics

### Santa Barbara Herb Clinic

A general practice founded and directed by Henry Han, O.M.D., who was trained in both Chinese and Western medicine at the prestigious Beijing University of Traditional Chinese Medicine. Dr. Han often uses Western diagnostic laboratory tests in evaluating and monitoring patients' progress throughout the course of treatment. He clearly communicates with his patients, to make each one feel comfortable with their understanding of the disease and herbal treatment. His training in psychology gives him effective tools in treating and communicating with his patients.

The Santa Barbara Herb Clinic is comprised of two other Chinese-trained doctors, each with at least fifteen years of experience. Student interns from the Santa Barbara School of Oriental Medicine rotate through the clinic, acquiring clinical experience and supervision. The clinic has a fully stocked herb room with dried, granulated and patent herbal formulas. The practice offers herbal medicine, acupuncture, nutritional consultation, lifestyle consultation and other modalities of therapy that support the overall health and well-being of the patients, such as massage, acupressure, cupping and Qigong.

> *Henry Han, O.M.D.*
> Internal medicine
>
> *Xiang Jun Yang, O.M.D.*
> Internal medicine, An Mo Therapy and Tui Na
>
> *Jing Wa Zhao, O.M.D.*
> Acupuncture
>
> **Santa Barbara Herb Clinic**
> 3886 State Street
> Santa Barbara, CA 93105
> Phone 1-805-563-0222
> Fax 1-805-563-1870

### Tao of Wellness

A general practice comprised of five doctors, one massage therapist and six herbalists. The clinic has a fully stocked herb room with both dried and patent herbal formulas. From the time you enter the Tao of Wellness to the time you leave, you will experience every staff member as part of the healing team whose mission is to serve and provide you with a total healing experience. Each of the five doctors at the Tao of Wellness will personalize a health program to meet your needs.

*Maoshing Ni, Lic. Ac., D.O.M., Ph.D.*
Immunology, gastroenterology and longevity
*Daoshing Ni, Lic. Ac., D.O.M., Ph.D.*
General medicine, reproductive medicine and gynecology

**Tao of Wellness**
1131 Wilshire Boulevard, Suite 300
Santa Monica, CA 90401
Phone 1-310-917-2200
Fax 1-310-917-2204

## Colleges and Universities of Chinese Medicine

### Santa Barbara College of Oriental Medicine

SBCOM has been at the forefront of the integration of Eastern and Western medicine for over twenty years. The SBCOM clinic has between seven to ten doctors of Oriental medicine on staff. The clinic has eight treatment rooms, two patient counseling rooms and patent medicine, granules and raw herbs of all kinds. The SBCOM offers acupuncture, acupressure, nutritional counseling, lifestyle counseling and herbal treatments. SBCOM funds community health care projects in such areas as HIV/AIDS, drug detox, addiction, pain management and stress reduction.

**Santa Barbara College of Oriental Medicine**
JoAnn Tall, Lic. Ac., President
1919 State Street, Suite 207
Santa Barbara, CA 93101
Phone 1-805-898-1180
Fax 1-805-682-1864
www.sbcom.edu

### Yo San University

The Yo San University Clinic (YSU Clinic) provides effective, low-cost treatment for a wide variety of ailments using acupuncture and other healing modalities of Traditional Chinese Medicine. The YSU Clinic is a community-oriented teaching clinic established to provide Yo San University students with a professional setting in which to complete their internship requirements for the Master of Acupuncture and Traditional Chinese Medicine. Each intern is closely supervised by a highly educated and skilled acupuncturist. YSU clinic interns are in the last phase of a rigorous four-year program taught by experts in both traditional Chinese healing techniques and current Western medical practices.

Yo San University also offers a Chi Development Program aimed at teaching people the beneficial and enjoyable movements of Tai Chi and related disciplines.

> **Yo San University**
> Daoshing Ni, Lic. Ac., D.O.M., Ph.D., President
> 13315 Washington Boulevard
> Los Angeles, CA 90066
> Phone 1-310-577-3000
> www.yosan.edu

# Further Information on Chinese Herbal Clinics, Colleges of Oriental Medicine and Integrated Medical Facilities

## American Association of Oriental Medicine (AAOM)

The American Association of Acupuncture and Oriental Medicine (AAAOM) was formed in 1981 to be the unifying force for American acupuncturists who are committed to high ethical and educational standards and a well-regulated profession to ensure the safety of the public. Recently the AAAOM voted to change its name to better represent its membership. In recognition that acupuncture was just one part of the entire scope of Oriental medicine, the AAOM has streamlined its name to be the American Association of Oriental Medicine. AAOM members are regarded as the most highly qualified practitioners of Oriental Medicine in the United States. To locate AAOM members in your state: www.aaom.org/referrals.html.

> **American Association of Oriental Medicine**
> 433 Front Street
> Catasauqua, PA 18032
> Phone 1-610-266-1433
> Fax 1-610-264-2768
> www.aaom.org

## National Acupuncture and Oriental Medicine Alliance (National Alliance)

National Alliance offers over-the-phone personal referrals to herbalists and acupuncturists nationwide. Many of their acupuncturists are also licensed herbalists, but they do not differentiate between herbalists and acupuncturists. There are also referrals available on the Web site.

> **National Alliance**
> 14637 Starr Road, SE
> Olalla, WA 98359

Phone 1-253-851-6896
Fax 1-253-851-6883
www.acupuncturealliance.org


## Accreditation Commission for Acupuncture and Oriental Medicine (ACAOM)

The Accreditation Commission for Acupuncture and Oriental Medicine (ACAOM) (formerly the National Accreditation Commission for Schools and Colleges of Acupuncture and Oriental Medicine—NACSCAOM) was established in June 1982 by the Council of Colleges of Acupuncture and Oriental Medicine (CCAOM). Its mission is to foster excellence in acupuncture and Oriental medicine education. The commission acts as an independent body to evaluate professional master's degree and professional master's level certificate and diploma programs in acupuncture and Oriental medicine with a concentration in both acupuncture and herbal therapies for a level of performance, integrity and quality that entitles them to the confidence of the educational community and the public they serve. ACAOM does not provide referrals to individual practitioners.

*Accreditation Commission for Acupuncture and Oriental Medicine*
7501 Greenway Center Drive, Suite 820
Greenbelt, MD 20770
Phone 1-301-313-0855
Fax 1-301-313-0912
www.acaom.org


## California Hematology Oncology Medical Group and BIOS

BIOS stands for B'shert Integrative Oncology Services. *B'shert* is a Hebrew word that means "the path" or "God's way." For the treatment of cancer, BIOS integrates Western medicine with complementary medicines such as Chinese herbs, acupuncture, biofeedback, nutrition and many other services. Dr. Lorne Feldman gives patients a preliminary plan that involves the standard traditional approach with chemotherapy and/or radiation and/or surgery. He presents their information at a group meeting that includes the entire faculty of BIOS. He practices in two locations.

*California Hematology Oncology Medical Group and BIOS*
Lorne Feldman, M.D.
3400 W. Lomita Blvd., Suite 203
Torrance, CA 90505
Phone 1-310-530-9763
Fax 1-310-530-3154
www.chomg.com

6801 Park Terrace, Suite 130
Los Angeles, CA 90045
Phone 1-310-649-7222
Fax 1-310-649-7235
www.chomg.com

## The National Center for Complementary and Alternative Medicine (NCCAM)

The NCCAM at the National Institutes of Health (NIH) is dedicated to exploring complementary and alternative healing practices in the context of rigorous science, training complementary and alternative researchers, and disseminating authoritative information.

*The National Center for Complementary and Alternative Medicine*
P.O. Box 8218
Silver Spring, MD 20907-8218
Phone 1-888-644-6226
Fax 1-301-495-4957
www.nccam.nih.gov

## National Institutes of Health (NIH)

One of the world's foremost medical research centers, and the federal focal point for medical research in the United States. NIH's mission is to uncover new knowledge that will lead to better health for everyone. NIH works toward that mission by conducting research in its own laboratories; supporting the research of nonfederal scientists in universities, medical schools, hospitals and research institutions throughout the country and abroad; helping in the training of research investigators; and fostering communication of medical information.

*National Institutes of Health*
9000 Rockville Pike
Bethesda, MD 20892
Phone 1-301-496-4000
E-mail nihinfo@od.nih.gov
www.nih.gov

## North Hawaii Community Hospital

Earl Bakken, the inventor of the first wearable battery-operated, electronic pacemaker and the first implantable pacemaker, designed one of the first fully integrated hospitals in Hawaii. The full-service, fifty-bed, acute-care North Hawaii

Community Hospital opened in June 1996. In addition to the latest in advanced technology, equipment and diagnostic procedures, the hospital offers herbal medicine, acupuncture, chiropractic, guided imagery, healing touch, massage and naturopathy. Human touches such as soothing music and art, healing gardens and pets allowed in rooms provide a sense of security. Attending physicians consult with practitioners who are licensed and credentialed to provide holistic health care.

> *North Hawaii Community Hospital*
> 67-1125 Mamalahoa Highway
> Kamuela, HI 96743
> Phone 1-808-881-4425
> Fax 1-808-881-4404
> E-mail guilbejh@nhawaiipo.ah.org

## Oriental Healing Arts Institute (OHAI)

OHAI is a nonprofit educational organization dedicated to disseminating knowledge and improving the practice of Chinese medicine through the publication of the International Journal of Oriental Medicine, as well as books and other informational literature for health professionals, academicians and students. By making available English translations of these works, OHAI seeks to stimulate an interest in and an appreciation of Chinese medicine and to break down the barriers between Chinese and Western medicine. The Institute sponsors symposia and seminars/workshops, awards grants for students of Oriental medicine and supports pharmacognostic research.

Memberships (professional, associate and student) include subscription to the quarterly *International Journal of Oriental Medicine,* access to OHAI's medical reference library, consultation with health advisors and visiting scholars, discounts on books, seminars and symposia.

> *Oriental Healing Arts Institute*
> 1945 Palo Verde Avenue, Suite 208
> Long Beach, CA 90815-3444
> Phone 1-562-431-3544
> Fax 1-949-587-8967

## Western Health Care

### The American Academy of Antiaging Medicine

A not-for-profit medical society with ten thousand medical doctors as members that is dedicated to the advancement of technology to detect, prevent and treat age-related disease and to promote research into methods to retard and optimize the aging process. The academy hosts two antiaging conferences each year, one in the Chicago area in the summer and one in Las Vegas in the winter. Thousands of physicians attend the conferences to learn about ongoing clinical research to keep abreast of this quickly evolving and competitive field.

> *American Academy of Antiaging Medicine*
> 2415 North Greenview
> Chicago IL 60614
> Phone 1-773-528-4333
> Fax 1-773-528-5390

To find an antiaging clinic in your area log on to www.worldhealth.net.

## Great Smokies Diagnostic Laboratory

A laboratory dedicated to functional medicine. Functional medicine is the field of health care that employs laboratory assessment and early intervention to improve physiological, emotional/cognitive, and physical function. This health-care approach focuses attention on biochemical individuality, metabolic balance, ecological context and unique personal experience in the dynamics of health. Great Smokies Diagnostic Laboratory can refer you to a health-care provider in your area who can order the saliva, blood, hair and stool tests you may need.

> *Great Smokies Diagnostic Laboratory*
> 63 Zillicoa St.
> Asheville, NC 28801
> Phone 1-800-522-4762
> www.gsdl.com

# References for Further Reading

## Books and Journals on Chinese Medicine

*The Complete Illustrated Guide to Chinese Medicine: A Comprehensive System for Health and Fitness,* by Tom Williams, Ph.D., is a coffee-table guide to Chinese medicine.

*The Encyclopedia of Medicinal Plants,* by Andrew Chevallier, while not a book on Chinese medicine specifically, is a reference guide to more than 550 key medicinal plants and their uses.

*The Physician's Desk Reference for Herbal Medicine* is the most authoritative resource on herbal medicines with the latest scientific findings on efficacy, safety and potential interactions, among other important data.

*The Tao of Nutrition,* by Maoshing Ni, Lic. Ac., D.O.M., Ph.D., with Cathy Mc-Nease, B.S., M.H., explains the theories and philosophies of Chinese nutrition, describes over 130 common foods and their Energetic properties and therapeutic actions and gives recommendations for various medical conditions.

*The Web That Has No Weaver: Understanding Chinese Medicine,* by Ted J. Kaptchuk, O.M.D., is a thorough exposition on Chinese medicine suitable for deeper study.

*Velvet Antler: Nature's Superior Tonic,* by Alison Davidson, is a thoroughly researched reference book on the Chinese herb Deer Velvet Antler.


## Books on Natural Health

*Caffeine Blues: Wake Up to the Hidden Dangers of America's #1 Drug,* by Stephen Cherniske, M.S., a nutritional biochemist with more than twenty-five years of academic research, reveals the truth about caffeine and offers a step-by-step, clinically proven program to kick the addiction.

*Diet for a Poisoned Planet,* by David W. Steinman, is a well-researched, thoroughly documented book on the perils of environmental toxins.

*Ginger: Common Spice and Wonder Drug,* by Paul Schulick, is a thoroughly researched book on the benefits of gingerroot.

*Living Healthy in a Toxic World: Simple Steps to Protect You and Your Family from Everyday Chemicals, Poisons and Pollution,* by David W. Steinman and R. Michael Wisner, explains how you can further protect yourself from toxins.

*Medicinal Mushrooms: An Exploration of Tradition, Healing and Cultures,* by Christopher Hobbs, documents over one hundred species of edible fungi in the most complete work on medicinal mushrooms published to date.

*The Safe Shopper's Bible: A Consumer's Guide to Nontoxic Household Products, Cosmetics, and Food,* by David W. Steinman, M.A., and Samuel S. Epstein, M.D., contains extensive lists of brand-name products that you can use and those that are toxic and carcinogenic.

*The Schwarzbein Principle,* by Diana Schwarzbein, M.D., and Nancy Deville, is a comprehensive book on achieving a healthy metabolism and weight loss by eating balanced meals of real, whole foods. This book contains extensive carbohydrate guides for real foods.

*The Schwarzbein Principle Cookbook* and *The Schwarzbein Principle Vegetarian Cookbook,* by Diana Schwarzbein, M.D., Nancy Deville and Evelyn Jacob, focus on appetizing, easy-to-prepare balanced meat-based and vegetarian meals using real, whole foods.

*Tired of Being Tired: Ten Simple Solutions to Achieving Your Ideal Weight and Feeling and Looking Younger,* by Jesse Hanley, M.D., and Nancy Deville, offers a step-by-step guide to reversing adrenal burnout, feeling better and having more energy.

### Energy Healing and Positive Visualization

*Videos, CDs and Cassettes by Caroline Myss, Ph.D.* A pioneer in the field of energy medicine and human consciousness, Dr. Myss's work has helped define how stress and emotion contribute to disease.

*CDs by Belleruth Naparstek, L.I.S.W., B.C.D.* A nationally recognized innovator in the field of guided imagery and intuition.

# Bibliography

1

Bian, Zhiya (chief editor). *The History of Chinese Medicine.* Shanghai: Shanghai Science and Technology Press (1984).

Chen, Ke-ji. "The Research Progress and Developmental Projection of Traditional Chinese Medicine." *Reflection on the Development of Traditional Chinese Medicine.* Beijing: People's Health Press (1997):16–21.

Chen, Ruquan (chief editor). "The History of Integration of Traditional Chinese and Western Medicine." *The Methodology of the Integration of Traditional Chinese and Western Medicine.* Beijing: China Medical Science and Technology Press (1997).

Eisenberg, David, M., M.D., et al. "Trends in Alternative Medicine Use in the United States, 1990–1997: The Results of a Follow-up National Survey." *The Journal of American Medical Association* 280, no. 18 (11 November 1998).

Eisenberg, David, M., M.D., et al. "Unconventional Medicine in the United States: Prevalence, Costs, and Patterns of Use." *The New England Journal of Medicine* 328 (28 January 1993):246–252.

Huang Di. *The Yellow Emperor's Internal Classic.* The Big Collection of The Classics of Traditional Chinese Medicine. Changsha: Hunan Electronic Image Press (1998).

Qian, Chaochen. *The Study of the Yellow Emperor's Internal Classic and Taisu.* Beijing: People's Health Press (1998).

Tang, Shina. *The Difference, Interactions and Integration of Chinese and Western Medicine.* Beijing: People's Health Press (2000).

Veith, Ilza (translator). *The Yellow Emperor's Classic of Internal Medicine.* Berkeley: University of California Press (1949).

Wang, Qingren (Qing Dynasty). *Rectification of Mistakes in the Field of Medicine.* The Big Collection of the Classics of Traditional Chinese Medicine. Changsha: Hunan Electronic Image Press (1998).


# 2


Beinfield, H., and Korngold, E. *Between Heaven and Earth.* New York: Ballantine Books (1992).

He, Zhiguang (chief editor). *Traditional Chinese Medicine.* Beijing: People's Health Press (1997).

Hu, Qiaomu (chairman of editorial board). *Encyclopedia of China.* Beijing: Encyclopedia of China Press (1994).

Kaptchuk, Ted J. *The Web That Has No Weaver.* Chicago: NTC/Contemporary Publishing Group, Inc. (2000).

Ma, Binrong. *The Expert Systems of Traditional Chinese Medicine.* Beijing: Beijing Press (1998).

Wang, Qi. *The Zang Xiang Theory of Traditional Chinese Medicine.* Beijing: People's Health Press (2001).

Wang, Xinhua. *The Basic Theory of Traditional Chinese Medicine.* Beijing: People's Health Press (2001).

Wu, Dunxu (chief editor). *The Basic Theory of Traditional Chinese Medicine.* Shanghai: Shanghai Science and Technology Press (1994).


# 3


Chen, Zeling. *Studies of Tongue Diagnosis.* Shanghai: Shanghai Science and Technology Press (1982).

Dou, Hongtao. *Angels in the Company of Devils.* Beijing: Sunshine Press (1999).

Han, Xiangming. *Clinical Guide of Current Diagnosis and Treatment in Traditional Chinese Medicine.* Beijing: People's Health Press (2001).

Huang, Shiling. *A Study of Pulse Diagnosis of Traditional Chinese Medicine.* Beijing: People's Health Press (1997).

Lu, S., et al. "Detection of human papilloma virus in esophageal squamous cell carcinoma and adjacent tissue specimens in Lin Xian." *Chinese Journal of Oncology* 17, no. 5 (1995): 321–324.

Song, Tianbing. *Atlas of Tongue*. Beijing: People's Health Press (1998).

WGBS/BBC. *Cancer Detectives of Lin Xian*. New York: Time-Life Video (1980).

Wu, Xiufen. *Diagnosis of Traditional Chinese Medicine*. Beijing: People's Health Press (1995).

Xiao, Dexin. *Methodology of Traditional Chinese Medicine*. Chongqing: Chongqing Press (1988).

Zhang, Guangqi. *An Inquiry of Essentials of Etiology of Traditional Chinese Medicine*. Shanghai: Shanghai Science and Technology Press (2002).


## 4


Cheng, Xinnong. *Chinese Acupuncture and Moxabustion*. Beijing: People's Health Press (1998).

Guo, Xiaozong. *The Theory and Clinical Application of Acupuncture Points*. Beijing: People's Health Press (1995).

Jiao, Shunfa. *The Principle and Clinical Practice of Acupuncture and Moxabustion*. Beijing: People's Health Press (2000).

Yang, Jiasan. *Acupuncture and Moxabustion*. Beijing: People's Health Press (1998).

Zhang, Wenkang (chief editor). *The Meridians*. Shanghai: Shanghai Science and Technology Press (1994).

Zhao, Wurong. *The Method of Acupressure*. Beijing: People's Health Press (2000).


## 5


Bian, Zhiya (chief editor). "Mineral Intake, Alchemy and Medicinal Chemistry." *The History of Chinese Medicine*. Shanghai: Shanghai Science and Technology Press (1984): 43–44.

Chen, Chaozu. *Treatment Strategies and Formulas of Traditional Chinese Medicine*. Beijing: People's Health Press (1995).

Fan, Bitin (chief editor). *Pharmacopoeia of Chinese Herbal Medicine*. Shanghai: Shanghai Science and Technology Press (1983).

Hu, Qiaomu (chairman of editorial board). Section of Traditional Chinese Medicine. *Encyclopedia of China.* Beijing: Encyclopedia of China Press (1994).

Jiao, Shude. *Ten Lectures of the Insights in Clinical Practice of Herbology.* Beijing: People's Health Press (1998).

Lin, Yikui (chief editor). *Herbology.* Shanghai: Shanghai Science and Technology Press (1983).

Ma, Jixin. *Compilation and Annotation of Shen Nong's Herbal Materia Medica.* Beijing: People's Health Press (1996).

Shen Nong. *Shen Nong's Herbal Materia Medica.* The Big Collection of the Classics of Traditional Chinese Medicine. Changsha: Hunan Electronic Image Press (1998).

Wang, Mianzhi. *Studies of Herbal Formula.* Beijing: People's Health Press (1998).

Wen, Weiliang (chief editor). *Clinical Herbology.* Zhengzhou: Henan Science and Technology Press (1998).

Xu, Jiqun (chief editor). *Formula.* Shanghai: Shanghai Science and Technology Press (1983).

Zhang, Binxin (chief editor). *Practical Manual of Patent Herbal Formulas.* Beijing: People's Health Press (1996).

Zhou, Yanchang. *Business Management of Chinese Herbal Manufacturing.* Beijing: People's Health Press (1998).

## 6

Feng, Guanghua. *A Clinical Manual of Internal Medicine in Traditional Chinese Medicine.* Beijing: People's Health Press (1999).

Han, Xiangming. *A Clinical Guide of Current Diagnosis and Treatment in Traditional Chinese Medicine.* Beijing: People's Health Press (2001).

Leng, Fangnan. *Clinical Applications of Chinese Medicinal Food Therapy.* Beijing: People's Health Press (1996).

Su, Wei. *A Practical Manual of Therapies in Traditional Chinese Medicine.* Beijing: People's Health Press (1999).

Tierney, L. M., Jr., et al. (editors). *Current Medical Diagnosis and Treatment.* Stamford, CT: Appleton & Lange (1998).

Xiang, Ping. *A Clinical Manual of Common Chronic Illnesses.* Beijing: People's Health Press (1998).

## 7

Borchers, A. T., Stern, J. S., Hackman, R. M., et al. "Mushrooms, tumors, and immunity." *Proc Soc Exp Biol Med.* 221 (1999):281–293.

Feng, Guanghua. *A Clinical Manual of Internal Medicine in Traditional Chinese Medicine.* Beijing: People's Health Press (1999).

Gao, Y. "The evaluation of PSP capsules in clinical pharmacology." In: Yang, Q., Kwok, C., eds. *PSP International Symposium 1993.* Hong Kong: Fudan University Press (1993):209–215.

Han, Xiangming. *A Clinical Guide of Current Diagnosis and Treatment in Traditional Chinese Medicine.* Beijing: People's Health Press (2001).

Kidd, P. M. "The Use of Mushroom Glucans and Proteoglycans in Cancer Treatment." *Alternative Medical Review* 5, no. 1 (2000):4–27.

Shanghai Traditional Chinese Medical Literature Library. *A Compilation of Traditional Chinese Medical Literature on Common Illnesses.* Shanghai: Shanghai Science and Technology Press (2001).

Su, Wei. *A Practical Manual of Therapies in Traditional Chinese Medicine.* Beijing: People's Health Press (1999).

Xiang, Ping. *A Clinical Manual of Common Chronic Illnesses.* Beijing: People's Health Press (1998).

Xu, Yihou. *The Treatment of Skin Diseases by Traditional Chinese Medicine.* Beijing: People's Health Press (1991).

Yang, Q. "History, Present Status and Perspectives of the Study of Yun Zhi Polysaccharopeptide." In: Yang, Q., ed. *Advanced Research in PSP, 1999.* Hong Kong: Hong Kong Association for Health Care Ltd. (1999):5–15.

## 8

Chen, Chaozu. *Treatment Strategies and Formulas of Traditional Chinese Medicine.* Beijing: People's Health Press (1995).

Feng, Guanghua. *A Clinical Manual of Internal Medicine in Traditional Chinese Medicine.* Beijing: People's Health Press (1999).

Han, Xiangming. *A Clinical Guide of Current Diagnosis and Treatment in Traditional Chinese Medicine.* Beijing: People's Health Press (2001).

Meng, Shujiang (chief editor). *Febrile Disease.* Shanghai: Shanghai Science and Technology Press (1983).

Shanghai Traditional Chinese Medical Literature Library. *A Compilation of Traditional Chinese Medical Literature on Common Illnesses.* Shanghai: Shanghai Science and Technology Press (2001).

Su, Wei. *A Practical Manual of Therapies in Traditional Chinese Medicine.* Beijing: People's Health Press (1999).

Xiang, Ping. *A Clinical Manual of Common Chronic Illnesses.* Beijing: People's Health Press (1998).

Xiang, Ping. *Traditional Chinese Medical Treatment of Common Viral Infections.* Beijing: People's Health Press (2001).

Zhang, Xuewen. *Zheng and Treatment of Complex and Difficult Illnesses.* Beijing: People's Health Press (1997).

Zhu, Jianfang. *Treatment and Research of Complex and Difficult Illnesses.* Beijing: People's Health Press (1995).

# 9

Han, Xiangming. *A Clinical Guide of Current Diagnosis and Treatment in Traditional Chinese Medicine.* Beijing: People's Health Press (2001).

Su, Wei. *A Practical Manual of Therapies in Traditional Chinese Medicine.* Beijing: People's Health Press (1999).

Tierney, L. M., Jr., et al. (editors). *Current Medical Diagnosis and Treatment.* Stamford, CT: Appleton & Lange (1998).

Xiao, Dexin. *Methodology of Traditional Chinese Medicine.* Chongqing: Chongqing Press (1988).

Zang, Mingren. *Integrative Treatment of Mental Diseases by Traditional and Western Medicines.* Beijing: People's Health Press (1998).

# 10

Agrawal, P., Rai, V., and Singh, R. B. "Randomized Placebo-Controlled, Single Blind Trial of Holy Basil Leaves in Patients with Noninsulin-Dependent Diabetes Mellitus." *Int J Clin Pharmacol Ther* 34, no. 9 (1996):406–409.

Balter, M.B., and Uhlenhuth, E.T. "New Epidemiologic Findings About Insomnia and Its Treatment." *J Clin Psychiatry* 53 (1992):34–39.

Banerjee, S., Prashar, R., Kumar, A., and Rao, A. R. "Modulatory Influence Of Alcoholic Extract of Ocimum Leaves on Carcinogen-Metabolizing Enzyme

Activities and Reduced Glutathione Levels in Mice." *Nutr Cancer* 25, no. 2 (1996):205–217.

Bhargava, K. P., and Singh, N. "Anti-Stress Activity of Ocimum Sanctum Linn." *Indian J Med Res* 73 (1981):443–451.

Eddy, M., and Walbroehl, G. S. "Insomnia." *Am Family Physician* 59 (1999): 1911–1915.

Jin, Yiqiang. *Modern Research and Clinical Application of Zangxiang Theory in Traditional Chinese Medicine.* Beijing: People's Health Press (2001).

Rechtshaffen, A., and Kales, A. A manual of standardized terminology, techniques, and scoring system for sleep stages of human subjects. *NIH Rep.* no. 204. Bethesda, MD: Natl. Inst. Health (1968).

Sarkar, A., Lavania, S. C., Pandey, D. N., and Pant, M. C. "Changes in the Blood Lipid Profile After Administration of Ocimum Sanctum (Tulsi) Leaves in the Normal Albino Rabbits." *Indian J Physiol Pharmacol* 38, no. 4 (1994):311–312.

Sharpley, A. L., and Cowen, P. J. "Effect of Pharmacologic Treatments on the Sleep of Depressed Patients." *Biol Psychiatry* 37 (1995):85–88.

Shen, Ziyin. *Studies of the Essence of Kidney in Traditional Chinese Medicine.* Shanghai: Shanghai Science and Technology Press (1998).

Singth, S., Majumdar, D. K., and Rehan, H. M. "Evaluation of Anti-inflammatory Potential of Fixed Oil of Ocimum Sanctum (Holy Basil) and Its Possible Mechanism of Action." *J Ethnopharmacol* 54, no. 1 (1996):19–26.

Zu, Yunxi. *The Practical Acupuncture and Cupping.* Beijing: People's Health Press (1998).

## 11

Cherniske, Stephen. *Caffeine Blues.* Warner Books (1998).

Crinnion, W. J. "Environmental Medicine, Part One: The Human Burden of Environmental Toxins and Their Common Health Effects." *Alternative Medicine Review* (February 2000):52–63.

Crinnion, W. J. "Environmental Medicine, Part Two: Health Effects of and Protection from Ubiquitous Airborne Solvent Exposure." *Alternative Medicine Review* (March 2000):133–143.

Han, Xiangming. *A Clinical Guide of Current Diagnosis and Treatment in Traditional Chinese Medicine.* Beijing: People's Health Press (2001).

Ke, Xuefan. *Contemplation and Exploration of Complex and Difficult Diseases and Zheng.* Beijing: People's Health Press (1998).

Lu, Cheng. *Toxic Zheng*. Beijing: People's Health Press (1998).

Zhang, Xuewen. *Zheng and Treatment of Complex and Difficult Illnesses*. Beijing: People's Health Press (1997).


# 12

Fujiki, H., Suganuma, M., Okabe, S., et al. "Mechanistic Findings of Green Tea as Cancer Preventive for Humans." *Proc Soc Exp Biol Med* 220, no. 4 (April 1999):225–228.

Hamilton-Miller, J.M. "Anti-carcinogenic Properties of Tea (Camellia sinensis)." *J Med Microbiol* 50, no. 4 (April 2001):299–302.

Luo, H.W. "Observation of Long-Term Therapeutic Effect of Comprehensive Treatment of Intermediate and Terminal Stage Uterine Cervical Cancers. Compilation of Studies on Integrative Treatment of Prevalent Gynecological Diseases by Western and Chinese Medicines." *People's Health* (1979):12–17.

Picard, Dennis. "The Biochemistry of Green Tea Polyphenols and Their Potential Application in Human Skin Cancer." *Alternative Medicine Review* 1 (1996):31–42.

Sung, H., Nah, J., Chun, S., et al. "In Vivo Antioxidant Effect of Green Tea." *Eur J Clin Nutr* 54, no. 7 (July 2000):527–529.

Vinson, J.A. "Black and Green Tea and Heart Disease: A Review." *Biofactors* 13, nos. 1–4 (2000):27–32.

Weisburger, J. "Tea and Health: A Historical Perspective." *Cancer Lett* 114, nos. 1–2 (19 March 1997):315–317.

Zhang, Daizhao. *The Chinese and Western Medical Integrative Treatment of Toxic Reactions and Side Effects Caused by Chemo and Radiotherapies*. Beijing: People's Health Press (2000).

Zhang, Mingqin. *Clinical Applications of Anticancer Herbs*. Beijing: People's Health Press (1998).

Zhang, Xuewen. *Zheng and Treatment of Complex and Difficult Illnesses*. Beijing: People's Health Press (1997).

Zhu, Jianfang. *Treatment and Research of Complex and Difficult Illnesses*. Beijing: People's Health Press (1995).

## 13

Jin, Shi. *Diagnosis and Treatment of Viral Hepatitis by Traditional Chinese Medicine.* Beijing: People's Health Press (2001).

Xiang, Ping. *Traditional Chinese Medical Treatment of Common Viral Infections.* Beijing: People's Health Press (2001).

## 14

Enig, M. "Trans Fatty Acids in the Food Supply: A Comprehensive Report Covering 60 Years of Research." Silver Spring, MD: Enig Associates, Inc. (1995).

Feng, Guanghua. *A Clinical Manual of Internal Medicine in Traditional Chinese Medicine.* Beijing: People's Health Press (1999).

Feng, Jianhua. *Treatment of Endocrine and Metabolic Diseases by Traditional Chinese Medicine.* Beijing: People's Health Press (2001).

Huang, Chunling. *Diagnosis and Treatment of Coronary Heart Disease by Traditional Chinese Medicine.* Beijing: People's Health Press (2000).

Li, Qiyi. *Treatment of Heart and Brain Vascular Diseases by Traditional Chinese Medicine.* Beijing: People's Health Press (2001).

Lu, Zhizheng. *Clinical Rheumatology of Traditional Chinese Medicine.* Beijing: People's Health Press (1998).

Lu, Zhizheng. *Integrative Treatment of Diabetes and Its Complications by Chinese and Western Medicines.* Beijing: People's Health Press (1998).

Luo, Yuankai. *Gynecology of Traditional Chinese Medicine.* Beijing: People's Health Press (1997).

Srivastava, K. C., and Mustafa, T. "Ginger (Zingiber officinale) and Rheumatic Disorders." *Medical Hypotheses* 29, no. 1 (May 1989):25–28.

Srivastava, K. C., and Mustafa, T. "Ginger (Zingiber officinale) in Rheumatism and Musculoskeletal Disorders." *Medical Hypotheses* 39, no. 4 (December 1992):342–348.

Xia, Guicheng. *Clinical Gynecology of Traditional Chinese Medicine.* Beijing: People's Health Press (1996).

Xie, Keyong. "Treatment and Prevention of Postmenopausal Osteoporosis by Tonifying Kidney and Restoring Jing." *Collection of Outstanding Ph.D. Dissertations of Traditional Chinese Medicine.* Shanghai: Shanghai University of Traditional Chinese Medicine Press (1996).

## 15

Jin, Shi. *Diagnosis and Treatment of Viral Hepatitis by Traditional Chinese Medicine.* Beijing: People's Health Press (2001).

Leng, Fangnan. *Clinical Applications of Chinese Medicinal Food Therapy.* Beijing: People's Health Press (1996).

Patrick, Lyn. "Nutrients and HIV: Part One—Beta Carotene and Selenium." *Alternative Medical Review* (January 2000):13–23.

Patrick, Lyn. "Nutrients and HIV: Part Two—Vitamins A and E, Zinc, B-Vitamins and Magnesium." *Alternative Medical Review* (February 2000):39–51.


## 16

Chen, Keji (chief editor). *Reflection on the Development of Traditional Chinese Medicine.* Beijing: People's Health Press (1997):16–21.

Cohen, Kenneth S. *The Way of Qigong: The Art and Science of Chinese Energy Healing.* New York: Ballantine (1999).

Garripoli, Francesco Garri. *Gigong, Essence of the Healing Dance.* Deerfield Beach, FL: Health Communications, Inc. (1999).

Hua-Ching Ni with Daosing Ni and Maoshing Ni. *Mastering Qi.* Santa Monica, CA: Seven Star Communications (1994).

Huang Di. *The Yellow Emperor's Internal Classic.* The Big Collection of the Classics of Traditional Chinese Medicine. Changsha: Hunan Electronic Image Press (1998).

Liu, Guangrong. *The Basis of Qi Gong.* Beijing: People's Health Press (1996).

Liu, Yianjun. *Qi Gong Therapy of Traditional Chinese Medicine.* Beijing: People's Health Press (1999).

Song, Tianbin. *Qi Gong Therapy of Traditional Chinese Medicine.* Beijing: People's Health Press (1996).

Xiao, Dexin. *Methodology of Traditional Chinese Medicine.* Chongqing: Chongqing Press (1988).

Zhang, Qiwen. *Health Maintenance and Preservation: The Theory and Practice of Traditional Chinese Medicine.* Beijing: People's Health Press (1998).

Zhu, Shina, et al. *System Theory of Traditional Chinese Medicine.* Chongqing: Chongqing Press (1997).

## 17

Luo, Yuankai. *Gynecology of Traditional Chinese Medicine.* Beijing: People's Health Press (1997).

Shi, Yuguang (chief editor). *Infertility: The Summary of Clinical Strategies by the Leading Experts of Traditional Chinese Medicine.* Beijing: TCM Ancient Books Press (1999).

Xia, Guicheng. *Clinical Gynecology of Traditional Chinese Medicine.* Beijing: People's Health Press (1996).

Xie, Keyong. "Treatment and Prevention of Postmenopausal Osteoporosis by Tonifying Kidney and Restoring Jing." *Collection of Outstanding Ph.D. Dissertations of Traditional Chinese Medicine.* Shanghai: Shanghai University of Traditional Chinese Medicine Press (1996).

## 18

Wen, Weiliang (chief editor). *Clinical Herbology.* Zhengzhou: Henan Science and Technology Press (1998).

Wu, Lingsheng. *Sports Medicine of Traditional Chinese Medicine.* Beijing: TCM Ancient Books Press (1999).

Zhao, Yu. "Investigation of Ma's Troops." *Chinese Writer* (March 1995).

## 19

Chen, Ke-ji. *Study of the Medical Archive of Forbidden City from Qing Dynasty.* Beijing: China Press (1980).

Ding, Y. E. "Experimental Study of the Anti-aging Effect of Huan Jing Jian I: Influence on the Life Span of Lab Mice." *Shanghai Journal of Traditional Chinese Medicine* 12 (1985):39.

Ding, Y. F. "Influence of Huan Jing Jian on Body's Ability to Repair DNA Damages." *Chinese Journal of Integrated Traditional and Western Medicine* 11, no. 11 (1989):647–649.

Gong, B. "Experimental Study of the Anti-aging Effect of Huan Jing Jian II: Influence on the C-nucleotide in Lung and Liver Tissues in Aging Mice." *Shanghai Journal of Traditional Chinese Medicine* 1 (1986):43.

Li, C. S., and Hou, R. X. "A Review of Past Decade's Anti-aging Study in China: Effect of Herbs Through Employment of Life-Experiment and Senile Animal Models." *Journal of Traditional Chinese Medicine* 39, no. 11 (1998):690–693.

Li, Chunsheng. *New Anti-aging Chinese Medicine.* Beijing: People's Health Press (1998).

Li, Chunsheng. *New Materia Medica of Anti-aging Herbs.* Beijing: People's Health Press (1998).

Ling, S. M. "Clinical Study of Aging-Retarding Effect of Huan Jing Jian." *Chinese Journal of Integrated Traditional and Western Medicine* 11, no. 11 (1984): 655–657.

Liu, Changhua. *Practical Formulas for Tonification and Vitality Preservation.* Beijing: People's Health Press (1999).

Pan, Y. X. "Experimental Study of the Anti-aging Effect of Huan Jing Jian V: Impact on Hypothalamus Sex Hormone Receptors and the Functions of Serum Thymus Factors in Aging Mice." *Shanghai Journal of Traditional Chinese Medicine* 4 (1986):46–47.

Qiu, D. Z. "Efficacy Analysis of Huan Jing Jian Plus Hai Gou Pills Treatment Protocol in 161 Cases of Male Disorders." *Jiangxi Journal of Chinese Medicine* 25, no. 2 (1994):23.

Shi, Y. H. "Experimental Study of the Anti-Aging Effect of Huan Jing Jian IV: On the Changes of Histochemistry of Internal Sex Organs and Sub-cellular Structure of Liver in Aging Mice." *Shanghai Journal of Traditional Chinese Medicine* 3 (1986):46–48.

Shen, Z. Y., et al. "Clinical Observation of the Therapeutic Effect of Huan Jing Jian on 52 Cases of Original Hypertension Patients." *Shandong Journal of Traditional Chinese Medicine* 13, no. 10 (1994):447.

Yao, P. F. "On Anti-aging and Treating Geriatric Illnesses Through Tonifying Kidney Energy." In: Jing, M. Y., Zhang, J., editors, *Collection of clinical style and work by leading TCM doctors in Shanghai area.* Shanghai: Science, Technology & Education Press (1990).

Zhang, J. "A Review of the Research on Anti-aging Chinese Herbal Formula Huan Jing Jian." *Learned Journal of Gansu TCM College* 4 (1993):49–51.

Zhang, Qiwen. *Health Maintenance and Preservation: The Theory and Practice of Traditional Chinese Medicine.* Beijing: People's Health Press (1998).

Zhang, Y. Z. "Experimental Study of the Anti-aging Effect of Huan Jing Jian III: Influence on the Subsistence Rate of Lymphocytes in Vitro and Their Immune Functions in Aging Mice." *Shanghai Journal of Traditional Chinese Medicine* 2 (1986):47.

Zhao, W. K. "Study of the Effects of Huan Jing Jian on Sub-cellular Structure Thymus and Sex Hormone Receptors in Aging Mice." *Chinese Journal of Integrated Traditional and Western Medicine* 11, no. 4 (1987):226–228.

# Index

*Page numbers of illustrations appear in italics.*
*Main entries for health conditions appear in bold type.*

# About the Authors

HENRY HAN, O.M.D., was born in 1958 into a family of doctors in China. His mother was a surgical/oncological gynecologist, his father a dermatologist, and his grandfather a Chinese herbalist. Dr. Han's pre-college education is mostly self-taught. At the age of 8, during China's "Great Cultural Revolution," he was separated from his parents and sister. Unable to go to school, he continued his education on his own.

The Cultural Revolution officially ended in 1976 with the death of Chairman Mao, and Dr. Han was admitted to the prestigious Beijing University of Chinese Medicine.

From 1983 to 1985, he did a residency program in internal medicine in Beijing Dong Zhi Men Hospital, a hospital that specializes in the integration of Chinese and Western medicine. In September 1985, he was awarded one of two government scholarships to study psychology at the graduate level in the United States. Until June 1988, he studied clinical psychology and cognitive science at the University of California.

Since March 1989, he has been in private practice. He founded the Santa Barbara Herb and Wellness Center in 1998 and the Santa Barbara Herb Clinic in 1991. Over the years, Dr. Han has treated thousands of patients and is recognized as a master herbalist and diagnostician. He has a reputation for treating difficult and complex cases, and his practice attracts patients from all over the United States as well as other countries. He frequently gives talks and lectures and serves as an advisory or scientific board member of several companies.

GLENN E. MILLER, M.D., was born, raised and educated in the Midwest. Raised in a family of pharmacists, Dr. Miller has spent over twenty years developing and implementing professional and business models for a variety of medical and pharmaceutical ventures, as well as maintaining a private medical practice. He serves on the Board of Directors of Body Trends Health and Fitness, Inc. (www.bodytrends.com); chairs the Professional Advisory Board of Desert Health Products, Inc., a Scottsdale, Arizona–based multinational nutriceutical company; has been a consultant to the U.S. Department of Justice, Bureau of Prisons; has held an academic appointment with the University of California—Santa Barbara Graduate School of Education; and has served as an appointee of California Governor Pete Wilson from 1994 to 1997.

Dr. Miller received a B.S. Pharmacy degree with a minor in Business Administration from Drake University in 1978, and a Medical Doctorate from the University of Illinois College of Medicine in 1983, followed by a four-year residency at Northwestern University, McGaw Medical Center. Dr. Miller is a Diplomat of the American Board of Psychiatry and Neurology.

Dr. Miller currently resides in Santa Barbara, California, with his wife, Marjorie S. Gies, M.D., Ph.D., their daughter, Margaret, and son, Dillon.

NANCY DEVILLE is a medical writer and author with a talent for educating the layperson on issues related to medical science, alternative medicine and wellness. Her books unravel the complicated and often contradictory health and medical advice that can discourage and confuse the average reader. She is the co-author of the bestselling *The Schwarzbein Principle* and two companion cookbooks, which have helped over two hundred thousand people reverse accelerated metabolic aging through a simple nutritional plan. She is also the co-author of *Tired of Being Tired,* which offers commonsense solutions to exhaustion, illness and weight gain inherent in our stress-filled society.

Nancy Deville lives with her husband in Santa Barbara, California.

Printed in the United States
by Baker & Taylor Publisher Services